Praise for *Food Can Fix It*

"It was Hippocrates who once said, 'Let food be thy medicine, and medicine be thy food.' Both Dr. Oz and I first heard that in medical school many years ago. Now, with *Food Can Fix It*, Dr. Oz will teach everyone this valuable lesson and explain what it means and how to draw upon the amazing healing powers of food."

—Sanjay Gupta, M.D., Associate Chief
of Neurosurgery at Grady Memorial Hospital,
Chief Medical Correspondent at CNN,
and contributor to *60 Minutes*

"As a heart surgeon and early pioneer to some of the Blue Zones areas, Dr. Oz knows how to eat your way to a longer and stronger life. Fix what you eat, and you could very well fix your health problems. Dr. Oz explains how in this informative, accessible book filled with anecdotes, science, recipes, and guidelines for cooking, shopping, and eating out."

—Dan Buettner, author of *The Blue Zones Solution:
Eating and Living Like the World's Healthiest People*

"This extraordinary book by Dr. Oz is a must-read for anyone who wants to understand how food can be the best medicine and how you can evoke the body's natural healing mechanisms. Follow his simple plan and you'll be on a healthy journey for life."

—Deepak Chopra, M.D., F.A.C.P, Founder of the Chopra Foundation and Co-founder of
the Chopra Center for Wellbeing

"If you're aiming for virtuous good health, you'll certainly find a book to fuel your preoccupation . . . Dr. Mehmet Oz's *Food Can Fix It*."

—*The New York Times Book Review*

"Sprinkled throughout the book, making it not only an interesting but also a fun read, are tips and factoids to devour. We give Dr. Oz three cheers for his thoughts on how food should be thought of as even more than just good for the physical body."

—*Healthy Aging* magazine

"I am a firsthand witness to Dr. Oz's holistic approach to modern medicine and healing. When he performed my mom's heart valve replacement surgery, he asked her first to heal herself with food. His work gave me ten more years with my mom. In the years since, I have seen him live the life he preaches and the results. *Food Can Fix It* hits all notes of a nutritious and delicious lifestyle. I know from personal experience, food can fix it!"

—Rocco DiSpirito, award-winning chef
and author of *Rocco's Healthy & Delicious*

"*Food Can Fix It* elegantly reveals the science and wisdom that food can be a powerful medicine for the body."

—Mike Roizen, M.D., Chief Wellness Officer
at Cleveland Clinic and coauthor of *YOU: On a Diet*

"What we eat is one of the most powerful determinants of our health and well-being. In *Food Can Fix It*, Dr. Oz—America's doctor—has written one of the most authoritative yet user-friendly guides to foods that keep us healthy and vibrant that are also delicious, familiar, and fun. If you read only one book on nutrition this year, this is it. Highly recommended!"

—Dean Ornish, M.D., Founder and President of
Preventive Medicine Research Institute and author of
The Spectrum and *Dr. Dean Ornish's Program for Reversing Heart Disease*

"Experts have long known that food has remarkable potential as medicine to prevent, treat, and even reverse disease. Far too little, however, has been done with this crucial information. No one is better suited to fix this problem, deliver this empowering memo, and help millions add years to their lives and life to their years than Dr. Mehmet Oz."

—David L. Katz, M.D., M.P.H., Founding Director of
Yale University Prevention Research Center and
Founder and President of the True Health Initiative

ALSO BY DR. MEHMET OZ

*Healing from the Heart: A Leading Surgeon Combines Eastern and
Western Traditions to Create the Medicine of the Future*

**ALSO BY DR. MEHMET OZ
WITH DR. MICHAEL ROIZEN**

YOU: The Owner's Manual

YOU: Losing Weight

YOU: On a Diet

YOU: The Smart Patient

YOU: Stress Less

YOU: Staying Young

YOU: Being Beautiful

YOU: Having a Baby

YOU: Raising Your Child

YOU: The Owner's Manual for Teens

YOU(r) Teen: Losing Weight at Any Age

Food Can Fix It

The Superfood Switch to Fight Fat, Defy Aging, and Eat Your Way Healthy

Dr. Mehmet C. Oz

WITH TED SPIKER AND THE EDITORS OF
DR. OZ THE GOOD LIFE

SCRIBNER

New York London Toronto Sydney New Delhi

Scribner
An Imprint of Simon & Schuster, Inc.
1230 Avenue of the Americas
New York, NY 10020

First Scribner trade paperback edition November 2018

SCRIBNER and design are registered trademarks of The Gale Group, Inc., used under license by Simon & Schuster, Inc., the publisher of this work.

For information about special discounts for bulk purchases, please contact Simon & Schuster Special Sales at 1-866-506-1949 or business@simonandschuster.com.

The Simon & Schuster Speakers Bureau can bring authors to your live event. For more information or to book an event, contact the Simon & Schuster Speakers Bureau at 1-866-248-3049 or visit our website at www.simonspeakers.com.

Interior design by Kris Tobiassen of Matchbook Digital
Endpaper photograph by Yasu + Junko

Manufactured in the United States of America

10 9 8 7 6 5 4 3 2 1

Library of Congress Cataloging-in-Publication Data is available.

ISBN 978-1-5011-5815-5
ISBN 978-1-5011-5816-2 (pbk)
ISBN 978-1-5011-5817-9 (ebook)

*To moms, who have always
known that food can fix it*

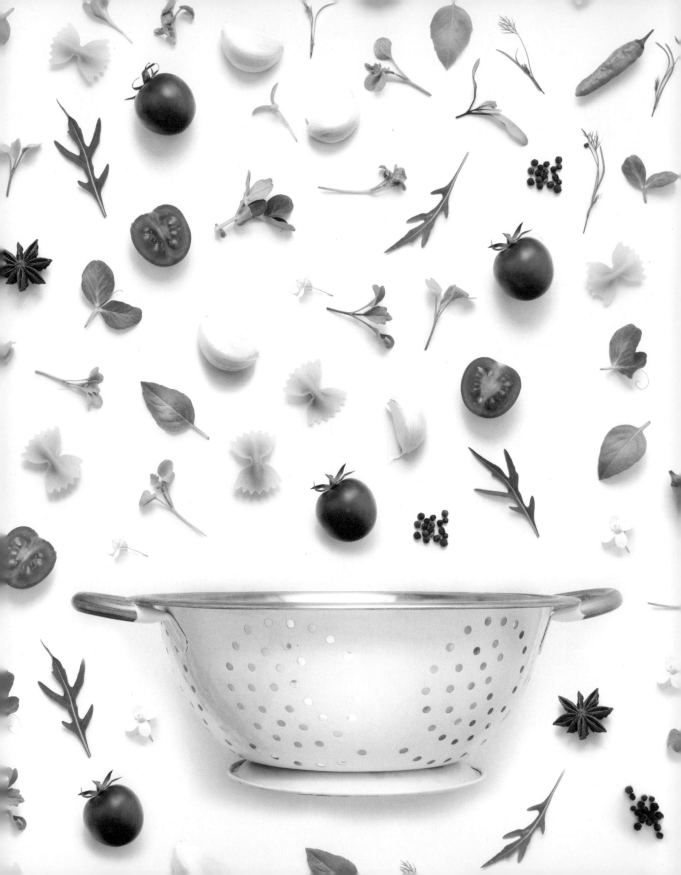

contents

PART 1: FOOD FOUNDATIONS

1. How Food Fixes You

Meals can work like medicine, or create mayhem in your body. Watch how it happens (and you may never eat junk again).

2. Your 5 Food FIXES

My easy-to-remember way of eating is your secret code to a longer and stronger life.

3. Strength in Strategy

These tactics will help you resist cravings and temptations by putting knowledge into action.

4. A Serving of Soul

As the backdrop for a million special moments in your life, meals pack more than just nutritional power.

PART 2: FOOD FIXES

PART 3: EAT IT, LOVE IT, LIVE IT

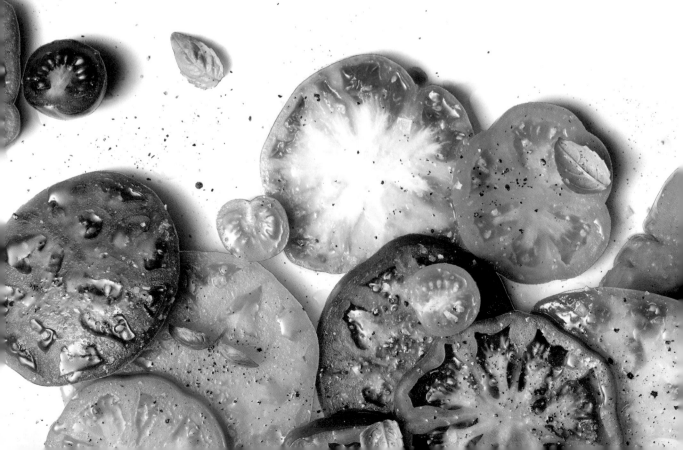

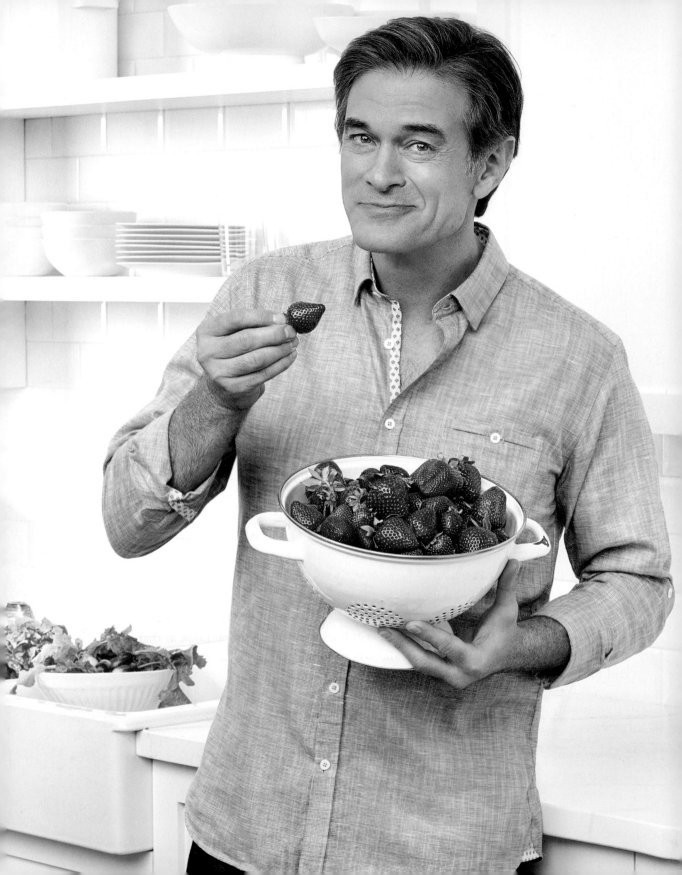

The Power of Your Plate

How food heals your body and energizes your life.

Right here, right now, I want you to stop what you're doing and think of the last thing you ate.

I don't care if it was healthy or unhealthy, homemade or plucked out of a vending machine, plain or smothered in cheese. Remember what it looked like and how it tasted?

Now think about this: Do you know what happened afterward?

Sure, you may understand in broad terms—some of it exited your body, some might have trespassed on your belly, hips, or thighs. Beyond that, do you understand how food interacts with your biological universe, in all of its mystery and majesty?

Every ingredient in every bite of every meal you eat is a passenger on a ride through the magical kingdom that is made up of your organs, cells, tissues, and various vessels. And they're not passive passengers who just *ooh* and *ahh* at the attractions ("Cool! Look at that colon rolling!"). These passengers participate in the way your body works—how you operate, how you feel, how you live.

Of all the personal choices you can make about your health, nothing holds greater influence than the food you eat. Yes, food can break you, but it also holds the power to fix your body, prevent some diseases, and reverse others. I wrote this book to help you harness that power and to share some of the lessons I have learned about food, eating, and life. I'll begin with my top five.

Food is medicine. In Italy, pharmacy is spelled *farmacia*, and there is a lot of truth embedded in how we read that word. Some of the world's best cures are grown on our farms and available in our supermarkets, ready to go to work in your body if you know what to reach for and how to prepare it. The right food can even replace that daily pill (and all the annoying side effects that come with it).

Food is an eraser that can wipe away past lifestyle lapses and health mistakes.

Food is the extension cord that energizes and lengthens your life. Science is only now advanced enough to prove what our ancestors may have figured out with trial and error, and scores and scores of new studies annually are reinforcing the power of food on longevity.

Food is sacred and historically has brought people together in a unique way. When you can unite good eating with good feelings, you reap tremendous biological, spiritual, and emotional rewards.

Food can fix it, and I want to show you how.

In this book, you will find a map—a way forward that lets food improve *your* journey. It begins with my 21-Day Plan (along with 33 recipes, plus snacks), a chance to retrain your body and your taste buds so that you can start a lifelong commitment to eating well— and loving every body-changing bite. I'm going to give you the knowledge, the tools, and the strategies to help you heal or prevent the problems you're most concerned about, because food can fix so many health issues, big and small, from your weight to your heart to your ability to fight off a nasty cold.

I call this approach a "superfood switch." Now, people throw around the term "super-food" a lot, sometimes implying that there's a single food with magical properties that can overhaul your health. No such food exists. I wouldn't even offer you a list of "Top 20 Super-foods" because a nutritious diet cannot be reduced that way. Instead, I will introduce you to an eating philosophy that emphasizes a *range* of healing whole foods, including hundreds of vegetables, fruits, sources of protein and fats, spices, herbs, teas, and more. They're *all* super-foods that work hard for your body, and when you embrace them, you'll not only reap their benefits but also crowd the bad stuff right off your plate. It's not a buy-this label or an eat-this checklist, but a superfood way of life.

Throughout my personal and professional journey, I have seen food change people. In fact, food has changed me. Let's take a quick look back at my childhood and I'll explain how.

In lots of kitchens, you'll find some kind of junk drawer. You know the one I'm talking about—it's filled with rubber bands, fourteen half-used tubes of ChapStick, some batteries, a recipe you tore out of a magazine, and various other random morsels.

When I was growing up, my mother kept a junk drawer. This one? Had nothing but candy.

Even now, I can see it perfectly—a little to the right of our kitchen sink. My mother kept it filled up like the car's gas tank. It never hit empty. Leftover Halloween candy? Went in the drawer. A handful of mints from a restaurant? Went in the drawer. Impulse chocolate buy from the supermarket line, lollipop from the barber, stick of gum from the bottom of a purse? Drawer, drawer, drawer.

That treasure chest was stocked, and my duty was to unstock it.

It's no wonder I had lots of cavities as a kid. Every day when I got home from school, I scooped out something sweet. Looking back at it now, I really was the poster child for the Pavlovian response: see drawer, drool, pop a treat.

I wish I could say that was my worst food habit. The first time I became aware of the effects of dumb eating came in fifth grade. I fell in love, and the object of my affection was Fluffernutter sandwiches.

White bread, peanut butter, Marshmallow Fluff.

I ate a couple of those gooey concoctions every day at lunch, and thought nothing of it until one afternoon in sixth grade, when a teacher came up to me in the cafeteria and said, "My, you've become a portly boy." Even though I didn't understand a lick about nutrition and had to look up the definition of *portly*, I sensed deep down that the Fluffernutters were probably to blame.

After this incident, I gradually started to pick up on the ways food could change you, but it really hit home once I started playing college football. There, we learned about nutrition as it related to performance—what we should eat to gain muscle, what we needed to do on game day, how to stay hydrated, and so on.

Coaches would warn us that all of our hard (and often painful) work on the practice field would be wasted if we made bad decisions in the dining hall. They made it seem simple. If I was going to push myself to lift weights, I should also skip the sweets so I wouldn't reverse all my training progress in the gym.

This was the first time I remember food being something that people talked about in a medicinal way, emphasizing how it could help our bodies. The message: Football wasn't just about making plays and lifting weights. It was about fueling ourselves to perform the best we could. That seems to me to be a truth that can apply to all of us in the stadium of life as well. We should eat to function, live, and perform as well as we can.

In medical school, I assumed my courses would teach everything I needed to know to diagnose and hopefully cure people. (As a kid, doctors were like Sherlock Holmes. Not only was my pediatrician all-knowing, he could even predict realities. Once he noted that I must be right handed because my left shoulder was higher than my right when I walked. I was stunned. Who notices this stuff?) I took classes in pharmacology, histology, physiology, pathology, every -ology you can think of.

Yet there was no food-ology.

We weren't offered any courses or material about nutrition. As president of the student body, I listened to what my fellow students wanted, and we agreed that we needed coursework on food's effect on health. Initially, the school developed classes on malnourished populations around the world, but we pushed for more on how vitamins and nutrients worked in conjunction with the body's systems. There wasn't much data available at the time, so I started to become more involved in research about food, working on papers about how nutrients functioned in the body (we did this by putting a needle in people's veins and feeding vitamins directly into the blood).

Later, as a cardiac surgeon and professor of surgery at Columbia University, I saw how nutrition was directly related to health and recovery. Yes, we could fix many problems with our scalpels and techniques. We were trained to heal with steel. But that approach wasn't all we needed to succeed. For example, when we did research on patients receiving artificial hearts, it turned out that one of the best ways we could predict their health outcomes was to look at how good their nutrition was before and after the operation. We were surprised to find that compared to major risk factors like the complexity of the operation or the type of machines we used, nutrition could also be an important predictor of how well they did.

My lightbulb moment: Our efforts in surgery wouldn't mean much if people opted back in to a life of gravy and doughnuts afterward.

I remember one young woman whose arteries were blocked and needed bypass surgery. After the operation, her husband brought fast food to her hospital bed as soon as she could eat. The scene hit me hard. He unknowingly helped her negate the work we had done. I've also seen it go in the opposite direction. Many patients have fully reversed their bad health situations, avoiding surgeries and other treatments, just by changing their diet.

Now, as host of *The Dr. Oz Show* and founder of *Dr. Oz The Good Life* magazine, I have had many unique opportunities to gather and share knowledge. Our team has published about one thousand articles and done some 1,500 shows (making up over ten thousand segments), and a large number of them have focused on our ever-changing nutritional world. I have interviewed some of the top thinkers in nutrition and food science—from universities like Harvard, University of Pennsylvania, and Stanford, as well as the country's leading hospitals, like Cleveland Clinic, Mayo Clinic, and my own New York–Presbyterian. It is my job to take my ideas as well as the thoughts of others and present them in a cohesive way that makes sense for my viewers and readers. I act like glue, piecing together some of the best ideas and tactics, even if they come from different sources.

My sources, by the way, aren't always scientists; I've also talked to athletes, celebrities, and regular folks who have experimented and found food strategies that have helped them improve performance or fight a disease or lose weight. On my show and in my magazine, we've listened to and learned from your struggles and your successes in the real world, where kids, spouses, and bosses are tugging at you for attention and where temptation awaits you under every neon sign.

Of all my nutritional influences, though, none has been more important than my wife, Lisa, and her family. When I met Lisa at age twenty-three, I experienced a life-changing education in what food *was*. Here I was eating steak and potatoes every night, and along comes this woman whose family operated on a totally different nutritional plane. Lisa's father, Gerald Lemole, M.D., was a heart surgeon as well, and so famous that he was the answer to a Trivial Pursuit question. My in-laws weren't farmers, yet they shared some of those same from-the-ground principles. The Lemoles grew lots of their own fruits, vegetables, and herbs, or sourced them locally. They made medicinal teas. They ate 100% whole-grain and Ezekiel bread. I went for white everything, but they chose grains I had never heard of. It was wonderful to learn about a whole new way of eating. I started sharing meals with them and loved not just the food, but also their different table traditions. Everyone gathered together and even shared "readings" at dinner—I grew up watching the news at our family dinners.

The Lemoles were ahead of their time, no doubt, as they instinctually linked nutrition and health together. It was fascinating to see them use food as their fountain of youth and vitality. And their six kids never seemed to get sick. Even their pets seemed healthier than normal.

This was the foundation for how Lisa and I raised our own family. Throughout these pages, I'm going to take you inside our family kitchen not just to pass along favorite recipes,

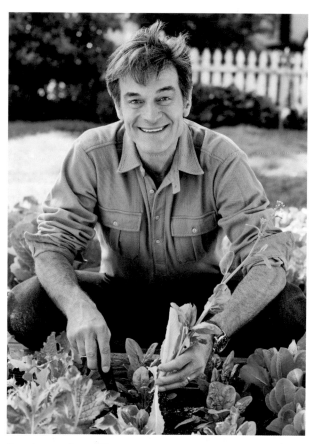

Fresh produce, like these greens in Lisa's parents' garden, is one of summer's best gifts. Fill up on it whenever you can.

but also because the kitchen is the focal point of our home. That's where big and small moments are celebrated, issues discussed (and resolved), and energy generated. I want the same for you. I want your kitchen to be a place of happiness and satisfaction.

My experiences in life and science have shaped my guiding principles about food and what it can (and can't) fix. The following seven principles serve as the foundation for much of what you will read in this book.

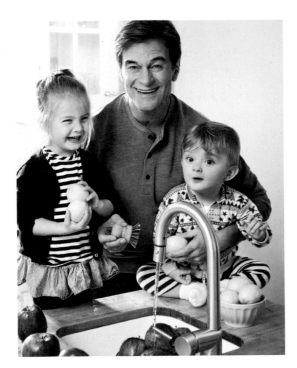

The kitchen island is where we all come together to laugh, connect, and prep meals. Yes, even our grandkids, Philomena and John, help out.

Food can be an answer, but it's not the only one. There is indisputable evidence that food plays a major role in how well our bodies work. You can use food to improve issues involving weight, heart disease, fatigue, and so many other ailments (you'll read about the biggies in the next section). But I also want to make this perfectly clear: Food cannot fix *everything*.

In some areas, we just don't know for sure what kind of an effect food might have. Also, I hope it goes without saying that while food indeed has superpowers, there are many ailments, diseases, and conditions that absolutely call for modern interventions—surgery, medication, or other treatments. Taking care of yourself often means tapping in to the latest developments in the health care field. After all, a salmon sandwich won't fix a bone-on-bone hip joint, but a hip replacement almost certainly will. That said, you can and should use food to prevent and improve many ailments—and doing so may mean you'll need fewer traditional interventions. You can actually heal with meals. That power you hold? Pretty amazing.

Many factors influence your health, but food is often the most important. Numerous variables play a role in determining how healthy you are, such as genetics, exercise, stress, and lifestyle choices (like smoking and other addictions). Your food decisions commingle with all those factors, amplifying some and counterbalancing others, and they all work in concert to determine your overall wellness. I won't refer to these other influences as much here, because I want the focus to stay on the potential power of food. But diet does not exist in isolation.

The goal isn't speed, but habit. This book is about bodily fixes, not magic bullets. It's not as if you can eat a bowl of walnuts and suddenly snap out of a bad mood or that three days of kale smoothies will make your heart stronger than a 747. But when you shift your dietary choices to delicious foods that become habitual and make you happy, you will slowly but surely reverse damage, restore your original body settings, and give yourself the best chance at living a strong and energetic life. That said, the effects deep down inside the body can kick in very quickly (at the biological level, things start shifting within two weeks). And changes in what you eat can make you *feel* different immediately.

You should use your body as a lab. The highest order of data—well-designed and peer-reviewed scientific studies—make up some of the evidence I will present. However, the most important studies about nutrition tend to be population-based—meaning that you can't say x *causes* y, but rather that there is a *relationship* between x and y. The takeaway for you: Plenty of nutritional evidence is revealing, but you also have to use individual experimentation to see how it works in *your* body. There's no perfect diet that can be applied to everyone,

but there are major principles that have been shown to work for many.

We can also take cues from communities that do some of their own experimentation, simply through the way they live. For example, I'll talk about the areas of the world where people live the longest. The insights from these populations can give us hints about food not yet covered thoroughly by traditional scientific research.

My basic approach is to take the best evidence that is available and translate it for my family and friends, with the understanding that it all goes back to the point I made above: You have to use your own body as sort of a mini lab. Try things, make adjustments, fine-tune, and experiment to hit on what works for you.

My goal? To provide a general field guide, so you know the basics about what to eat, how to eat, and why it matters. While we're all designed the same way, we don't all operate the same way. When you fiddle with the controls, you can zero in on what helps you feel better, live healthy, and heal when necessary.

You can't learn if you aren't willing to exit your comfort zone. The great musician and philosopher (well, sort of) Frank Zappa once said, "A mind is like a parachute. It doesn't work if it's not open." So I ask you to open your mind to new foods, to retry foods you think you don't like, and to give new ways of eating a shot.

In college, I roomed with a bright 6-foot-5 basketball player. One night he was rummaging around our fridge (tall men call these armrests), discovered a banana on top, and asked me what one tasted like. I couldn't believe my ears: Had this full-grown man never eaten a banana? He said that he remembered trying the fruit as a young child and not liking it, so he never tried it again, even though he knew the potassium would come in handy after long practices. We wrestled with the banana (literally) until I got him to taste it. That bite went over pretty well, and he ate bananas daily for the rest of our college days together. I tell this story because many people do what my roommate did: They say "never again" to foods they've sampled only once. I'm hoping you will follow along for a gastronomic ride in which you take some new routes, see new sights, and perhaps expand your world to options that you never considered before.

Good food doesn't have to be boring. Nowadays, people equate fun eating with helpings the size of sand castles and a Friday night date with a log of cookie dough. The flip side is that healthy eating must involve sad violin music playing as you nibble on four nuts and a baby carrot. Over the years I've tried to change the narrative about healthy eating, and this has been one of the most frustrating challenges. Can you trust that eating can *be* good for you and *taste* good to you? When you believe that both are possible, that's the real recipe for success.

Healing foods help to heal the planet. If your body could talk, it would tell you to eat the way this book suggests, fueling up with foods that provide sustainable energy and maintain your biological balance. And guess what: If the planet had a voice, it would cheer for the choices you'll be making. That's because you'll be cutting back a bit on red meat, though you'll never miss it, with all the luscious plant-based foods heaped on your plate. Anytime one of us replaces an animal protein with something grown from the ground, we do the environment a giant favor. My friend David Katz, Director of the Yale University Prevention Research Center, points to a recent study that suggests we could meet half or more of the greenhouse gas reductions pledged in the Paris Accord just by swapping beans for beef on a regular basis. It's that simple to help repair our environment while you rejuvenate your body.

The main ingredient in as many meals as possible: laughter. This is at the heart of the book you are holding: You should not only love the foods you eat, but also love the people you eat with. That way, meals become memories. As often as you can, make meals a time for building relationships, bonding with old and new friends, and learning about life. Above all, if healing with meals feels like a chore or makes you sad or doesn't send jolts of joy onto your tongue and down into your belly, then something's not right, and I want to fix that—so that food can fix you.

This isn't a cookbook, though you'll find plenty of delicious recipes here. This isn't a diet book, though my plan will help you lose weight if you need to. And this isn't a textbook, though I hope you learn a lot. In a way, *Food Can Fix It* is a bit of a stew that includes all of these things.

Here's what you'll find inside:

Part 1: Food Foundations. Right from the start, I will take you through the basics about how food interacts with your body, for better or worse. The biological principles we'll cover will explain why you're eating what you're eating in my 21-Day Plan. I will also include everyday tricks and strategies to help you eat well, because I understand that *knowing* the material isn't the same as *living* it. Finally, I will spend a few pages talking about the more spiritual and sacred elements of eating and why those play a role in helping you heal. In order to make the most of your meals, you have to really think about the biological, practical, and *soulful* elements of food. You'll get the big picture of all three to help you understand the biology of your body, make smart food decisions, and automate your great new habits.

Part 2: Food Fixes. The book's bread-and-butter (which is not a food fix, by the way), this section covers some of the most common and feared ailments, and gives you the main eating approach for improving problems or preventing them in the first place. You can focus on only the individual ailments that are most concerning to you, but I recommend that you read them all to get a whole-body picture of how food acts as medicine.

Part 3: Eat It, Love It, Live It. This section explains how to put your nutritional know-how into action. My program includes the 21-Day Plan with 33 recipes and snacks, a 3-day optional cleanse, and strategies for eating well forever. Here you'll find more than 100 recipes as well as ideas to put this plan into action every day, including when you're dining out. You'll start the process of healing your body—fortifying yourself against a host of health threats—and, perhaps most important, you'll have fun doing it.

Throughout, I'm going to pepper your reading with bits of trivia about food. Some of them might make you smile, or just inspire an *I-never-knew-that* head shake. I'm not prepping you for an appearance on *Jeopardy!* or tossing out cocktail-party fodder; I have simply loved learning about all the different ways that food is grown and prepared, and how it nourishes us. I want to share some of the cool facts I've learned about coffee, chicken, wine, fruit, and more, because when you know about the origin and preparation of food, you understand why your choices matter. Plus, it just makes eating more interesting.

Before we get started, it's worth asking yourself one question:

What's your version of the candy drawer?

I want you to clean it out, whatever it is. Because we're going to create a new one filled with nourishing ingredients, easy and delicious meals, and a new way of thinking about nature's most powerful—and pleasing—medicine.

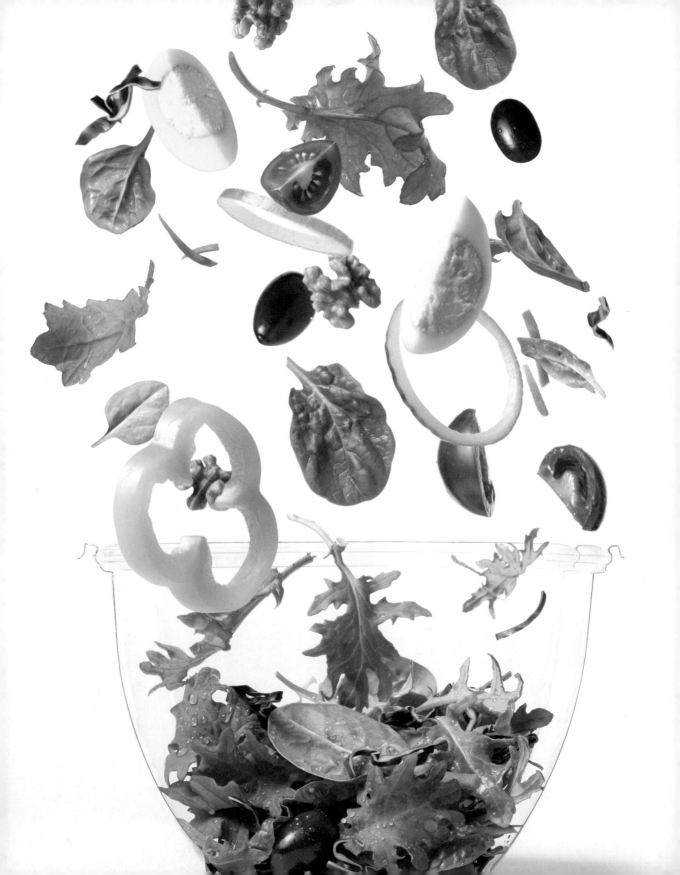

PART 1

FOOD FOUNDATIONS

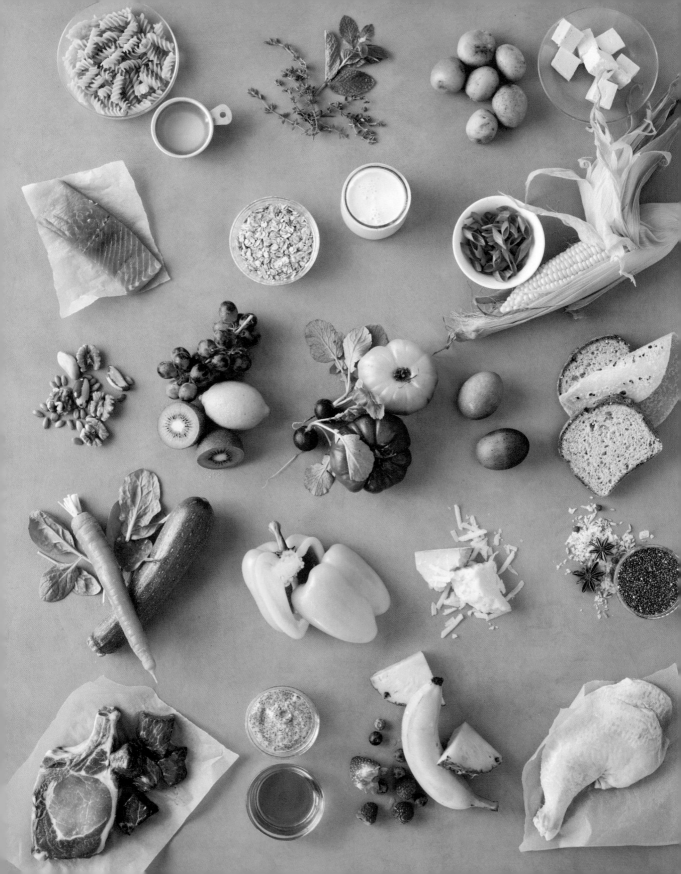

How Food Fixes You

Meals can work like medicine, or create mayhem in your body. Watch how it happens (and you may never eat junk again).

In this day and age, the collective medical bag of tricks is overflowing. We use robots to help perform surgery. We can transplant hearts and replace joints. We laser corneas to restore perfect eyesight, freeze off suspicious skin spots, and design prosthetic limbs worthy of an Olympian.

The scientific and medical communities have worked together to improve the length and quality of our lives. I am proud to have played a small part in this effort, but I am also a staunch believer in low-tech, patient-powered solutions. When it comes to food, I want you to have your own sort of medical license—a license to strengthen your body through the most effective tool that *you* control.

As you already know, candy, meat, potatoes, and ice cream made up most of my childhood diet. I've come a long way since then. When my eating habits changed, *I* changed. I had more energy, I had more stamina, I was in a better mood, I didn't get run down or suffer from colds and long streaks of blahness. I found enjoyment by living a healthy, zestful life, not from eating processed marshmallow goo.

That's *my* story. There are thousands of others who have discovered that you don't always need fancy interventions; you can direct your own well-being, largely through how you nourish yourself. Of the many guests who have been on my show to talk about their transformations, a few stand out. For example, a woman named Jenny, who told me she once weighed over five hundred pounds. Sometimes she would eat six bowls of pasta in a day. There were many things she couldn't do with her children, and she got angry when her family tried to help her. But her eye-opening moment came when she saw a picture of herself with her daughter. She started to cry. That was the moment, she said, when she realized she was a "double woman, living half a life."

Soon after, she embarked on a new food journey—changing what and how much she ate—with the encouragement of her husband and mother-in-law. She had two goals: to lose 250 pounds and to ride a bike again, something she hadn't been able to do for a long, long time.

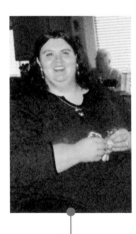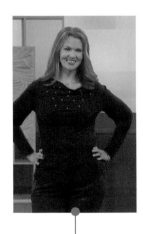

Jenny at her peak weight of 509 pounds . . .

. . . and after she lost 311 pounds.

She cut her portion sizes, for sure, but also made the superfood switch. She replaced foods that hurt with foods that healed. She found that healthful foods could taste good, give her energy, shrink her body, and soothe her soul. It took several years, but eventually she was able to ride that bike. And she lost more than three hundred pounds. Wow.

While Jenny's story is extreme, the takeaway is the same for anyone: Change the food you eat, and you change your body. It may take some time, but along the way, you will feel differences in your energy and happiness—and you will see the results in a stronger, fitter, healthier life.

I know it's not easy. Temptations, stresses, and various other hurdles mess with our good-eating intentions. But the picture gets clearer and simpler when you view it through this filter: Your body deserves for you to eat respectfully. And you can do that while enjoying delicious meals. But the first step is learning how food functions in your body so you can comprehend how it *fixes* your body. Understanding motivates change.

The thirty-thousand-foot view: Everything we eat and drink is measured by calories—the unit that represents how much energy a particular food gives us to fuel our organs and systems. Those calories get processed and distributed throughout the body. Too few calories? That's like running on an empty tank of gas—it just won't work. Too many calories? Well, you already know that's what triggers weight gain in the form of fat storage. But I don't want you to count every calorie or obsess about them. I'd much rather you concentrate on the *kinds* of foods you eat—and what they're made of.

That's because a calorie is not a calorie is not a calorie. They all interact in your body in ways that can be either messy or medicinal. Consider a small portion of food—say, 100 calories of cooked black beans (about ½ cup) versus 100 calories of jelly beans (about 25). The black beans have all sorts of things that are good for you, like fiber and protein. Your body breaks them down during digestion and takes those nutrients and puts them to good work. But because the candy is pure sugar, there's not a lot of nutritional value in it for your body. Your brain is searching for nutrients rather than calories. Give it empty calories, and your brain has you rummaging through the fridge for more nutrients. But if you give it nutrients, calories become an afterthought.

Food is made up of three macronutrients—protein, carbohydrates, and fat. Most foods aren't wholly one or the other, but rather a combination of the three. Some foods are considered "carbs" or "protein" or "fat" because they're predominantly made up of one of those macros, and that's how you will come to think of them.

In the next chapter, I will take you through each of these macros so you can see what constitutes low-quality food and high-quality food—the kind that will help you live longer and stronger. As you learn about them, keep this golden rule in mind:

The closer you can get to eating foods the way they appear in nature, the better off you will be.

Eat grilled fish, not fish sticks. Eat orange slices, not orange soda.

Think of it this way: The more "process" a food goes through *outside* your body, the higher the chance it will mess up the processes *inside* your body.

After you decide what goes from your fork to your mouth, that food essentially hits a fork in the road. During digestion, it will go one of three ways: Your body will use it, toss it, or store it.

Use It: Your body takes the calories you consume and turns them into glucose—sugar that circulates in your blood. That glucose is shuttled through a series of highways. The hormone insulin transports glucose into your cells to provide energy that will keep everything working. Some glucose goes to your muscles, some will help rev your brain, and so on.

Toss It: Bathroom breaks, basically. Your body knows it needs to eliminate some of what it doesn't immediately need, so it does so via our waste systems. After foods and drinks are digested through the stomach and intestines, some of the excess moves down and out.

Store It: Your body is smart, so it keeps a system to store some of your glucose. It knows you may not always have food on hand to give you energy (this was a need long ago, when we experienced periods of famine), so it holds on to some in reserve. Your body stores those extra calories as a substance called glycogen. This backup fuel tank isn't very large (only about 300 calories are in there), but it does come in handy; glycogen allows you to keep functioning even if it's been hours and hours since your last meal. The trouble comes when you eat more than your glycogen tank can store. That overflow? It gets stored in the form of fat cells. An excess intake of about 3,500 calories adds up to approximately one pound of fat. So if you are twenty-five pounds overweight (the average in America), you could be storing about 87,500 calories in fat.

To truly understand the effect of food, though, you have to parachute down from the thirty-thousand-foot view and look around in the weeds at all the chemical interactions that happen in your body day after day after day. Let's start with two more detailed scientific scenarios—one in which food plays the villain and another where food comes to the rescue.

Meals Making Mayhem

For this part of our journey, we need to cast an archenemy—that is, a sinister meal on a mission to sabotage your body. A number of culprits could take on this role (one look at a mall food court should give you a few ideas), but I'll stick with the All-American antagonist: a cheeseburger, a bucket of fries, a soda, and a sundae.

Even if you think you don't know diddly about nutrition, you're probably aware that this combo is often equated with weight gain, clogged arteries, and general body breakdown. In fact, some food joints get right to the point, calling their craziest burger platters the 9-1-1 or the Widow-Maker. You're about to see that there's *truth* to that menu-speak. This heaping helping of toxicity features all kinds of nasties

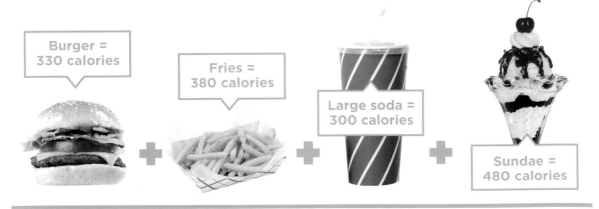

Burger = 330 calories + Fries = 380 calories + Large soda = 300 calories + Sundae = 480 calories

= 1,490 CALORIES IN ONE MEAL!

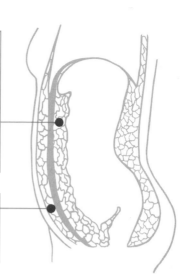

VISCERAL FAT is stored deep in the belly and wraps around organs. It is also stored in the omentum, the fatty tissue that covers and supports the intestines and other organs in the lower abdomen. Excess fat deposits here are associated with a number of health conditions.

SUBCUTANEOUS FAT, the kind you can pinch, is less dangerous.

that work against us—from bad fats to refined sugar to wacky chemicals. So let's give the scoundrel our own name: the Body Breaker.

What makes the Body Breaker a bad guy like no other? It lures you in, then turns on you.

That's because it tastes *good*. Fat has nice mouthfeel, and sugar pleases the tongue and mind (literally by hitting our brain like crack cocaine). As you dig in, you feel immediate satisfaction. But while the Body Breaker romances you with taste and texture, it vandalizes your insides. Let's take a look at all the things that are happening as this meal moves through your biological universe:

It gets stored as fat. A Body Breaker meal can have upward of 1,500 calories, which is more fuel than most people need for an entire day. Your body converts those calories into blood glucose and machine-guns it into your bloodstream. Because there's too much for you to use, your body decides some needs to be socked away. Through a complex chemical process, that glucose can eventually get converted into fat. Your body—via your genetic programming—will decide whether to store that fat in your belly, hips, thighs, or backside (usually some special combo of all four). Extra fat taxes your body's systems, which can contribute to heart and arterial problems. The most dangerous kind is stored deep in the belly—that's called visceral fat. Why is it so harmful? Fat releases toxins and stress hormones. Because the belly is so close to your vital organs, the toxins can damage those organs.

It puts you at risk for developing diabetes. Your pancreas produces insulin, which is your body's Uber driver, taking glucose where it needs to go. But when you overload your system with glucose (in the form of too much food and too many simple sugars that can't be used immediately), your body can't always produce enough insulin to keep up. The result is a condition called insulin resistance—and that means there's no vehicle to take the glucose around the body. The extra glucose hangs around, and those stranded sugar molecules float through your system looking for something to do. Diabetes happens when you have too much of that circulating blood sugar (officially defined as 126 milligrams per deciliter) and affects nearly 10 percent of us. Prediabetes (defined as 100 to 125 mg/dL) afflicts one-third of Americans. The excess glucose winds up looting your body by damaging blood vessels and organs, which also contributes to the next problem.

It nicks and clogs your arteries. Of all the crimes the Body Breaker commits, roughing up your arteries may be the scariest. This is the damage associated with life-changers like high blood pressure and other heart and arterial disease, as well as life-enders like heart attacks. Here's how it works: Your arteries are made up of various layers—the outer layer protecting the inner ones. The Body Breaker, which sends all of that extra glucose floating around, acts like a graffiti artist, leaving its mark all over the inside walls of the arteries in the form of nicks and scratches (FYI: Cigarette smoke vandalizes similarly). Your body picks up on the damage and wants to do anything it can to protect the inside of the artery from further harm. So it covers the wound and forms a scab like it would anywhere else that's hurt (for example a skinned knee). But the only plaster your body has is cholesterol. Some foods (including that burger) lead to increased LDL cholesterol (the

HOW PREDIABETES WORKS

1. Your digestive system breaks down carbs into molecules, including glucose, that enter your blood through the intestinal wall. In your bloodstream, the glucose is called blood sugar. 2. When your blood sugar level rises, the pancreas releases insulin into the bloodstream. It helps unlock your cells so the blood sugar can enter and be used for energy. 3. When you have prediabetes or type 2 diabetes, the body doesn't make enough insulin or can't use it properly—so the muscle cells can't take up enough sugar from the blood. All those sugar molecules build up in your blood and go floating around your system like vandals on a crime spree, damaging blood vessels and organs and raising your risk of cardiovascular disease, stroke, kidney disease, blindness, and amputation.

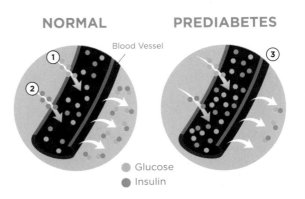

NORMAL   PREDIABETES

Blood Vessel

● Glucose
● Insulin

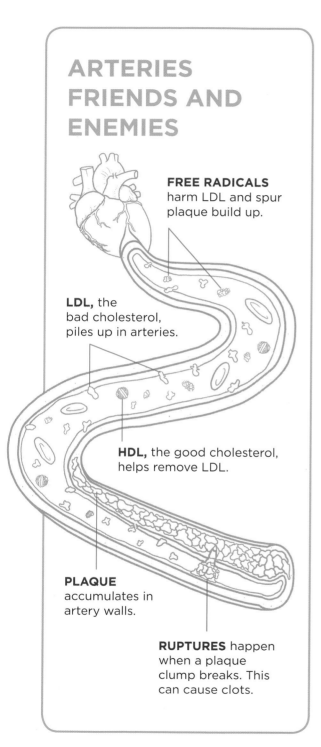

ARTERIES FRIENDS AND ENEMIES

FREE RADICALS harm LDL and spur plaque build up.

LDL, the bad cholesterol, piles up in arteries.

HDL, the good cholesterol, helps remove LDL.

PLAQUE accumulates in artery walls.

RUPTURES happen when a plaque clump breaks. This can cause clots.

bad kind—think *L* for Lousy), which burrows into those nicks and cuts in the arterial wall and eventually turns into plaque. The resulting clot means you risk cutting off blood flow in the artery. No blood flow is *no bueno*, because that's what causes heart attacks, strokes, kidney issues, impotence, and more. It's a process that started with having too much blood sugar from eating too much food and the wrong kinds of food. And it got helped along by having a lot of LDL "plaster" around, from saturated fats in stuff like red meat. Make Body Breaker meals a regular habit, and your body just can't keep up.

It creates a systematic riot in the form of inflammation. Your body is smart enough to recognize the Body Breaker and its team of hooligans, out to make trouble, and it has a police force in the form of immune cells. Their jobs are to heal damage and to bring peace to biological riots. Whenever your body is damaged—let's say you twist an ankle or cut yourself—your immune cells come in to protect the area. The resulting action is inflammation. It's the sign of the fight: the ankle swelling after you twist it, the skin scabbing after you cut it. Immune fighters come in, do their job, and go back to their headquarters to fight another day.

But the inflammation process happens deep inside your body as well, and can do more harm than good. When too many Body Breaker meals cause plaque to form in your arteries, inflammation happens there and raises your risk of heart trouble. And the fat those

Body Breakers add to your hips? It triggers inflammation, too. Fat cells don't just sit there; they actually contain and release chemicals that are toxic to nearby organs. Immune soldiers migrate to fight them off, and that brings on—you guessed it—more inflammation. When inflammation is elevated, immune cells are in overdrive, keeping your body in a constant state of stress and hyperactivity. It's called chronic inflammation, and it contributes to all-over destruction—not just heart damage, but brain decline, GI trouble, and more.

It makes you feel like garbage. Okay, so maybe that's not a clinical term you'll find in any medical text, but you know exactly what I'm talking about. While the Body Breaker may give you an immediate flavor high during the seven minutes you're gobbling it down, what you feel for the next twenty-three hours and fifty-three minutes is far more powerful. Pretty quickly, you'll want to hit the couch. Your stomach is weighed down with leadlike bad fats that take a long time to break down and digest, making your body feel sluggish and heavy. Then there's the sugar crash, which works as follows: The Body Breaker is full of simple carbohydrates and refined sugar (hello, white bread bun, soda, and hot fudge sundae), all of which get converted quickly into glucose and dumped into your bloodstream. To get glucose out of your blood and into the cells that need it, the pancreas cranks up the production of insulin. That major surge of insulin delivers blood sugar to the cells, which squirrel away what

4 NUMBERS YOU NEED TO KNOW

These blood tests are a crucial tool because they give you an indication of what's happening inside your arteries. You can raise or lower your scores (and risks) via the foods you eat. Find out your . . .

LDL cholesterol (ideal = less than 100 mg/dL): Your body naturally produces this waxy fat—your cell membranes and some of your hormones need it. But eating too much of the wrong things can push production beyond what's good for you. That's why we call it the bad cholesterol (remember, **L** is for Lousy).

HDL cholesterol (ideal = 60 mg/dL or higher): The body's sanitation worker, this stuff picks up cholesterol and shuttles it off to the liver to be disposed of. Exercise and eating the right foods help your body make more HDL (**H** is for Healthy).

Blood sugar (ideal = less than 100 mg/dL): The amount of circulating glucose. The higher the number, the more inflammation, fat storage, and damage can be done. A blood sugar reading of 126 mg/dL or higher indicates diabetes, while 100 to 125 mg/dL is prediabetes.

Blood pressure (ideal = lower than 120/80 mm Hg): The higher it is, the more damage can happen to your arterial walls as blood attempts to travel through your arteries. High blood pressure leaves little scars on delicate artery walls, which become inviting homes for plaque and inflammation. Plus, your heart has to put out extra effort to manage the high pressure, which can weaken the organ over time.

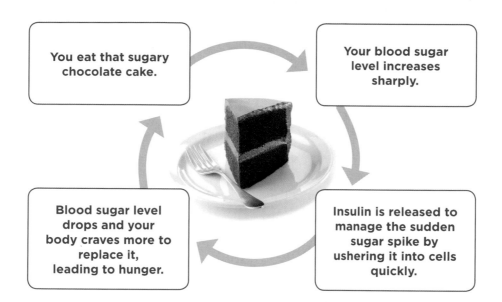

You eat that sugary chocolate cake.

Your blood sugar level increases sharply.

Insulin is released to manage the sudden sugar spike by ushering it into cells quickly.

Blood sugar level drops and your body craves more to replace it, leading to hunger.

they don't use. Suddenly, your brain can't find much sugar in your bloodstream anymore—so you may experience brain fog, low energy, and a strong desire to nap.

It makes you want to eat more. Your brain, sensing the abrupt drop-off, sends out a message: "Hey, eat something that will raise blood sugar fast!" You feel this as a craving to scarf down a snack, preferably a sweet one, ASAP. That may prop you up for a bit, but if you choose junk, the cycle starts all over again. Another dose of simple sugars goes through the same process you just read about—more energy highs and lows, more fat storage, more potential for damaged arteries. It's mayhem, folks.

You know these effects inherently because you *feel* them. Research backs up your experience with proof that criminal foods are related to bad moods, high stress, fatigue, and more. Much of that is caused by the dips and spikes in your blood sugar, yes. But there's another reason: When you fill your stomach with foods that fail you, you're not leaving room for foods that fix you, energizing and healing your body throughout the day.

Meals as Medicine

You just met a powerful foe, capable of crossing many of your biological wires. The result: damaged arteries, increased inflammation, added fat, ugh, ugh, ugh.

Now let's envision a more heroic meal. Many foods could fit the bill, but let's pick from the vast superfood menu a juicy piece of grilled chicken covered in, say, a peppery salsa or a mango relish. Sidekicks include a big-as-you-want serving of your favorite vegetable brushed with some olive oil and dotted with garlic, as well as a handful of baked sweet potato fries. *Ooh*, and there's a slice of avocado dressed with a squirt of lemon and a dash of red pepper flakes nestled onto your dish. The meal is packed with a bounty of flavors, satisfying portions, and vital nutrients.

The whole shebang would come in at around 416 calories, by the way. We'll call our hero the Hearty Healer. It works by calming all kinds of body chaos and maintaining biological equilibrium. How?

It slows digestion. The Hearty Healer contains nutrients that take longer to break down, which helps you avoid hunger highs and lows. For example, the nice hit of fiber in the sweet potatoes and vegetables takes longer to empty out of your stomach than foods made with simple sugars. That keeps you feeling full, which means you'll be less likely to overeat (and thus less likely to flood your bloodstream with extra glucose). And since none of the Hearty Healer foods is made with simple sugars, overpro-

cessed ingredients, or refined carbohydrates, they won't be immediately converted to glucose and shuttled into your bloodstream. They'll take time to transit through your body as it digests the healthy fats, proteins, and complex carbohydrates in this meal.

It keeps your blood flow moving. Remember what happens when the Body Breaker starts to funk up your arteries? Extra glucose causes nicks, which encourage the buildup of LDL cholesterol and plaque. Two elements of the Hearty Healer make it great for reducing damage in your arteries. One, the avocado contains healthy fats, which promote HDL cholesterol (the good kind—think *H* for Healthy). HDL sweeps away gooey cholesterol molecules. And two, the meal doesn't have lots of bad ingredients that can contribute to the buildup of LDL cholesterol, like the loads of saturated fat found in the Body Breaker, meaning that there's less cleanup work for the healthy cholesterol to do.

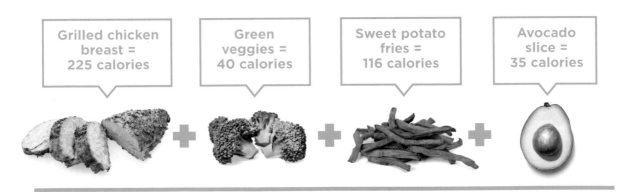

Grilled chicken breast = 225 calories + Green veggies = 40 calories + Sweet potato fries = 116 calories + Avocado slice = 35 calories

= 416 CALORIES

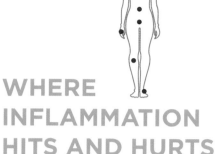

WHERE INFLAMMATION HITS AND HURTS

Sneaky inflammation may be at the root of many troubles.

↓

THE BRAIN
Alzheimer's, brain fog

↓

THE LUNGS
Allergic asthma

↓

THE HEART
Plaque buildup, hardening of the artery walls, heart attack, stroke

↓

THE GUT
Ulcerative colitis, Crohn's disease, irritable bowel syndrome (and the pain, gas, and bloating that can come with it)

↓

THE SKIN
Acne, rosacea, psoriasis, eczema

↓

THE JOINTS
General pain and arthritis

↓

ALL OVER
Diabetes, cancer, fatigue, feeling "meh," and low-grade depression

It quiets the inflammation. Inflammation happens when your body tries to heal some kind of conflict. Well, what happens when there's less conflict (fewer nicks in arteries, less plaque buildup)? Yup, there's less inflammation. So when you have a balanced meal in reasonable portions, there's no reason for your body to fight. Quiet the inflammation, and you'll quiet a whole host of potential issues.

It gives you zip and zest. Besides all the ways good foods work to stabilize your systems and reduce the chances you'll develop or worsen diseases and ailments, the Hearty Healer will just plain make you feel better. Why? Because a balanced diet with a steady supply of protein, healthy fats, and slow-digesting carbohydrates ensures that energy is provided to you steadily throughout the day, not in roller-coaster highs and lows. That also means you'll eat less—because you won't be reaching for sugary carbs to bring you up when you feel down. Welcome to a new, virtuous cycle: You eat to feel good, and feeling good helps you eat well.

The Hearty Healer works the way all nutritional superheroes do: strongly, quietly. In the next chapter, you will meet these heroes—and get a closer look at how their strength can become your strength.

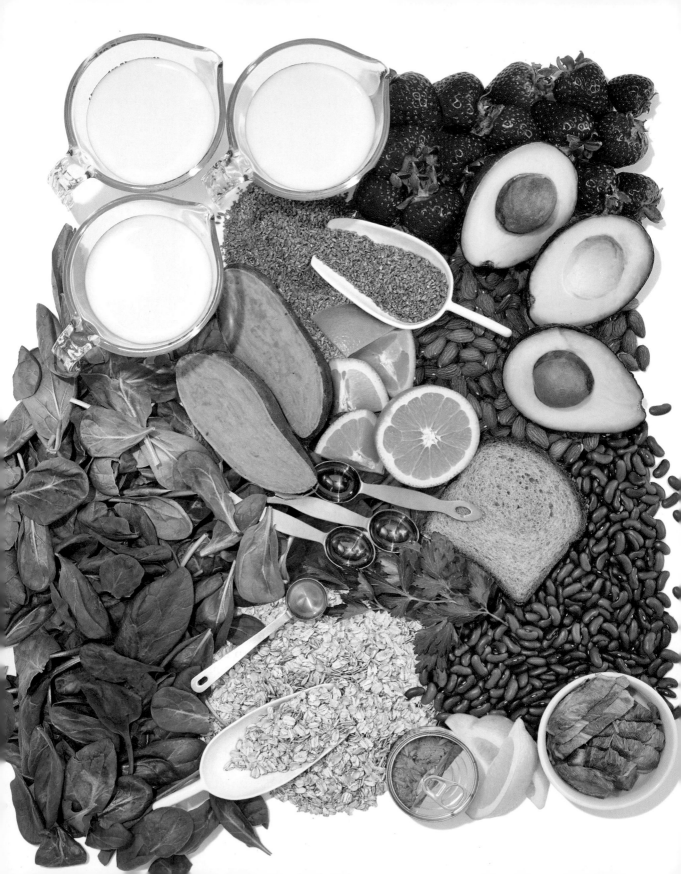

2

Your 5 Food FIXES

My easy-to-remember way of eating is your secret code to a longer and stronger life.

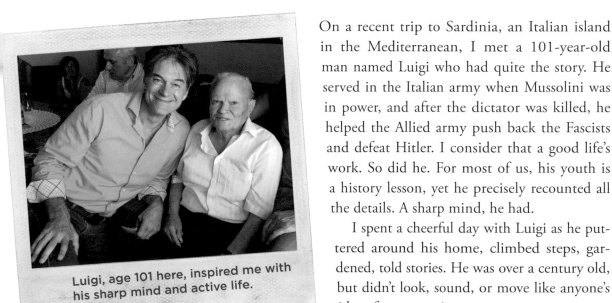

Luigi, age 101 here, inspired me with his sharp mind and active life.

On a recent trip to Sardinia, an Italian island in the Mediterranean, I met a 101-year-old man named Luigi who had quite the story. He served in the Italian army when Mussolini was in power, and after the dictator was killed, he helped the Allied army push back the Fascists and defeat Hitler. I consider that a good life's work. So did he. For most of us, his youth is a history lesson, yet he precisely recounted all the details. A sharp mind, he had.

I spent a cheerful day with Luigi as he puttered around his home, climbed steps, gardened, told stories. He was over a century old, but didn't look, sound, or move like anyone's idea of a centenarian.

I was visiting Sardinia because I wanted to learn more about the habits of the world's longest-living people. A couple of decades ago, a doctor and scientist named Gianni Pes was the first to identify Sardinia as one of the five places on earth where people enjoy the greatest longevity. He called them Blue Zones, and the term was popularized in a book of the same name by Dan Buettner. The other four areas are in Greece, Japan, Costa Rica, and the communities of Seventh-Day Adventists in California. There is even a Blue Zones company that teaches communities how to achieve similar longevity, and it's quite revealing when you learn the commonalities that cross from one part of the world to another. Half of them center around social habits—knowing your purpose, spending time with those you love, and having some kind of faith all seem to help people live longer, healthier lives. The other half? They revolve around food choices. Blue Zoners eat lots of plants, beans, and fish, and limit their meat and sugar. They also have some wine every day (except the Adventists).

That's how Luigi ate. That's how his friends ate. That's how people throughout the region ate. And that seems to be a main reason why these folks outlive most of us.

They certainly didn't follow a diet book, and nobody gave them an instruction manual or doctor's orders. People in Blue Zone cultures don't overthink their food. It's part of

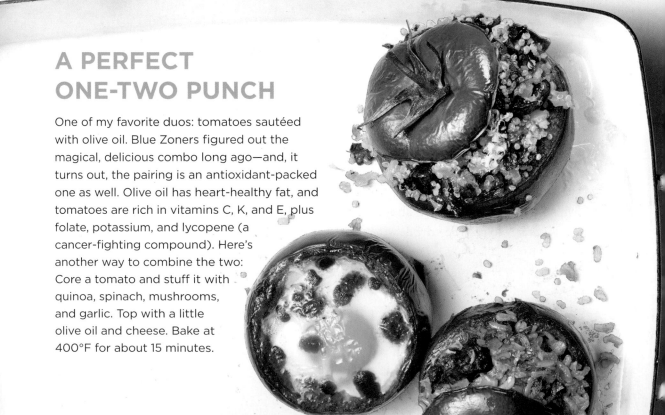

A PERFECT ONE-TWO PUNCH

One of my favorite duos: tomatoes sautéed with olive oil. Blue Zoners figured out the magical, delicious combo long ago—and, it turns out, the pairing is an antioxidant-packed one as well. Olive oil has heart-healthy fat, and tomatoes are rich in vitamins C, K, and E, plus folate, potassium, and lycopene (a cancer-fighting compound). Here's another way to combine the two: Core a tomato and stuff it with quinoa, spinach, mushrooms, and garlic. Top with a little olive oil and cheese. Bake at 400°F for about 15 minutes.

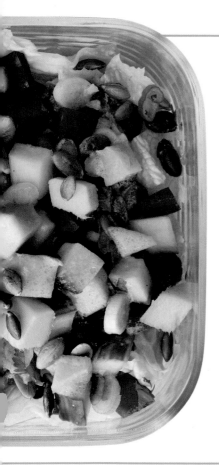

PACK YOUR FOODS SO YOU DON'T PACK ON THE POUNDS

It's not just *what* Blue Zoners eat, but *how* they eat that makes a difference. For example, their meals are essentially gorge-proof because their portions are small. One of the reasons? People carried their meals to work, so they couldn't bring a seven-course extravaganza.

I didn't even know it, but I practiced this Blue Zone technique early in my career. When I was first starting out at Columbia University, I rode my bike to work. It was much easier than driving in New York City traffic. I brought my lunch with me. Anything I wanted to eat I would have to carry, which meant I packed lightly. Small portions, by necessity.

Blue Zone eating habits—while all healthy—were automatic. It's how they lived. They didn't waste valuable mental energy figuring out what they were going to have morning, noon, and night. Packing light on the way to a place where there were no vending machines or food courts was natural and meant they would eat light as well. Automation was their stealth strategy.

Pre-prepped meals make good eating deliciously decision-free.

their lives—a happy part—but not the only part. They work, laugh, share, eat, and drink. They organize their days around food to reinforce a daily rhythm, but they don't obsess about it the way our modern culture does.

The Blue Zoners look to the wisdom of their ancestors for guidance about what belongs on their tables. They drink wine, but they don't imbibe with the goal of getting a buzz or forgetting about stresses. They figured out a long time ago that tomatoes and olive oil worked pretty well together in a sauce—it was simple and tasty—and they didn't find a need

to overprocess it. (By the way, it turns out that heating the tomatoes in oil is the best way to absorb the valuable antioxidant lycopene they contain. This was an antiaging trick before there was even a thing called antiaging.) They dotted their soups and pastas with meats, but felt no need to inhale pounds of beef at each sitting. And they carried those ways of life from one generation to the next without giving any thought to changing what was already working.

These people eat what is considered to be the classic Mediterranean diet and it's helped them live a very long time.

Longevity is one of the medicinal benefits of a superfood diet. The right foods are like high-octane fuel, increasing the efficiency and function of all your body's engines so they're less likely to break down. Remember all those systems I talked about in chapter 1? Healthy food helps to squash chemical chaos so everything works properly, and for a long time.

A second way in which healthy food works to heal you: On a chemical level, it acts a bit like body armor, protecting you against life's insults. Let me give an example.

I remember being a general-surgery resident and operating on a man who had colon cancer. He wasn't obese, but he didn't eat well. In many ways, he followed the junk-laden, standard American diet or SAD (which is often how we feel after consuming it). His health history showed that he didn't have many bowel movements, which partly explained why it took a while to detect his cancer. Poor nutrition meant that he wasn't regular, so when the colon cancer caused even more irregularity, he didn't pick up on the problem.

Our team operated on him, successfully cutting out the cancer and reattaching his intestines. Medically speaking, he should have been cured and lived for many years after that. But the man's wounds never healed. He died after a month in the hospital—not because of the cancer, but because his immune system couldn't overcome the insult of surgery. When we reviewed his case, we confirmed that his diet had played a role: Two very important markers in his blood—albumin and total protein, which are indicators of proper nutrition—showed that he was deficient in many nutrients and that his immune system was compromised.

WHY WINE WORKS

Wine may be the best example of how the plant kingdom relates to the animal kingdom. Grapes grown in hard conditions produce more of the compound resveratrol, which helps the grapes live longer—so they can survive the environment. When you take in resveratrol (by drinking wine or having foods that contain it—see page 102—it helps contribute to your longevity, because the antiaging benefits that the grape obtained are passed along to you. (This isn't license to glug-glug-glug the bottle, just insight into the origins of the health benefits of wine. While I don't want you to drink on my 21-Day Plan, after that, a glass of wine a day is fine.)

HOW TO READ A FOOD LABEL

Oftentimes, food labels are meant to distract you. Words that sound official—like *fat-free* and *healthy ingredients*—can be misleading. Fat-free can mean a food is packed with sugar, and just because a food contains healthy ingredients doesn't mean unhealthy ones aren't hiding in there as well. Plus, it can be difficult to interpret some of the numbers you see in the nutrient calculations. So keep these things in mind when looking at foods:

- In general, fewer ingredients is better. And if you don't recognize an ingredient, there's a good chance it doesn't come from Mother Nature.

- Don't just take calories into account; consider the size of a serving as well. If a can of food has 100 calories, that may not sound like a lot—until you see that it contains 3.5 servings and you had planned on eating the whole thing.

- Keep sugar (especially added sugar) to less than 4 grams per serving (see page 53 for a list of all of sugar's alter egos).

- Check for sodium and total carbohydrates (especially if they come from sugar). Look to see what percentage of the daily recommended value of each is in a serving.

- Be aware of jargon, like "100% all-natural." That sounds good until you remember that sugar is all-natural, too.

Clearly healthy eating is important not just to prevent diseases so you live longer, but to fortify your body to handle the inevitable moments when "stuff happens." At those times—maybe you break a leg, develop a heart problem, whatever—your body will need to call in reinforcements. If you've been eating powerful foods, your immune system is at the ready.

Your army wants to work for you. Let's find out how to feed it right.

VITAMIN POWER

Ideally, your meals will provide perfectly balanced nutrition, but life doesn't always work that way, and sometimes creating the ideal concoction of nutrients isn't possible. I do recommend taking a multivitamin every day to ensure that you get the daily recommended amounts of vitamins and minerals.

Your 5 Food FIXES

You may have a basic idea about what qualifies as healthy food and what doesn't. Onions = good. Giant Bloomin' Fried Onion appetizers = good for the job security of paramedics. Other foods, it's hard to judge, and with the millions of choices out there, *what to eat* becomes a complicated proposition.

If you stick to my golden rule—mainly eat foods that look the same as they do when they come out of the ground—that will serve you well. In addition, I created a way of *thinking* about eating that will guide you without calorie counting or complex rules. Those are stressful, and I want eating to make you happy—not only because you love how nourishing foods taste, but also because you know how good these foods will make you feel.

Best of all, everything you will read in this book—including the 21-Day Plan—will serve as the way to think about food for the rest of your life. You'll come away with a nutritional backbone that promotes healing and health. I will walk you through the specific food plans when we get there, but I also want you to be comfortable in uncharted territory ahead, once you're living with the plan. FIXES will be your guiding acronym, a torch that illuminates the sometimes serpentine path to healthy eating. So think FIXES and live FIXES.

Fats with Benefits

Ideal Proteins

Xtra Fruits and Veggies

Energizing Carbohydrates

Special-Occasion Sugar

MIXING FIXES

Most foods are made up of a combination of nutrients, not strictly one or another. So several superpower foods show up under two headings in my FIXES formula. For example, fish and nuts contain both protein and healthy fat. That's a good thing—an indication of their multifunctional medicinal benefits.

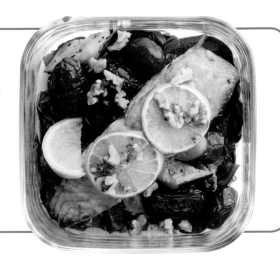

Fats with Benefits

Avocados

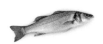

Fish

Nuts
(especially
almonds and
walnuts) and
low-sugar nut
butters

Olive oil and
vegetable oil

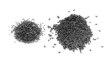

Seeds
(chia, flax,
pumpkin,
sesame,
sunflower)

For years, the mainstream thinking about fat sounded like a line that could appear in a nursery rhyme—*Don't want to* be *fat? Better not* eat *fat.* But that statement is actually false on two levels. You need fat. As one of the three macronutrients, it's a pillar of well-balanced nutrition. Your brain, for instance, is composed of 60 percent fat (we are really "fat heads"), so you require the dietary kind to support memory and clear thinking, and your body uses fat as energy throughout the day.

The trick is to get fat from the right sources, because dietary fats come in several forms. The ones you really want are found in the foods listed above because they're unsaturated fats.

Saturated fats are solid at room temperature (think butter), and they've been associated with heart disease. (Red meat contains saturated fat but this can be a tricky area, because grass-fed cattle deliver some healthy fat, but red meat also contains a compound called L-carnitine, which may lead to clogged

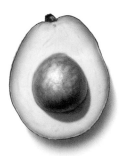

Make most of your fats the unsaturated kind, like what's found in avocado, nuts, and fish. The American Heart Association recommends eating between 25 and 35 percent of your daily calories in food fats. For example, one half of an avocado contains 12 grams and about 117 calories.

A handful of **pistachios** has as much fiber as ½ cup of broccoli.

Resveratrol in peanuts helps protect you from heart disease.

Hazelnuts lower bad cholesterol and raise the good kind.

Vitamin E in **pecans** helps support your immune system.

Walnuts can decrease the risk of colon cancer.

IN A NUTSHELL: Each variety of nut comes with multiple benefits as well as providing a good source of unsaturated fat.

arteries.) Small amounts of saturated fat appear to be okay. I don't want you to obsess about counting nutrients, but the recommendation is no more than 7 percent of your total diet should come from saturated fats—that's 14 grams on a 2,000-calorie day.

Trans fats are found in processed foods and made when hydrogen is infused into vegetable oil. These are enemy number one among all fats because of their association with many health problems, but they're being phased out of food manufacturing. I anticipate that they will be less of a worry in years to come, though they are still worth looking out for and avoiding whenever you can. Check labels and nutrition info on restaurant websites.

Fix-It Functions: Dietary fats play a vital role in your health primarily because of their effect on blood flow. Remember the process that leads to the formation of plaque and the clogging of arteries (the description on page 18)? Well, fats with benefits—unsaturated

BUT, BUT, BUT . . . BUTTER!

It tops pancakes and potatoes. It's the classic dip for lobster. It's a staple of homemade cookies. And, well, it just plain tastes good. Butter is one of those foods that the scientific jury has debated over the years, and it's gotten flak for its high saturated fat content, which has been linked to heart disease. However, the tide is shifting a bit. Unsaturated fat—like the kind found in olive oil—is generally better, but if you want to have an ounce or two of real butter occasionally, that's okay. The rest of the time, consider some alternatives to gussy up everything from a spud to a lobster (which, by the way, is great eating because it's high in omega-3 fatty acids, protein, and calcium).

- Mix lemon juice, olive oil, chives, and pepper.

- Mix plain Greek yogurt, chopped cilantro, lime juice, and red pepper flakes.

- Mix soy sauce, rice vinegar, fresh ginger, and minced garlic.

- Use ghee. Also called clarified butter, it's the trendiest butter out there right now. When butter is simmered, the pure butterfat and the milk solids separate. The clear yellow fat is poured off and the milk solids are discarded. Since the milk solids have been removed, ghee is good for the lactose-intolerant, and because you can heat it to higher temperatures (the milk solids make butter smoke at lower temperatures), it's good for sautéing.

ones—work to lower your levels of clog-happy bad cholesterol (LDL). The other fats—saturated and trans fats found in fatty meats (like most red meat), whole-fat dairy products, butter, and some oils—are linked to higher levels of bad cholesterol. This is why many diet plans suggest that you limit saturated fats.

Science backs up that suggestion. A recent report from the World Heart Federation determined that healthy sources of fat reduce total cholesterol and bad cholesterol, both of which put you at risk for developing heart disease. Another study conducted by Harvard University and the Cleveland Clinic

A CLINIC ON MAYO

Over the years, mayonnaise has gotten a bad rap. During the era when high-fat foods were demonized, mayo was right in the thick of things because it contained fat. To respond, manufacturers lowered the fat and added a whole bunch of junk to make it taste okay. But here's the thing. Mayo has good omega-6 fats, so you should go ahead and have the full-fat version if you choose—just pair it up with something with omega-3s (like tuna) to get the most nutritional benefit. (You can even make mayo yourself by whisking together eggs and a dash of lemon juice or vinegar, then slowly drizzling in oil while whisking so it emulsifies with the egg. Add a pinch of salt and/or a little mustard to taste. But store-bought kinds with simple ingredients lists are fine, too.)

AVOID FISH FRAUDS

Some studies have found that seafood may be mislabeled 25 to 70 percent of the time. Labels for common species like Atlantic cod, red snapper, and wild salmon are swapped with versions of fish that are cheaper or less desirable. For example, tilefish can be labeled as red snapper and escolar is presented as white tuna, primarily in sushi venues. (Escolar is a type of snake mackerel, not even a tuna at all, and its oily flesh can cause digestive problems in some people when they eat more than a few ounces.) It's difficult for you as the consumer to investigate every piece of fish you eat (and more regulation of the seafood industry is needed), but you can do a few things. Ask questions about the origin of the fish. If your retailer or restaurant is not able to give answers about the seafood it is selling, you may want to make a different choice. And if the price is too good to be true, it may be a sign that you're looking at mislabeled fish. Also, buy the whole fish whenever possible. You can ask for it to be cut into fillets at the store. The more processed your fish and the more hands it passes through, the more opportunities for a bait and switch.

looked at more than 125,000 people over a thirty-year span, and found those with higher intakes of healthy fats had significantly lower rates of heart disease.

Bottom line: I don't want you to think fat is evil, because many food sources contain the kind you want and need. Moreover, fat goes a long way in helping you feel satisfied. But this may be one of the more confusing nutritional areas because fat comes in so many forms from so many sources, and because the thinking on it has been in flux over the past several decades. To make it easy to understand fats, use this guide:

Fat Friends or Foes?

FRIENDLY FIX-IT FATS

Monounsaturated/Polyunsaturated Fats: Dominant in avocado and avocado oil; corn oil; fish oils; olives and olive oil; peanuts, peanut butter, and peanut oil; canola oil; nuts, nut butters, and nut oils; safflower oil; seeds; sesame oil; and sunflower oil. Omega-3 and omega-6 fats are forms of polyunsaturated fats—omega-3s come from fatty fish and some nuts, while omega-6s come from seeds, nuts, and the oils extracted from them. We tend to get a lot more omega-6s, but increasing omega-3s is important for overall health.

IN-MODERATION FATS

Saturated: Found in butter, poultry skin, red meat, dairy products. One note: Saturated fat in the form of coconut oil and in coconut-based products does not seem to have the same downside as saturated fat from animal products, likely due to its chemical makeup.

FOOLISH FATS

Trans Fats: Found in partially hydrogenated oils, processed foods. The deadline for trans fats to be taken out of processed foods is 2018. Some believe that this change in regulation could prevent twenty thousand heart attacks a year.

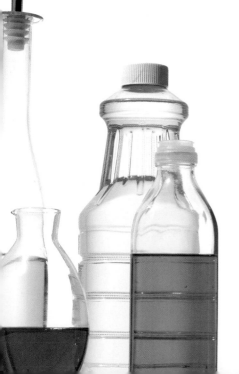
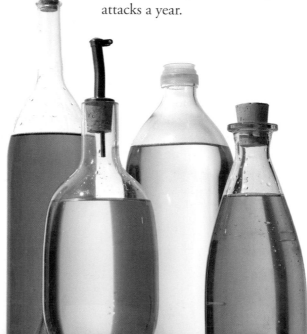

Ideal Proteins

Beans and legumes

Chicken

Dairy
(milk, cheese, yogurt)

Eggs

Fish and shellfish

Lean pork and some lean
cuts of red meat (look for
"loin" or "round" on the label
for the lowest-fat versions)

Nuts and low-sugar
nut butters

Tofu and tempeh

Turkey

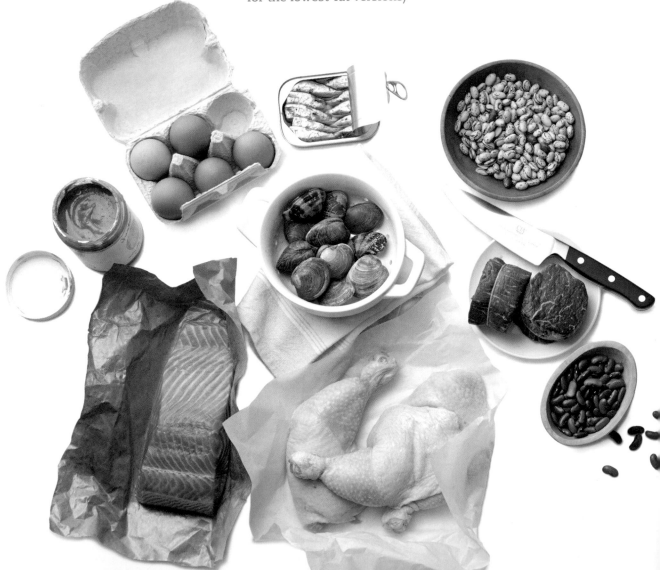

Simply said, you gotta have protein. That's because it's made up of amino acids, the building blocks for your body's tissues. The human body produces some of those amino acids on its own, but the primary source of them is through food. And when your body is under stress or development—think infancy and childhood, pregnancy, any time you exercise intensely, or just a run-around day—you especially need to replenish those building blocks.

Protein, which you will get plenty of in the 21-Day Plan, delivers the compounds that repair, maintain, and strengthen your anatomical infrastructure. It also plays a vital role in staving off weight gain and all the health problems that come along with extra pounds.

Why? First, protein curbs hunger throughout the long time it takes your body to process it. And protein helps to build up muscle tissues that make for a faster metabolism. That's because muscle tissue is metabolically more expensive than fat—meaning that your body burns more calories to feed muscle than it does to maintain fat. Protein is also inefficient to digest, so we spend more energy converting it into calories compared to when we eat carbs and fats. That nets us, in essence, a discount on the protein calories we consume.

SHOULD YOU EAT TURKEY OR VEGGIE BURGERS?

Turkey burgers have been around since the 1930s, but they didn't hit the mainstream until the 1970s—as a way to address the "fat is making you fat" mantra of the time. Are they a good substitute for red meat? Maybe. Turkey comes in lower on calories and saturated fat, true, but it has less protein than beef, which also has higher amounts of omega-3s. Ground turkey breast is the best option, but ground turkey often includes dark meat and skin, which bump the fat content to as much as 20 percent. So pay attention to the label to make sure you're getting only the light meat. Bottom line: It can be a bit of a wash, because often turkey burgers are plumped up with other ingredients to make them tastier. If you crave a beef burger, go for it, but stick to once a week. As for veggie burgers, they do have a nice name to make you think they're healthier, but they, too, are often overprocessed and filled with other ingredients to plump up their taste. To get the healthiest version, make sure the first three ingredients are vegetables and the label says that the burgers are USDA-certified. A bean burger is another great option because of the protein and fiber it contains. See one that has just black beans, vegetables, and spices as its ingredients? You're good to go.

YOUR BEST CHEESE CHOICE

Without question, my top cheese choice is cottage cheese. It has lots of protein and fewer calories than yogurt, and it's something you can use in a variety of ways. I like to eat it with nuts stirred in. But you can also put a thin layer of it on some avocado toast. Try mixing in a tablespoon when you scramble eggs, too.

POWDER POWER

It's best to get your protein from whole foods, but protein powder can be a nice and easy addition to smoothies. Powders often contain sugar and artificial sweeteners, so be on the lookout for options with 14 to 21 grams of protein and less than 5 grams of sugar per serving. "NSF certified" on the label means that it's been tested for contaminants. And skip ones made with collagen, a cheap filler protein with little nutritional value.

GOT MILK? KNOW THIS.

Within two hours of standing in daylight, milk loses between half and two-thirds of its vitamin B content. By the way, it takes, on average, 345 squirts from a cow's udder to yield one gallon of milk. In case you were wondering.

WHAT EXACTLY IS *LEAN* MEAT?

It's meat that has fewer than 10 grams of fat, 4.5 or fewer grams of saturated fat, and less than 95 mg of cholesterol per 3.5-ounce portion. Your leanest meat options are turkey (white or dark meat without the skin), chicken breast (without the skin), pork tenderloin, and red meat that is top sirloin or bottom round.

Steak is fine in moderation. Just shop for lean cuts and watch your servings. Note that the American Institute for Cancer Research suggests that you consume no more than 18 ounces of red meat a week. That's equal to six 3-ounce servings (3 ounces is about the size of a deck of cards). I prefer to eat red meat no more than two or three times a week, and very rarely is the portion larger than the size of my palm.

Yes, it's possible to overeat protein (true of almost any kind of food, with the exception of certain vegetables), because whatever is not used is stored as fat. But the bigger challenge is making sure that you get steady sources of the right kind throughout the day.

Fix-It Functions: As I've said, macronutrients don't work in isolation. You don't go to the meat counter at the market and pick up a package of protein. You pick up a cut of some kind of meat—which has both high concentrations of protein and some form of fat. It's one macro paired up with other macros. So what makes a protein "ideal"? The simple way to think about it is this: Proteins that are low fat or have high amounts of healthy fat should be on your list. The ones with higher amounts of saturated fats are typically associated with adverse health effects, and those should be every-so-often indulgences. Remember, Luigi and his long-lived comrades eat red meat, but sparingly, and not daily. All meats should be grilled, baked, or roasted, not fried, because the coating and frying of these foods usually includes some kind of saturated fat or other processed ingredients.

The most recent data suggest that red meats (particularly processed red meats, like sausage and bacon) are associated with increased heart disease, stroke, and cancer deaths. Poultry is not. One study found that a higher intake of red meat was linked to a 22 percent increase in risk of breast cancer, while two other studies found women who ate lots of vegetable protein (seeds, beans,

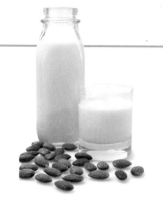

OTHER'S MILK

If you have trouble with dairy, it's worth looking into different forms—almond milk, hemp milk, sheep's/goat's milk, soy milk. They lack one of the chemicals (a sugar molecule) that causes the digestive disagreement.

and soy) had a 30 percent lower risk of heart disease and 18 percent lower risk of type 2 diabetes. All of this illustrates how important it is to look at food holistically. Just because something has protein doesn't mean that it's always perfect. You have to examine other things that a food might contain, such as the kind of fat in it or the way it's processed.

The trouble with red meat comes from a compound found in it called L-carnitine, which I mentioned above, that messes with your gut bacteria. (See chapter 13 for more on the power of the bacteria in your gut.)

Dairy, which contains saturated fat, is often considered a tricky area; for a long time, people argued you should have low-fat or nonfat versions of milk, cheese, and so on. But a recent paper published in the journal *Circulation* suggests that people who eat full-fat versions of dairy do better than those who eat nonfat versions. The thinking is that the low-fat version may not be as satisfying, so people respond by having more sugary foods to compensate. Plus, when you take fat out of milk, you are left with mostly sugar, which affects your hormones adversely. Remember, you need some fat in your diet. That's why I recommend the 2% fat version of dairy products.

WHY GRANDMA'S CHICKEN WAS BETTER

If you think chicken doesn't taste the way it did when you were a kid, you're right. On our show we looked at the reasons why. Chickens—our number one protein source—are no longer raised on farms and in pastures where they live outside, eating grass, bugs, and other natural elements. Instead, most are packed into farmhouses, eating a bland mix of corn, soybeans, and minerals—so that they grow quickly and cheaply. (Chicken-growing contests in the 1940s helped inspire folks to perfect the plumping-up process.) It turns out that what chickens eat affects the way they taste. And we learned that some processing techniques leach the flavor from the birds. Today only a small percentage of chickens are free-range, meaning they have space to eat and roam while they grow. We found that the farm-grown chicken that took fourteen weeks to mature was still 50 percent smaller than the chicken that was speeded up in the modern farming process to grow up in six weeks. The old-time, farm-raised chickens mature more slowly—and in the end, are tastier.

SURPRISING SOURCES OF PROTEIN

Meat, eggs, beans, fish, and nuts aren't your only options. Check nutritional labels and you'll discover some who-knew ways to get your protein quota, including these:

Avocado
1 gram per half

Whole wheat bread
4 grams per slice

Sun-dried tomatoes
2 grams per ¼ cup

Whole wheat spaghetti
7 grams per cup

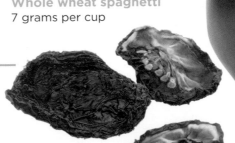
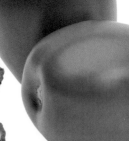

Xtra Fruits and Vegetables

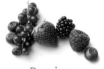

Berries

Citrus fruits

Cruciferous
vegetables
(like broccoli
and cauliflower)

Greens

Melons

Just about everything you find in the produce section!
(See the complete list on page 172.)

As you read this book, you will see the phrase *more fruits and vegetables* over and over. Sorry to be a broken record, but casting fruits and vegetables in a leading role—not just a cameo appearance—is the most pivotal shift you can make in your diet. Do that, and you've taken a big step toward healing your body and protecting against disease.

I could spend many pages singing the praises of these superfoods (and I will, as you'll see them throughout the book and as a major part of the 21-Day Plan). First, when you eat them, they still look like you just picked them, which follows my golden rule. (This is why I also consider nuts and seeds to

be baby fruits and vegetables—cousins, if you will.) And they bring these primary benefits to the party:

- **Fiber:** A healthy form of carbohydrates, fiber helps slow digestion, which is a good thing for satiety, cholesterol levels, and blood sugar management.

- **Vitamins:** These essential micronutrients are found naturally in your body and are associated with good health. Fruits and vegetables are packed with vitamins (you know them by letters A, B, C, E, and so on) to help replenish the vitamins you naturally lose as you age.

- **Minerals:** Minerals are also micronutrients, but they're not organically found in the body, so you *have* to get them through foods. A handful of examples of mineral-rich veggies and their benefits: Chromium in broccoli helps manage blood sugar. Magnesium found in beets helps your body fight stress. Zinc in spinach keeps your immune system strong. Potassium in papayas and bananas helps keep your muscle spasms and blood pressure under control.

- **Antioxidants:** Found in many fruits and vegetables, antioxidants are powerful disease-fighters. How? They go up against chemicals called free radicals, some of which help bad LDL cholesterol inflame our arteries and thus put you at more risk for sudden clogs. Antioxidants mitigate some of that damage and help to lower inflammation in the body. The color of each vegetable we eat comes from specific pigments designed to protect the plant against the sun. We harvest the protective antioxidants when we

THE JUICE TRUTH

Of course juice must be healthy—"It's fruit," you say. But not if it's packed with more sugar than a toddler's birthday party. I don't care if the label says "real" or "fruit" or "all-natural," you have to read the ingredients if you're going to buy juice. Some things to keep in mind:

- **Watch out for sugar.** Just say no if you see any sweeteners (see page 53 for a complete list) in the first three ingredients. And even if the juice doesn't have any added sugars, most fruit juices load in 20-plus grams of natural sugar per pour. (For perspective: One 8-ounce glass of grape juice contains more sugar than 1.5 pounds of grapes.) Try to go for actual fruit instead—it's fiber-rich, which helps to fill you up for fewer calories. If you're really craving the liquid version, stick to a half-serving, or dilute it with sparkling water.

- **Looking at a vegetable drink?** Good thinking. They're better for you than fruit drinks because they generally have a lower sugar content. If you have the choice, pick one that looks darker in color. Those often contain kale, spinach, beets, tomatoes, and/or carrots, which have more minerals and vitamins than juices filled with lighter-hued veggies like cucumbers and celery.

- **I'd rather you concoct your own fruity drink.** Make a big jug of ice water and slice some fruit into it. If you want a little more sweetness, you can also stir in a teaspoon of stevia. Or you can buy juice from the store and dilute it with equal parts water to cut the sugar in half while still maintaining the volume. In either case, you'll satisfy a sweetness craving without going near the soda machine.

consume this produce, as long as we prepare the veggies correctly (boiling may leach out elements in some foods, so it's often best to eat them raw or steamed).

Fix-It Functions: Piles of evidence point to this basic premise: Eat your fruits and veggies to build a more resilient body. A recent Chinese and Harvard University review of sixteen studies involving nearly a million people found that those with a higher consumption of fruits and vegetables (a modest five servings a day) had a lower risk of *all* causes of death. Researchers pointed to the vitamins, antioxidants, and other compounds as the likely reason why.

Now, it is worth discussing the two biggest questions I get when it comes to fruits and vegetables. One, doesn't fruit contain sugar and isn't sugar bad? It is true that fruits contain a simple sugar called fructose. With sugar, however, we're most concerned with the kind *added* to foods, not the sugar that naturally comes *in* food like fruits. So dumping sugar in your coffee isn't great. Same with sugar-loaded foods like ice cream and soda and cookies. But naturally sweet watermelon? A-OK.

That said, I typically advise people to tilt in favor of fruits with lower natural sugar content, like berries, and not to eat too many servings of sugary fruits, like bananas, grapes, and pineapples. It's advice that falls under the "too much of anything is bad" rule. But if you're having three servings a day of any fruit,

THE FALLOUT FROM FRUIT?

How do plants protect themselves against possible invaders, like insects and mammals (including us!)? They produce chemicals that work to beat them back. One of those chemicals, called lectin, is found in skins and seeds and protects the fruit. It prevents us from eating them before they're ripe—and gives plants enough time for their young seeds to drop and grow into a new plant. The effect in us? Some evidence suggests lectin can trigger an inflammatory response in the gut and poke little holes in the intestinal lining. Maybe that's why Italians knew instinctively that removing the seeds and skins of tomatoes was the smart way to make sauce. It's not that you should avoid fruits and veggies; just a theory worth considering. To easily peel tomatoes, immerse them in boiling water for about thirty seconds. Or spear tomatoes on a long fork and rotate them over the flame of your gas burner. Do the same with peppers until they blacken, then place them in a paper bag to cool. The skin will easily peel off.

that's just fine, and it's certainly better than other sweet, processed options. Plus, the fiber in fruit slows the absorption of sugar, and that's a good thing, because it prevents that sudden spill of glucose into your bloodstream.

The second question I get is similar: Aren't there some starchy vegetables we should avoid, like potatoes and corn? Those are higher in

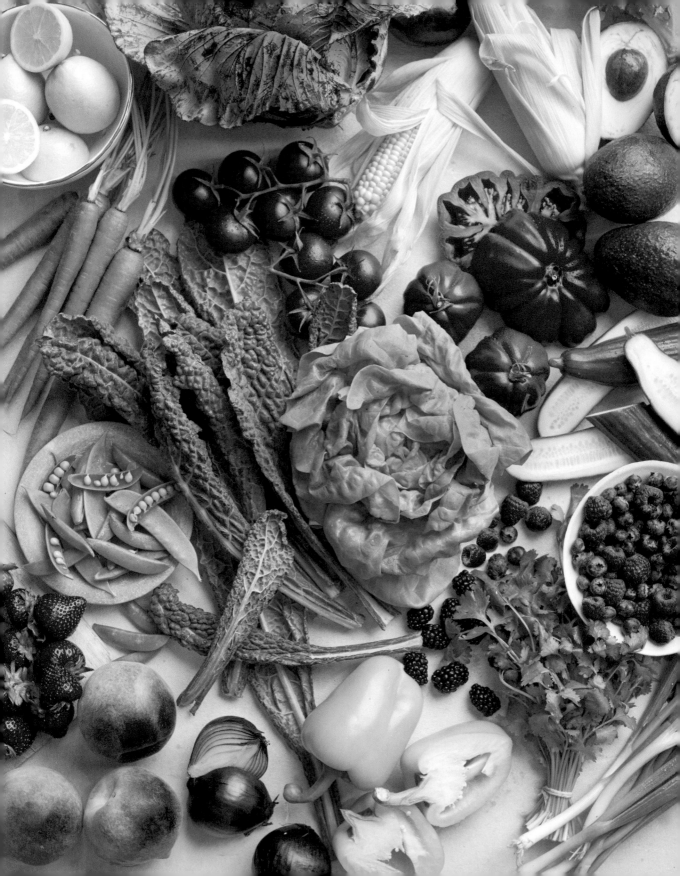

carbohydrates, yes, but unless you're eating them in jumbo amounts, they're good choices. They contain minerals and other compounds that are good for you, and they meet the golden-rule test—you eat them in their natural form. So while it's smart to be aware of starchy vegetables (for a reason you'll see in a moment when I explain the glycemic index on page 48), these are another food to take off the can't-eat list. Just don't go crazy on the French fries, okay? Their prep makes them high in fat—sometimes the saturated kind. Eat your taters baked or roasted, drizzled with olive oil, and dusted with spices for a healthy side dish.

Bottom line: There's little risk of you overeating produce, though there are always extremes (my friend Mike Roizen of the Cleveland Clinic once told me he had a patient who gained weight because she downed seventy-five servings a day of fruits and vegetables!). The simple approach is to fill half your plate with veggies for almost all of your meals and integrate fruits as snacks and sweet-tooth satisfiers.

WHAT'S COOKING?

Certain compounds in tomatoes and carrots get unlocked from their fibrous plant cell walls when heated. That makes it easier for your body to absorb the good stuff, like lycopene from tomatoes and beta-carotene in carrots. Some other heating tips:

- Boiling veggies may leave most of the vitamins behind in the water; steam them instead.

- Roast vegetables in big chunks because the smaller you cut them, the more of their healthy ingredients will get lost to heat and air.

THE VEGGIE WHISPERER

If you've always avoided vegetables, you can start the journey to loving them with a little help. Vinegar is the perfect salad dressing—not just because it's lower in calories and junky ingredients than processed salad dressing, but also because it helps lower the glycemic index of foods. That means it helps you metabolize sugar better so it will be less likely to wreak havoc in your system. So if you want to spice up your vegetables, a little vinegar is the way to go. You can mix it with olive oil for a mellower taste, or try apple cider vinegar, which is milder.

Eat More Fruit and Veggies. Two leaves of lettuce on your sandwich or a couple of berries in your morning cereal bowl aren't going to cut it. Go for volume instead. Make one meal each day a salad with lots of greens and your favorite veggies. Then add a piece of fruit to your breakfast and afternoon snack, and you're on your way.

Energizing Carbohydrates

| 100% whole-grain breads and pastas | Beans and legumes (like lentils and chickpeas) | Fruits and vegetables | Nuts and seeds | Popcorn (unbuttered) | Sweet potatoes and yams | Whole grains (like barley, brown rice, oats, and quinoa) |

Oh, carbohydrates. There are dieters who have demonized you. *Carbs make you fat!* There are athletes who have thanked you. *I need to carbo-load!* Same nutrient, opposing points of view. What's a person supposed to believe about pasta and pancakes?

First, this shouldn't be an all-or-nothing discussion—that is, you either eat carbs or you don't. Your policy should be based on an understanding of what carbs are and what they do. They take many forms—fiber is one and so is sugar—and the form dictates how they work in the body. All forms of carbohydrates serve as an immediate source of energy. When your body needs to get calories to your brain, heart, muscles, and more, it takes quickly accessible carbohydrates and converts them to energy. So that's good. But when you have too much of that fast-track-carb-turned-to-glucose, you're suddenly at risk for all the issues I talked about in chapter 1—insulin problems, too much circulating blood sugar, fat storage, and more.

So the way to think about carbohydrates is to separate them into two groups. Complex carbs are the ones that take a long time for your body to break down and digest. Simple carbs are the ones that your body converts to blood sugar in a New York minute.

How do you know which is which? The foods rich in carbs that come in their natural form are complex—beans, 100% whole grains, vegetables. The foods that are processed with added sugar or are stripped of some of their minerals (meaning that they're not 100% whole grain) are the ones you want to avoid. Stuff you'd order at a diner breakfast comes to mind—French toast, pancakes, muffins, biscuits, and so on. This group, of course, includes ultra-processed carbs like candy, chips, and cookies.

GET THE WHOLE-GRAIN TRUTH

Whole grains contain more fiber and nutrients than refined carbohydrates. That's because they contain the whole kernel—the bran, endosperm, and germ of the kernel. Brown rice, barley, quinoa, and other whole grains are better choices than foods made with refined white flour (white bread, white pasta) since you digest them more slowly and the fiber helps you feel full for a longer period of time after a meal. A half-cup serving at each meal is a good guideline for weight loss. With refined grains, many of those power-packed parts of the kernel are stripped out. If the label does not say "100% whole-grain," check the ingredients list for refined culprits in the "not whole grain" list here.

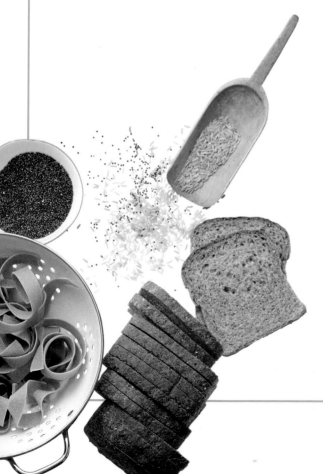

WHOLE GRAIN

Brown rice
Buckwheat
Bulgur or cracked
   wheat
Millet
Quinoa
Sorghum
Teff
Triticale
Wheat berries
Whole-grain barley
   or pearl barley
Whole-grain corn
Whole oats or
   oatmeal
Whole rice
Whole rye
Whole spelt
Whole wheat

NOT WHOLE GRAIN

Corn flour
Cornmeal
Degerminated cornmeal
Enriched flour
Pumpernickel
Rice, white
Rice flour
Rye flour or rye
Stone-ground wheat
   (if whole grain, label
   should say "stone-
   ground whole wheat")
Unbleached wheat flour
Wheat
Wheat flour
Wheat germ
   (it's not a whole grain,
   but its vitamin E and
   folate content makes
   it healthy)

THE 30-SECOND CRACKER TEST

I don't normally think you should eat processed crackers; many don't have much nutritional value. But you can use one to determine your "carb type"—that is, how well you tolerate carbs (why some people gain weight at the mere bite of a carb, while others could eat a bagel every morning and never gain weight). Dr. Sharon Moalem, a geneticist, developed this test: Coat your mouth with as much saliva as you can. Eat one plain, unsalted cracker, setting a timer as soon as you start chewing. Note the time it takes for the cracker to start to taste differently than when you first started chewing. Go ahead and swallow it after you note the change. If you reach thirty seconds, you can stop and swallow. Do it two more times and note your average time. If you stopped the time at fourteen seconds or under, it means you can tolerate more carbs, while thirty seconds means you can tolerate fewer carbs. The middle area is, well, the middle area. The test is a proxy for identifying how your genes break down carbohydrates. While not the be-all and end-all marker, it gives you some insight into the role carbs should play in your diet.

TAKE A LOAD OFF

The glycemic index (GI) gauges how dramatically various foods raise blood sugar. A low score means the food delivers glucose to the blood at a slow, steady rate; a high one means it dumps its load of glucose into the blood more immediately. It lets researchers compare how much your blood sugar jumps when it gets 100 grams of one food versus the same amount of another. But it's not very helpful to the average person, since you might eat 100 grams of bread (one slice) but not of arugula (10 cups). So scientists developed a related measure, the glycemic load, that takes into account the serving size to get a real-world picture of what a normal portion will do to blood sugar. Foods that score 10 or under are low GL foods (that's good); anything above 20 is considered high. Some examples:

Low GL Foods: Whole-grain bread, apples, steel-cut oatmeal, chickpeas, whole-grain spaghetti, brown rice, Greek yogurt

High GL Foods: Raisins, instant oatmeal, white spaghetti, white rice, low-fat yogurt

You can change the glycemic load in the way you prepare your foods. For example, how potatoes are cooked matters. If you cool them after you cook them, the glycemic index is reduced. Same goes for rice, especially when cooked with a little coconut oil (the fat slows down the blitz of glucose). Al dente pasta (which is firm) is processed more slowly than soft noodles.

Another way to determine the value of a carb is to check what's called the glycemic index (GI), a measuring tool that determines how long it takes a carb to be digested. You're looking for low glycemic index foods. It's a good guide, because you can easily see that choices like chickpeas are low, while baked potatoes are on the higher end. That doesn't mean potatoes aren't good for you, as we've discussed, but in the spectrum of carbohydrates, they take a shorter time to digest, and our goal is longer. (Learn more in the Take a Load Off box at left.)

Fix-It Functions: While carbohydrates tend to be the most controversial of our nutrients, there is good evidence to suggest that whole grains do help lower the risk of diseases associated with blood pressure, high cholesterol, and the like. For example, a 2013 Australian review of studies looked at the effect of whole grains on the body, and found that eating more of them was associated with a lower incidence of heart disease, colon cancer, and inflammation. The effect could be related to fiber, minerals, or other characteristics of complex carbohydrates.

The other reason why carbs play such a crucial role in your health revolves around the E in our FIXES equation: Energizing. The kinds of carbs you choose will drive how you feel throughout the day. Eating simple sugars and carbs leads to extreme highs and head-on-your-desk crashes. Complex carbohydrates will slow down your body's digestion and energy-distribution process so that you run on a strong, steady engine all day.

THE WORST THING SINCE SLICED (WHITE) BREAD . . .

White bread has become a public health enemy. The slices of refined carbs have little nutritional value, but they sure are convenient vehicles for carrying sandwich innards, so we eat a lot of them. Modern wheats don't have much flavor or nutritional value, and sometimes, even whole wheat products are processed so quickly that they stimulate an aggressive insulin response. I buy sprouted grain or Ezekiel bread for the most nutritional punch. It's tasty, filling, and has the complex carbs that give you sustained energy. Other breads worth trying are made with different kinds of flour, such as tapioca, which is derived from the yuca plant, and coconut. The history of slicing our bread is actually pretty interesting. American inventor Otto Frederick Rohwedder came up with the idea for a bread-slicing machine in the early 1900s. But it wasn't always considered the greatest thing, because sliced bread would also go stale quickly. That's when plastic wrap packaging came into play.

Special-Occasion Sugar

Treat yourself to it in small doses, but also learn the secret weapons that can satisfy sweet cravings, healthfully.

One of the most common questions I get (at least in October) is: "What do you do on Halloween, Dr. Oz?" My answer: I do what everybody does. I have and give out—*shocker!*—some candy. You don't have to eat healthy every minute of every day, and there's a lot of emotional value that comes with diving into your favorite foods, even if they're not part of the first four letters in my FIXES foundation.

Foods with added sugar (from cookies to Frappuccinos) top the bad-for-you list. Because sugar comes in condiments, desserts, alcoholic drinks, and many processed foods, it's pervasive. And the reality is that our overconsumption of sugar may very well be our biggest nutritional problem today. We eat too much, and it sparks numerous biological processes that cause inflammation, heart troubles, fat storage, and more. The average American eats more than 150 pounds of sugar a year, and that's just too much.

Yes, we need sugar for energy, but very, very, very few of us are active enough to immediately burn all the calories in the sugar many of us consume. And if sugar calories are not used quickly, they get stored as fat, wreak havoc on your insulin response, and send your energy levels on a roller coaster through the day.

Sugar is like a powerful drug, and therefore it should be used with caution. Have it irregularly, and only when you really want to enjoy the food and/or the wonderful occasion that surrounds it. This isn't a free pass, just permission to tap into sugar now and then, when it makes you feel happy, connected, and engaged with people around you. In other words, a special occasion. The problem occurs when you abuse the "drug"—when you have too much, when you rely on it, when you have a steady drip of sugar into your system. *That's* what causes mayhem in your body.

Sugar addiction is real: Brain scans show that heavily sugared foods stimulate the brain's rewards center in the same way that cocaine and heroin do. Keep eating them, and you've trained your brain to crave more and more. One study even found that rats preferred to get their feel-good hits from sweet drinks rather than cocaine. Over time, we get desensitized and need a bigger sugar fix to get the same satisfaction.

Your body pays a heavy price. A 2015 review of studies by the University of California found that excess sugar is associated with increased risk of developing heart disease and diabetes. Extra sugar is linked to high blood pressure and triglycerides (a blood fat that's associated with heart disease). Eating 25 percent more than the recommended amount of sugar *triples* the risk of dying of heart disease. That's because too much sugar in your bloodstream leaves damage behind as it blasts through the linings of your arteries, which puts you at risk of heart attack and stroke.

Fix-It Functions: Because sugar has little nutritional punch, I am asking you to pull way back on it in my 21-Day Plan, so you can recalibrate your body a bit. Your antisugar weapon: Eating fat and protein together.

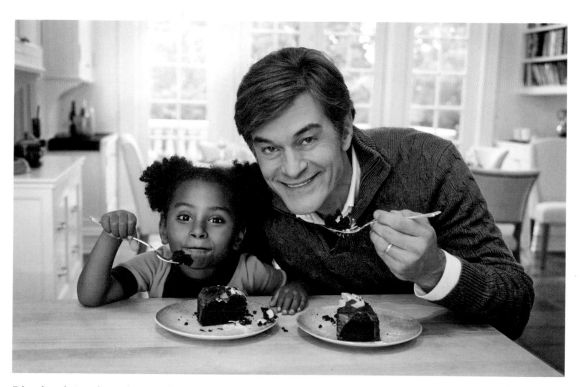

Digging into chocolate cake with my niece Charlotte at the holidays. That's special-occasion sugar in my book.

Fat will keep you satiated and protein will even out your blood sugar so you have fewer crashes and cravings for sweet foods. After twenty-one days off the "drug," you won't feel like you need or want sugar the way you do now. You'll reset your sweet tooth so you can enjoy the superfood deliciousness of fruits and will hardly need a sugar fix from other

THE CASE AGAINST SODA (EVEN DIET SODA)

A single soda a day raises an adult's chances of being overweight by 27 percent and a child's by 55 percent. And choosing the artificially sweetened kind won't solve the problem. Artificial sweeteners may confuse your body with a sense of false satisfaction, so you may end up reaching for more sweet foods to find the energy your body's missing. Sweeter than sugar, these sweeteners dull your palate and prevent you from enjoying naturally sweet foods, like fruits. So you may be more likely to fulfill your sweet fixes with high-calorie and overly processed foods. Another reason to skip diet sodas: A recent study found that drinking them is associated with a higher risk of both stroke and dementia. That glass of water infused with lemon is looking pretty good, right?

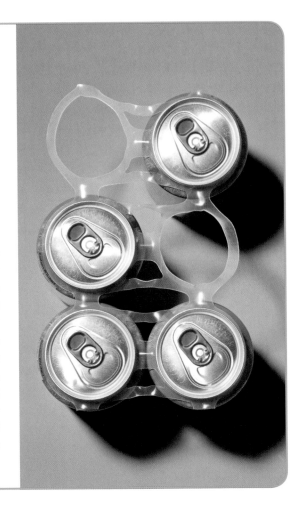

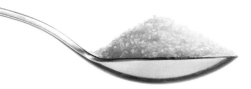

Women should aim for 6 teaspoons of sugar a day or fewer, which is the recommendation of the American Heart Association and the World Health Organization. Men can go up to 9 teaspoons. But lots of people eat more than *double* that—on average, women have 15 teaspoons a day, and men have 20. Whoa!

sources. A drizzle of honey and a perfectly ripe strawberry? Wow.

When you return to enjoying treats, make sure you do it in modest amounts. Also consider these ways of satisfying your sweet tooth with the least amount of sugar damage:

- Dark chocolate that's at least 60 to 75% cacao. (It's sweet, but bitter enough that you won't feel like eating a whole bar. If you're tempted to gobble more, start buying 80% cacao or even the pure source, cacao nibs.)

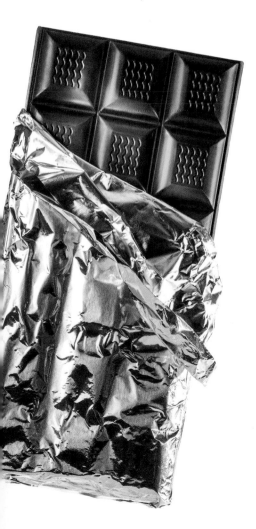

SUGAR PSEUDONYMS

Sugar is like a most-wanted criminal; it has a lot of aliases. But the thing is, your body processes all forms of sugar the same way. So if you're reducing the amount of added sugar in your diet, you need to check food labels for these:

Agave

Brown rice syrup

Cane crystals

Dextrose

Evaporated cane juice

Fructose

Fruit juice concentrate (such as grape or white grape)

High-fructose corn syrup

Honey

Lactose

Maltose

Malt Syrup

Molasses

Raw sugar

Sucrose

Syrup (any kind)

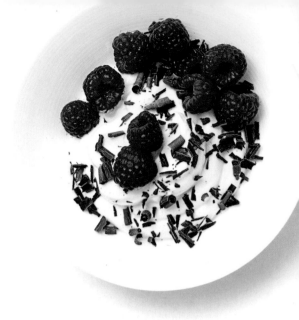

- A bowl of plain Greek yogurt with berries, sprinkled with honey, and a few dark chocolate chips or shavings.

- A smoothie made with unsweetened almond milk, a scoop of almond butter, plain Greek yogurt, and chocolate protein powder (your healthy milk shake!).

- Mixed nuts with a few semisweet chocolate chips (roasted with spices also works).

- Roasted cinnamon chickpeas: Rinse, drain, and coat chickpeas with olive oil and cinnamon. Bake at 375°F for 25 minutes.

IN DEFENSE OF HONEY

Honey is one of the rare foods that does not spoil (some uncovered by archaeologists in the tombs of Egyptian pharaohs was found to still be edible). To produce a pound of the golden stuff, bees must visit two million flowers. In some parts of the world, it's still used to treat wounds, because it won't hurt your cells, but will kill invading bacteria. Our family has three hives that make about seventy pounds of honey a year, and I have trouble giving it all away! In place of added sugar, a drizzle of honey can deliver sweetness with some health benefits, such as:

Controlling blood sugar: Diabetic patients who swapped out sugar for honey had more stable blood sugar levels. Add it to tea or oatmeal.

Calming a cough: Adding some to a cup of tea has been shown to reduce coughing. Honey works by soothing the throat, while methylxanthine, a stimulant in caffeine, may expand airways, helping to reduce the hack.

Soothe burns: Some honey has bacteria-battling power because of a high concentration of a compound called methyglyoxal. You can put it on burns or minor wounds. Look for labels with a Unique Manuka Factor of above 10; that means it's both medical-grade and edible.

YOUR SECRET SUGAR STASH

Your go-to sweet treat when you need a fix: Dark chocolate containing greater than 60% cacao. It's full of a group of anti-oxidants that has been linked to reduced risk of blood clots, decreased blood pressure, better moods, and memory boosts, among other benefits. It also contains magnesium and may have some cancer-fighting properties. Because the kind with 60% cacao or more is made of cocoa butter, and not palm or coconut oils, it's been shown to have a neutral effect on cholesterol, unlike those two oils. Have a square of dark chocolate (an ounce or so). You'll get that sweet fix, but not such a sugar rush that you feel the need to gorge on a lot.

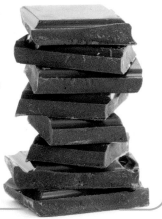

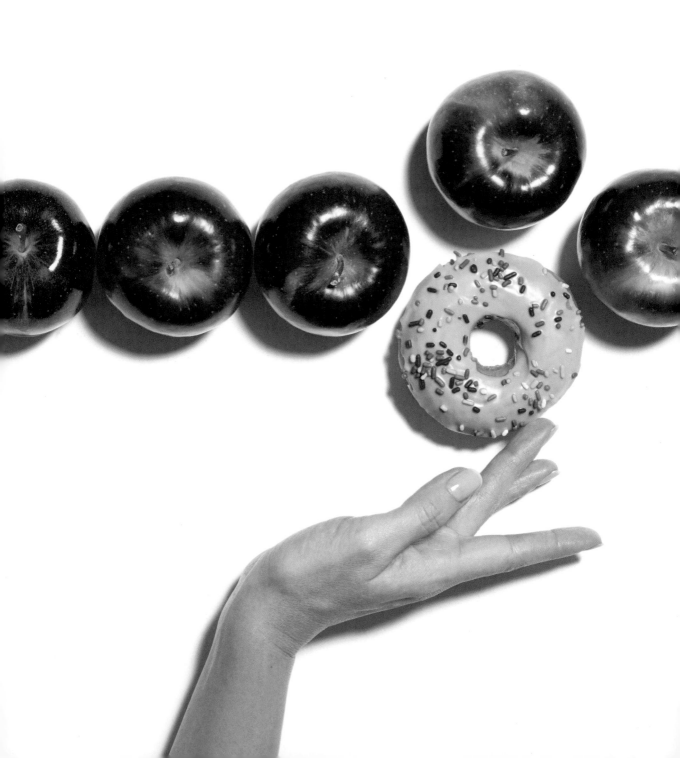

3

Strength in Strategy

These tactics will help you resist cravings and temptations by putting knowledge into action.

Having talked to thousands of people—including close friends and relatives—who struggle with food choices, I understand the tug-of-war that happens nearly every time you eat.

On one end of the rope is your inner nutritionist, reminding you about all the food fixes I explained in the last chapter and pulling you toward those veggies and that delicious salsa-smothered chicken breast. On the other end, there's a puff-pastry doughboy with a come-hither finger, reeling you in to a land of bakery shop temptation.

These everyday moments are where the weight and health battle is won or lost, one decision at a time. Information isn't always enough to steer your nutritional choices in the right direction. Neither is motivation. Sometimes, no matter how smart, driven, inspired, or even desperate you are, the slice of cake wins. Sometimes, when you're hungry or sad or out-of-your-mind mad, you will comfort-binge on leftover linguine. Sometimes, you need reinforcements to support your best intentions.

This is where strategy comes in.

For food fixes to work, they have to be automatic, almost mindlessly easy to put into practice. Your goal is to get to where you're not struggling with decisions but instead eating right because that's *just what you do naturally.*

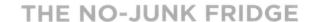

THE NO-JUNK FRIDGE

Juice. For the best health payoff, look for veggie-based blends with no added sugar.

Eggs. These have plenty of protein to curb cravings.

Milk. Its protein can keep you feeling full longer.

Nuts and Nut Butters. Healthy fats and protein are super satiating. These help you stave off hunger.

Leafy Greens and Veggies. Loaded with nutrients and low in calories, these are a healthy-eating staple.

Beans. A versatile source of filling fiber and protein. (Try eating these in place of meat for dinner once or twice a week.)

Yogurt. Healthy bacteria in many yogurts (labeled "live and active cultures") may ease irritable bowel syndrome and keep food moving smoothly through the GI tract.

Meat. Think of it as a side dish, not the main event. (See page 38 on portion size.)

Water. Sparkling or still, it's always a smart choice.

Fruit. Eat the rainbow for more antioxidants. The high water content will help fill you up.

Avocados. Rich in healthy unsaturated fat to keep you satiated.

Freezer: Stock it with frozen fruits, veggies, and cooked whole grains.

In this chapter, you'll tune in to your habits around food. You'll reinforce positive choices, nix damaging patterns, and learn new tricks so you never have to give your good choices a second thought.

Strategy 1: Commit to an Environmental Makeover

If you want to succeed with food, make it easy to do the right thing. Create personal environments that are full of healing options. Your fridge, your freezer, your pantry, your kitchen counters, and your bag should be well stocked with foods that can sustain you through a day's arc of hunger pangs and emotions.

Think about it: How many times do you reach for organ-strangling foods just because they're closest? It happens when you walk by an open cabinet and see that orange box, beckoning you to crunch some crackers. (There's a reason that manufacturers make boxes so brightly colored—they say "eat me!" loud and clear.) It happens when that nice lady brings in cupcakes for the volunteer crew. It happens when you didn't think ahead about lunch, one o'clock rolls around, and the closest thing to you is the Chinese buffet—a great deal at $5.99. But at 3,000 calories and who knows how much deep-fried fat, that buffet is the furthest thing from a bargain. It happens all the time. (By the way, you *can* make good choices in a Chinese restaurant, and I'll show you how on page 258.)

I've learned so much from food researchers who have done fascinating work in the area of mindless eating—how subconscious cues get us to eat more and choose poorly. For example, researchers at Cornell University, led by Brian Wansink, have done some wild experiments in which they show how visual cues have a huge impact on how much we eat, using things like bottomless bowls of soup (soup is pumped up through the bottom of the bowl so the eater has no idea more is being added). And they have looked at factors like noise and light levels to see how they influence food decisions. They found that a lot of factors *unrelated to hunger* nudge us to eat more and more and more.

The two keys to thwarting those forces are planning and creation. Have you planned for thin-ice moments—times when you're most vulnerable to overeating or flooding your bloodstream with enemy ingredients? And have you created simple solutions that let you eat, snack, graze, and treat yourself the healthy way?

Picture this and you'll see what I mean: It's ten at night, you've had a hard day, the dishes are washed, and you finally get a chance to kick back and watch an episode of your guilty-pleasure reality TV show. Quiet time. De-stress time. Me time. Time, you might think, for a heaping bowl of vanilla ice cream scattered with chocolate chips that you can roll your tongue around for the next little while. Three minutes later, that bowl is on your lap, the remote is in your hand,

Take a small bag of nuts with you to work or on the go. Add-ins like chickpeas and curry powder take them way beyond basic. See the recipe on page 273.

and before long, your insulin response team has dialed a biological 9-1-1.

Now, what happens if you have nothing that even begins to resemble ice cream in your home? You're certainly in no mood to get in the car, drive to the convenience store, pick up sweet supplies, then drive back. Not worth it. So instead—because this is what's sitting in your fridge—you fill a bowl with plain Greek yogurt, add a generous scoop of berries, and shave some dark chocolate over the top.

My prediction: The show will be just as fun and the snack just as satisfying, while the health outcome is so much better. Prepare yourself and your kitchen for times when you would typically grab ice cream (or whatever junk food you go for), and you'll change what's going on in your body just by letting superfoods do their good work.

Once you get started, you'll always be tweaking your environment for the better.

Spicy-Smoky Hummus satisfies those hunger cravings deliciously. See the recipe on page 241.

Recently at my home, we moved our veggies and salad ingredients out of the crisper. It was harder to see them there, so they'd often go bad before we used them. While we're generally conscientious about eating enough fruits and vegetables, this change made a big difference. Instead of our having to consciously root around for healthy produce, it looks us in the eye as soon as we open the refrigerator.

Lisa makes a wonderful brothy soup (see page 302) we always have on hand. It's great for nights when I don't feel like having a big dinner, but I do want *something*. A bowl of that soup is a life-saver. I get nourishment and feel satisfied, but I don't load up on food for no reason. If it wasn't there, I'd probably end up eating more than I want. We keep lots of healthy options ready to go, including dinner staples in the freezer—fish, for example—so we're never more than an hour away from a feel-good meal. I'd rather determine my own health destiny than leave it up to a pizza delivery person.

Just the other day, I was on a work call at noon. I had been busting it all morning,

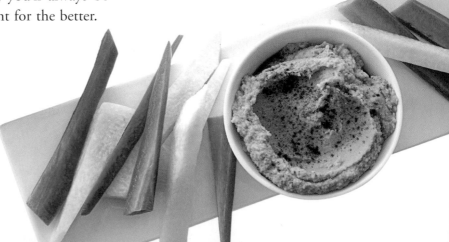

5 TRICKS TO AUTOMATE YOUR ENVIRONMENT

- Take an hour and clean out your pantry. Get rid of processed junk. Make a shopping list to include food FIXES. The grocery list for the 21-Day Plan is on page 181.

- Plan your lunches for the week and pack them to take to work or wherever.

- Make Sunday a meal-plan, meal-prep, and meal-making day. Cook a big batch of something healthy that you can use for several lunches and dinners. Use the day to cut up veggies and have them ready to go as snacks and sides.

- If you stash junk food in your home for other people to eat, put it on the top shelf of the pantry (and behind other items). The harder they are to see and reach, the less likely you are to dig for them when a momentary urge strikes.

- Keep a small bag of nuts in your car, purse, or briefcase. It'll save you in a hunger emergency.

and I was really hungry—truly sand-in-your-bathing-suit uncomfortable—but I had to keep plugging away.

I'm famous for always carrying nuts, and this day was no exception. So I noshed on those, even though, to be honest, I wasn't really in the mood for them. That held me over until I could get lunch. I would have had a cookie if some were nearby. And you can be sure that I would have cannoned down a cupcake if I'd been making the call next to a plate of them.

Here's the bottom line: We are products of our environments, and we make choices not based on what we know, but on what's in front of us. This plays out every day: Graz-ing while making dinner, nibbling in front of the TV with a bottomless bag of something crunchy, stopping at the vending machine because the urge strikes at four P.M., finishing the last scoop of potatoes because, well, that's just not enough to pack for leftovers. These mindless habits—when they're unhealthy—defeat many of us. To win, we have to create new environments and experiences and auto-matic behaviors that capitalize on the health-ful joy food can give us.

To quiet a rumbly stomach, we eat what we see. We eat what's close. The drive to satisfy hunger is stronger than any drive to hold out thirty minutes for the carrots and hummus. So you have to be prepared to handle your hunger and

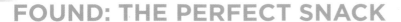

FOUND: THE PERFECT SNACK

Nuts are packed with good fat and satiating protein, and some research suggests that they may help lower levels of inflammation, which can help you stave off various diseases and conditions. It's an impressive cast of characters:

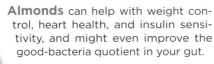

Almonds can help with weight control, heart health, and insulin sensitivity, and might even improve the good-bacteria quotient in your gut.

Brazil nuts contain selenium, a mineral that can improve thyroid and immune function.

Cashews have immune-boosting zinc, as well as copper, which increases your ability to make red blood cells—crucial for ferrying oxygen throughout your body.

Hazelnuts have folate, which can help you build strong bones and lower bad cholesterol while raising the good kind.

Macadamias are high in calories, yes, but they have more of the good monounsaturated fat than any other nut and even avocados.

Peanuts which, strictly speaking, are a legume, pack even more protein than nuts and are a great source of phytosterol, which helps control cholesterol.

Pecans have a special type of vitamin E that keeps your brain healthy and could help lower levels of bad cholesterol.

Pistachios boast fatigue-fighting potassium, as well as lots of fiber.

Walnuts have the most of the plant version of healthy omega-3 fats (called ALAs).

your temptations. This is why it's so important to pack snacks in the morning so you reach for the good foods, rather than the ones that will tinker with your blood sugar and energy levels later in the day. (See more stress-busting and satisfying snacks on page 133 or 239.)

One more time: Control your food environment. Make it easy to do the right thing.

Strategy 2: More Yes, Less No

Recently, a group of us were playing a coed volleyball game. A guy on the other team served as the de facto leader. He yelled, clapped, tried to fire up his team. When their play turned south, he implored them to do better. His preferred mode of coaching: "Just stop doing that!"

You know what happened next: His teammates couldn't do anything right. When told what *not* to do, that's all they *could* do, and they missed the ball again and again.

This is exactly the way our diet culture works. Again and again, we hear, *Just stop doing that!* Stop eating pie. Stop snacking. Stop carbs. Stop dreaming of a naughty interlude with that hot Italian, fettuccine Alfredo.

We live in an opposite-of-Nike dieting environment. Just *don't* do it.

But the more you're told what not to do, the more tempted you are to rebel. That's not because you're naturally defiant (though defiance certainly plays a role). It happens for a couple of reasons—for one, your brain doesn't always hear the "no." For example, when a child's brain is exposed to the words "don't run," it processes the word "run." A better imperative is "walk." By changing up the messaging, you're imploring your brain to *do* something, instead of *not* doing something. It also works because your brain needs to have some action to perform; it wants to be occupied. So the smarter move is to find an understudy for a habit you want to change, a behavior that gradually replaces it.

Your brain learns a new behavior with practice. It lays down neurological wiring so it knows what to do easily. It may take some time at first, but eventually your brain just flips the switch and you act accordingly. When you replace bad habits with healthy ones, you're laying down new track to hide the old ones.

So how does it work, practically speaking?

Let's say your vice is a bag of chips every afternoon around five P.M. You crave the crunch, you crave the salt, you crave that ritual of eating and relaxing.

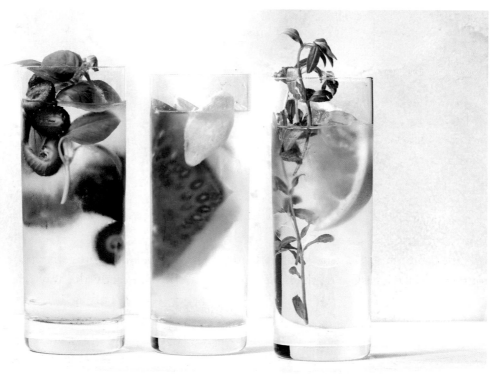

Sip seltzer with fruit slices instead of soda and save 10 teaspoons of sugar. Or try these refreshing flavor combinations: strawberry and basil, watermelon and ginger, pink grapefruit and tarragon.

Now, after what you've read so far, you want to give up the chips, or you at least know you *should*. But sit at your desk in the witching hour with nothing to munch on, and you'll still feel the magnetic force of the crinkly bag. The way to counteract that very real pull is to find an adequate substitute. When you're ready to make the change, you fill a bowl with something else that crunches (maybe a bag of air-popped popcorn with some sea salt or paprika sprinkled on top). Now you're off and munching away. Your stomach and mind are both satisfied—and your body is better off for it. (Note: You also don't need to go cold turkey. You could start with a bowl of carrot sticks and half a bowl of chips, then steadily decrease the amount of chips you have over a few weeks.)

Apply the same principle to any of your lightning rod foods. Soda, for instance, is a biggie. Maybe you sub in bubbly water with fruit, so you still get some sweetness and the carbonation.

Remember that you're not giving up your favorites forever; as I said in chapter 2, you do get special-occasion sugar. But you *are* retraining your brain so that healthier behaviors are the general rule and unhealthy ones are the once-in-a-while exception. The positive side effect of going off bad foods for a bit? You won't crave them nearly as much afterward, and life won't require as much willpower.

Strategy 3: Customize Your "Rules"

We all have to live by somebody else's rules when it comes to school, work, or the community swimming pool. I just don't think you should have to live by anyone else's food rules. Instead, I want you to come up with your own internal monitoring system, because you know your individual pressure points best and can invent unique ways to address them. These solutions become your nutritional constitution, guiding you when it's time to make decisions.

Here are some examples that work for me. Borrow anything that seems helpful, or get inspired to write your own.

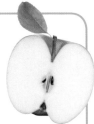

THE EASIEST WEIGHT-LOSS TRICK EVER?

People who leave fruit and veggies out on the counter have a lower body mass index compared to those with none in sight.

- I have a soft spot for sweet spots. Give me some chocolate ice cream, and I'm like a kid in, well, an ice-cream store. I know better, but it's not as if I have a will of steel. So I've created two main principles that I live by when it comes to dessert: One, I don't eat it at home. We don't keep desserts around, so I just don't have them. And two, if we're eating out as a family, we may order one special dish to share, and we'll each have one or two bites. It's enough to enjoy the intense sweetness every once in a while, but not enough to stretch waistbands to the breaking point.

- My nickname should be King of the Doggie Bag. I will take home anything that's left after a meal out, even the smallest portion. That's because my tendency to overeat comes from guilt about wasting food. (I was raised in that classic home environment where grown-ups told you to clean your plate because there are starving children around the world.) Now I plan to bring food home with me, so I don't feel pressure to hoover everything on my plate.

- If I taste something I really like (see *ice cream, chocolate*) and know I might go down a bad road, I quickly look for some kind of palate changer. So I have a breath mint or brush my teeth if I can. At a party I'll eat an olive, which has a strong enough taste to erase the mouthfeel high I might be getting from something unhealthy on the buffet table. That immediately and effectively roadblocks my keep-eating reflex.

See how they're not really rules, per se? I could very well say "no desserts in the home, don't finish the plate, no more than two bites of bad food," but I don't think that's the effective way to handle eating.

Look at your own life and figure out where it's difficult to eat well. Maybe you graze when you cook or you clean your child's plate so

YOU MAKE THE RULES: ONE EASY TRICK FOR GAINING CONTROL

Researchers have studied the power of a simple word swap when it comes to behavior change. When you're giving something up, say "I don't" rather than "I can't." As in: "I just don't eat pie," rather than "I can't eat pie." This is different than someone telling you not to do it; this is you making a decision about what you do and don't do. That simple shift, researchers found, flips the narrative of control. You're the one in charge, not some diet plan—and this leads to more successful outcomes.

you don't waste food. Identify some of your danger zones, then create some strategies for dealing with them. Ask yourself, "How can I make it easier to do better in those situations?" It's all about smart systems and diversionary tactics that empower you instead of needling you.

Strategy 4: Consider Food Shopping a Quest

The supermarket can be a tricky place, a confusing circus of food choices that make it hard for you to decide between brands, look at prices, decipher labels, and avoid temptations. But with a solid understanding of nutri-

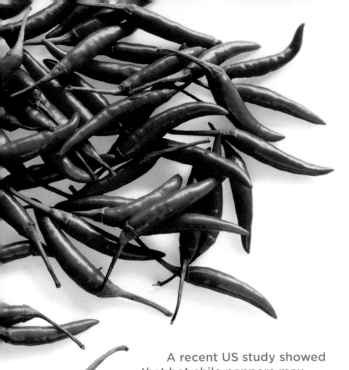

A recent US study showed that hot chile peppers may help reduce risk of heart disease and stroke. Cut out the core and seeds, then add the peppers to any dish that needs a kick—chili, soups, homemade salsa, tacos, etc.

tion, you can get past food-marketing lingo, find fix-it foods, and avoid trouble zones. The healthiest foods in a supermarket, like produce and fresh seafood and meats, are usually on the perimeter, while the less-healthy, more processed ones are in the middle aisles. The best time to shop? After a meal, so your brain, not your belly, makes the decisions.

Another rule of thumb: When you shop, choose foods with the fewest ingredients listed on the label. The smaller the number the better. It's an easy guide to remember as you start your journey, and before you dive into more advanced-level thinking about nutrition.

But the big lesson isn't that you have to avoid cartoon characters selling snacks; it's that food shopping can be *fun*. Think of it as a challenge and an adventure, not a time-sucking chore. Explore the store and see what

DON'T FALL FOR "FLAVORS" ON FOOD LABELS

Are natural flavors really better than artificial flavors? The bottom line: They're really not that different. And those "natural flavors" can actually contain synthetic chemicals. The main difference between a natural flavor and an artificial one is the origin of the flavor chemicals. Natural flavors must be derived from plant or animal material. Artificial flavors are synthesized in the lab. The actual chemicals in these two kinds of flavors may be exactly the same, and in many cases, they're both engineered to make you addicted to them. They may also dull your senses to the flavors that are in real food. I avoid both "synthetic" and "natural" flavors when I can by minimizing my consumption of processed foods.

you can discover, whether it's a different kind of nut or fruit or something untried at the fish counter. Visit farmers' markets or ethnic grocery stores. See what's out there and experiment with healthy ingredients that add flavor to your plate and joy to your cooking. There's a payoff, too: A Cornell University study found that women who ate adventurously—meaning a wide variety of uncommon foods—weighed less than those who ate more conventional diets.

Strategy 5: Eat Write

If you're contemplating a 180-degree diet change or seeing that the scale is nowhere near where it needs to be, start by keeping a food journal. Writing down everything you eat has been shown to be an effective tactic for several reasons. One, it holds you accountable (even if it's just you reviewing the day). Two, it makes you think twice about popping a handful of gummy candies if you know you're going to log them later. Three, even a few extra bites here and there while you're preparing dinner add, on average, 25 calories to your daily intake. If you record every bite, it will help you resist that habit.

I also love the idea of meal mapping: You write down what you're *going* to eat that day before you get started. It's sort of like an exercise-training program; you devise a plan and you aim to stick to it. Decisions no longer get made in the heat of the moment, and you can look at the day as a whole, fitting in as many food FIXES as possible.

For either method, pen and paper or a computer document works just fine. Many smartphone apps, like MyFitnessPal and Fooducate, make it easy to record your daily intake. To me, it's not about counting calories, per se, but more about having an awareness of things that you may not even realize you're consuming throughout the day. I recommend trying it for two weeks, but you may find you like journaling and make it a lifelong habit.

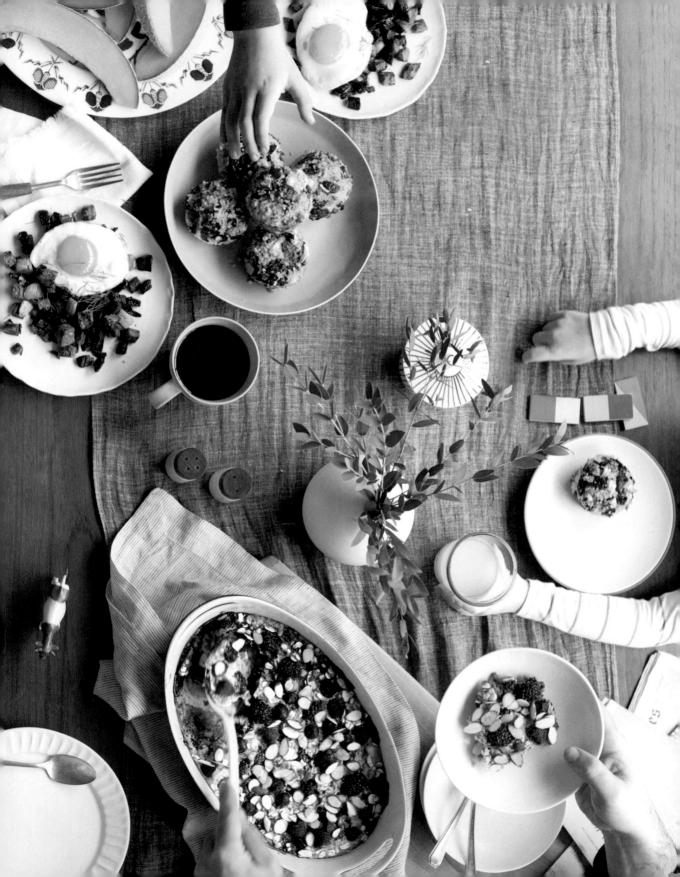

4

A Serving of Soul

As the backdrop for a million special moments in your life, meals pack more than just nutritional power.

What is the hub of your home? For many of us, it's the family room or living room. Heck, their very names beg us to hang out there. Family? Living? *That's where we should be.*

Trouble is, these spaces invite us to plop down on the couch with our eyeballs on the TV, our phone, or a laptop. While there's nothing wrong with relaxing, working, or tapping four hundred emojis a minute, I urge families to move the focal point of their household to the kitchen and dining table—a place where eyeballs zigzag to people, not pixels. Too often, when it comes to meal prep, the assigned cook is left to chop, stir, bake, and clean alone, while the rest of the clan is off somewhere else with their fingers woodpeckering on keyboards.

But what happens if the kitchen and the table serve as the "sun" of your household—the center around which everything else revolves? Life gets a little fuller and more buoyant with talking, laughing, doing. Meals become a powerful source of familial energy. No matter how big or small the kitchen. No matter if the meal takes twenty minutes or an hour to prepare. No matter if your home includes two people or ten.

Lisa and I made a conscious effort to ensure that salads wouldn't be the only things tossed in our kitchen. We also tossed around ideas, stories, questions, issues, and laughter with each other, and later, with our children from the time they were babies. The result: The space where we cook and eat has become our family's Grand Central Terminal, the place where we connect. While one or more of the Oz crew is prepping food, others join in and chat, and the conversation continues right into the meal. I want all of us to recapture the spiritual benefits of mealtime and relearn some important truths:

Food helps you bond with others.

Food strengthens your family.

Food sets the stage for meaningful exchanges, passing on traditions (like Grandma's incredible tomato sauce recipe), and sharing lessons with the people you love.

We've established that food is about science, yes, but it's also about soul—the humanity that is revealed during intimate gatherings at the table. That element actually has healing power in its own right, helping you decrease anxiety, improve mood, and lead an overall healthier life. No wonder a small study from New Zealand looked at the effect of family meals and found that they improved people's health and relationships.

So as you embark on your food-fixing journey, spend a few moments thinking about how to get your crew to engage actively in the kitchen, instead of simply showing up at the table, waiting for food to appear. Start small—cooking one family dinner together each week, or proposing a Sunday tradition where everyone works as a team to assemble lunches for the week, or having once-a-month surprise meals where one member of the family prepares a new dish. Over time, and by piloting little ideas like these, the kitchen becomes a place of creation rather than one of obligation.

There is value in food above and beyond macros and micros. That value comes in the form of moments. Let me share a few from my life.

ROLE OF SOUL 1:
The Missing Ingredient in Many Meals Is Connection

Growing up, I spent my summers in Turkey with my relatives. When we visited, my extended family would have a feast once a week. The table was covered with all kinds of Turkish delicacies, like baklava and baba ghanoush (a rich eggplant dish). One aunt made dolma, or stuffed vegetables, such as

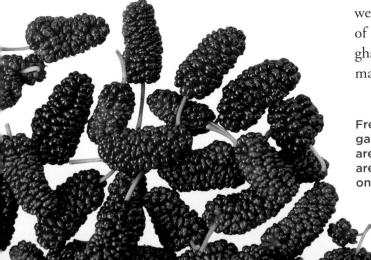

Fresh mulberries like the ones I gathered and gobbled as a kid are tough to find, but dried ones are readily available at many online retailers.

zucchini filled with rice and meat. Another aunt had a mulberry tree. I would climb up and shake the berries off the branches. We'd collect the delicious mulberries by the bushel and bulldoze through them, licking our fingers. (Dried mulberries, by the way, are sweet like figs but have two-thirds the sugar of raisins. And they're a nice source of fiber and antioxidants.)

While we were all feasting—the meal lasted an hour and a half or so—the kids would play hide-and-seek and the adults might play poker or some other card game. I didn't think about these rituals at the time. We enjoyed the food. Nothing was expensive or difficult to make, and everything was fresh and healthy. It was just how we lived.

Now that I'm many years removed from those summers, I look back and see more than berries and baklava. Our eating was entertainment. Our eating was social. Eating meant time together.

Too often these days, schedules and stress have fostered an on-your-own eating environment, and we've lost this communal and multigenerational spirit. In our house, we try to resurrect the tradition of family feasting as often as we can, even as our kids head off in different directions with school, work, and their own lives.

When my granddaughter, Philo, was a baby, she used to sit on my lap during meals. Partly this was to give her mom, Daphne, a break, and it kept her from scooping up a knife when she began to grab things willy-nilly. But mostly we just wanted to include her in our meals instead of putting her aside while the adults ate. Philo, now a three-and-a-half-year-old, will sometimes still sit on my lap at the table—not because she needs my help, but because it's one of the ways that we eat as a family. It's been fascinating to watch *her* watch everyone. When someone laughs, she stares and processes it all. You can see her little cerebral wheels turning, trying to figure out what made that person crack up. And then she laughs, too. The dinner table has been a wonderful place to watch her grow and learn, right before our eyes.

At these family meals, passing plates is just a proxy for passing along wisdom, memories, ideas, and questions. (That's one of the reasons we don't allow digital devices at the table. Lisa and I wanted to establish the importance of eliminating distractions so we can be present for each other.) One of my favorite family traditions involves something that happens when we're at my in-laws' home. The dinners include all kinds of fresh dishes and natural ingredients. They're full of flavor—really tapping into the taste of umami, that magical essence of certain savory foods on your tongue. While I've always appreciated the meals that my mother-in-law, Emily Jane, makes, there's something I love even more about those dinners.

She brings a reading to share.

They can be readings about love, about friendship, about the world around us. They're not long, but they're always thought-provoking and get the conversation going in a way that makes us appreciate each other's viewpoints and feelings. It's not a kumbaya exercise that Mom likes to do. It's a way to honor the sacredness of the family gathering at the table.

Now, I don't think every meal needs to have a script or sermon, but I want to challenge you to rethink how you eat as a group of family members, friends, or colleagues. Conversation doesn't always have to revert to things like office politics or today's headlines, though there's a time and place for that. Try simple conversation starters like asking every-

THE SINGLE SECRET TO A HEALTHIER HOME

Studies show that people who eat eleven to fourteen home-cooked meals per week are 13 percent less likely to develop type 2 diabetes than those who eat six or fewer meals per week at home. You don't have to log Julia Child hours in the kitchen: Many recipes in my 21-Day Plan come together in half an hour.

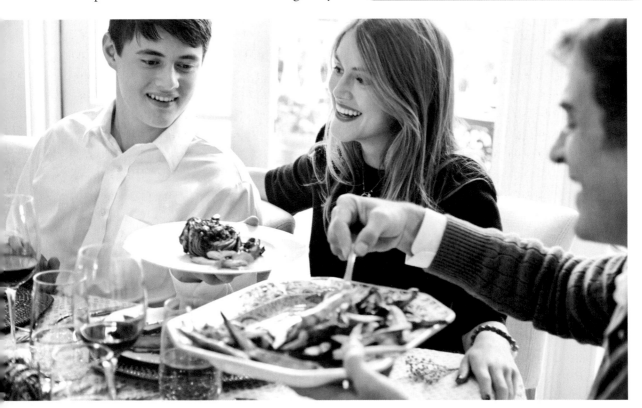

There's lots of love at the Oz family table—especially for Lisa's cooking!

one to name a movie they'd take if stranded on a desert island. Or have everyone tell a story about their favorite teacher. Or ask each person to share the nicest thing they saw that day. If you do it right, the discussion and joking around linger at the table and last in your memories.

That bonding is crucial to the soul of food, and there's no doubt it helps the body, too. A University of Texas review of studies looked at the link between social ties and health. One study in that review, for example, found that those who were socially isolated had double the death rate from heart disease than those who had stronger social circles. Other research links fewer social ties to a greater risk of high blood pressure, a weaker immune system, difficulty recovering from cancer, and a higher risk of inflammation. And that's not even including the psychological effects: Lack of social ties puts people at greater risk for anxiety and depression (which, in turn, are associated with many health problems).

Conversely, the more social connections you have, the more likely you are to live healthy and happy. Makes a lot of sense, and it also makes sense that food sets the stage for relationships to thrive.

In practical terms, what do I mean? I mean that not every family dinner should be a rush job. If you live alone, make an effort to plan get-together dinners with neighbors and lunches with friends or coworkers (they don't

have to be meals "out"; brown baggers in the nearby park are great, too).

The combination of soulful thought and energy-giving nutrients is at the heart of my message about food. Realize that meals are a chance to feed your emotions, your intellect, and your spirit when you break bread with the people closest to you.

Open your mouth. Open your mind. Open your world.

ROLE OF SOUL 2:
Redefine Emotional Eating

Recently, my son Oliver and I went on a fishing trip. That day, everybody was catching a lot of fish except Oliver, even though he tried every kind of tempting bait and cast it gently and stealthily into the river. A friend who was with us explained why: At that moment, the fish were swimming upstream to spawn, so they had no interest in eating. If they took the bait, it was because the fisherman had slapped his line into the water, causing a ruckus and irritating the fish. The fish that were biting were doing so because they were annoyed by the distraction from their journey, not because they were hungry.

Sound familiar?

Emotional eating—the idea that we often nosh because we're feeling angry or stressed or sad—is a common theme among those who struggle with diet and weight. Many people mindlessly chomp away just like those fish did. They get emotional, so they reach for the first thing they can bite down on. A few seconds of eating relief comes with long-term consequences.

Eating *should* be emotional—but I want the emotions tied to food to be positive and productive, not negative and reactive. Instead of attacking a tub of ice cream because somebody sent you a snarky text or tucking into an entire pound of pasta because life is tough, I want eating to enhance your relationships and grow your joy.

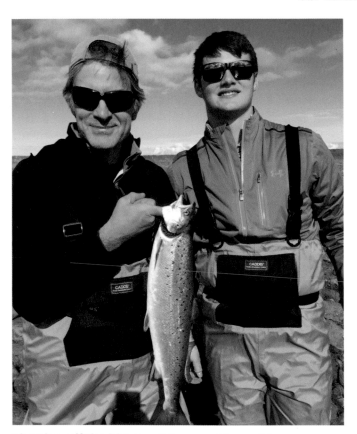

Showing off the big one Oliver and I caught.

This is another reason to team up for mealtime as much as you can. Destructive emotional eating tends to be a solitary affair; add a supportive friend or partner and you're less likely to use food for comfort. Wherever we travel, Lisa and I like to taste the local food and carve out some slowed-down alone time together. We'll gather up picnic supplies and head out to a park or a beach or even a city bench. Salads, cheeses, honey . . . It's not just about what we're eating, but that we're together. We talk about our kids, our goals, our challenges. Surely that happens at other times, too, but some of our nicest memories stem from these simple meals.

Positive emotional eating can happen when you're one-on-one, or when the gang's all there. Every fall, for example, our family travels to an orchard to pick apples. We bring dozens home for ourselves and friends to enjoy and make pies with the leftovers. On the way to the orchard, we stop at a Renaissance fair, eat turkey legs with our hands, ravaging them Henry VIII–style. Our kids know these traditions, and they're an important part of our lives and memories. They make us happy.

Everyone loves their foodie customs at holidays, birthdays,

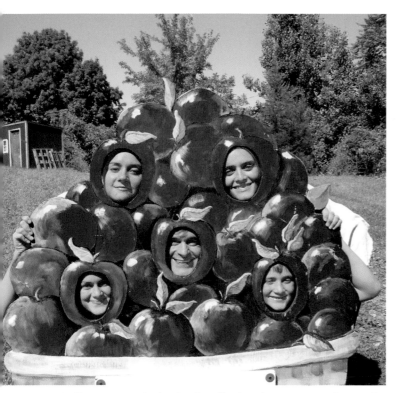
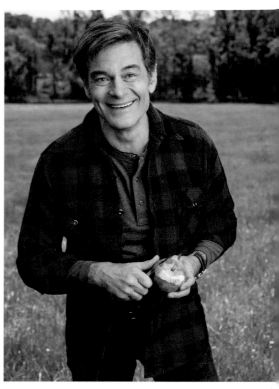

Call us an apple-lovin' family: Each year we take a trip to an orchard together to pick bunches of them. Yes, I've been known to sample the fruit right there, and if there's a chance for a silly photo op, we're in!

THE EASY TRICK TO DIVERT EMOTIONAL EATING

Many of your best tactics to avoid binges tied to anxiety, depression, fatigue, or stress are the ones you saw in chapter 3, where I discussed removing bad food from your environment. I also find that if you can remove *yourself* from a situation momentarily—by taking a brisk walk or doing a set of squats or a one-minute stretch, for example—the immediate craving will subside enough to allow your brain to make a good decision, rather than a purely reactive one. The physical task will help your body overpower the emotional response.

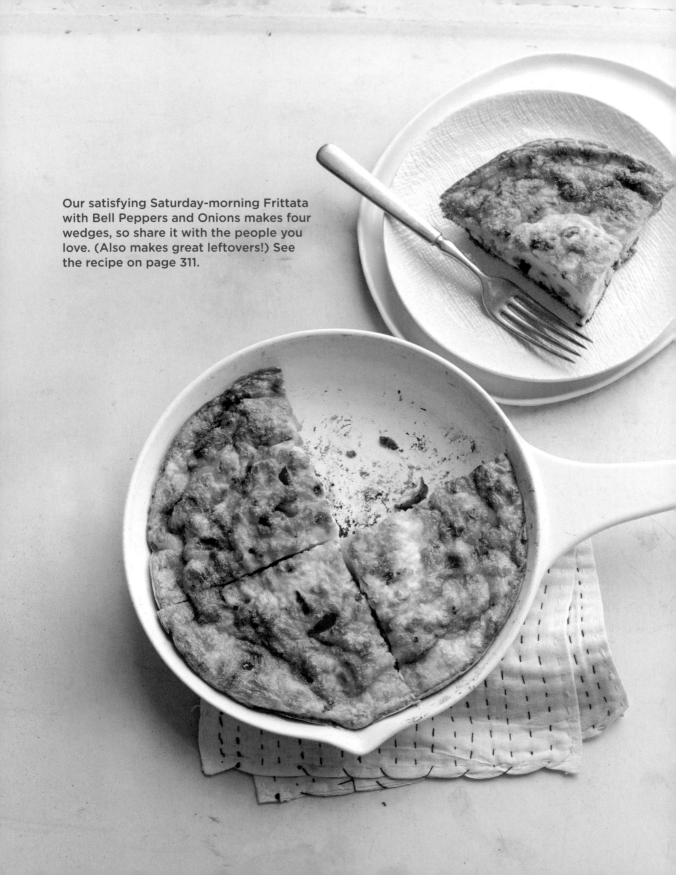

Our satisfying Saturday-morning Frittata with Bell Peppers and Onions makes four wedges, so share it with the people you love. (Also makes great leftovers!) See the recipe on page 311.

or big-game days. But let's start to think of family food traditions not as something you do just five or six times a year, but more regularly. For example, we have Sunday meals after we worship, and it's the one time of the week that we all get together (which is even more meaningful as the kids have moved on with their lives). A family feast for you might happen the night before the first day of school; whenever Grandma visits; or every Saturday morning, with a delicious frittata.

Hey, how about potlucks with the neighborhood crew on the first Friday of the month?

Doesn't matter *what* you do. It just matters *that* you do.

ROLE OF SOUL 3:
Be Mindful of the Experience

I'll admit I have a few skills I'm proud of. I'm a good listener, have a decent-for-my-age backhand in tennis, and can still finesse my way around a chest cavity in the OR. But here's a skill I've had to develop over the last decade or so: I practice what it means to be *really* aware of what I am eating. I'm not talking about counting every calorie or gram of sugar in my meals; instead, I try to go deep into the sensory wonder of food.

This is what's called mindful eating—the ability to slow down, savor the flavors, shut out distractions, and really embrace food as more than just sustenance, but as an experience.

Mealtime should be the ultimate smell-the-roses moment, when you stop to engage all your senses. Smell and taste are no-brainers. But so is sight—I try to appreciate what good food looks like, too. Fun fact: A study published in the journal *Appetite* looked at people's enjoyment of meals with the exact same

THE 24-HOUR MINDFULNESS CHALLENGE

One day in the next week or so, I want you to do four things every time you eat:

1. Your eyes must be on your food and other people (not on a screen of any sort) when you eat. Really savor as you chew and swallow. Take a bite and put your utensil down. Take another.

2. Think about at least one other sense besides taste. What's the texture and temperature? How does it look on the plate, and what do you smell?

3. Have one healthy ingredient or food you haven't eaten in ages (or never tried). Maybe pick up a new-to-you piece of fruit at the market and have it after your lunch, or sprinkle an exotic-sounding spice onto a grilled chicken breast.

4. Before bed, gauge how you felt eating and how you feel now that you're done. Like it? Try it again the next day.

ingredients where one was presented more attractively than the other. It's no surprise that study participants said the artfully plated meal tasted better.

In addition, you may also want to appreciate the texture of what you eat. The crisp crunch of fresh snow peas? Sublime. Don't just taste for flavor, but zone in on how foods feel different, too.

When I put all these senses in play, I find my eating experience is richer and I eat more slowly, and that means I eat less. It also makes me think about what I *don't* enjoy. And if I don't like it, I push it away. I no longer (or at least, rarely) chomp on foods simply because they're there.

Research backs me up: One review of studies published in the journal *Appetite* found that eating more mindfully can help promote weight loss, which, as you know, comes with a slew of health benefits.

Being mindful doesn't take the focus of a fighter pilot, but it does mean saying goodbye to distracted eating. What do I mean by that? No more shoveling your meal into your mouth with your eyeballs glued to your phone, laptop, or TV. Dine at a table with others—actively participating, listening, and appreciating different flavors (of food and people). And when you eat alone, just sit and enjoy what's in front of you. This won't require a ninety-minute breakfast—just a little awareness that will slow the moment.

ROLE OF SOUL 4:
Diets Are Lonely. Don't Be Lonely.

I talk to a lot of people about weight loss, diets, and food plans. Some are experts and some are friends. Many are guests on my show. The thing I hear over and over about why people resist the switch to healthier eating isn't that they all despise broccoli or refuse to give up soda or can't live without lasagna. It's that diets make them feel like they're on a desert island (when they would really rather

THE ORIGINAL CULINARY ART

When you look at cave paintings from our ancestors—ones done thirty thousand years ago—you'll see images of animals and rituals and all kinds of things that represented meaningful parts of a community. Lisa and I once visited some cave paintings in Spain, and I was amazed at how prevalent the pictures of fish were, even though the caves were some one hundred miles from the ocean. Though we don't really know if fish was depicted as food or just a symbol (no recipes were included, after all), it was clear to me that protein sources have always been a special thread in people's lives.

be on a dessert island). Nobody is around, they're hungry, and the food options are strictly limited.

In a survey we did for my show with famous pollster Mike Berland, we found that 60 percent of all respondents reported feeling lonely, and that feeling is magnified when they're dieting. After all, when you're "on a diet," you can't partake in parties, happy hours, and nights out because you're handcuffed to a stalk of celery while everyone else is clinking glasses and licking their fingers.

While some food plans might suggest you simply need willpower to resist or you have to just say no while others say yes, my take is a bit different.

Don't miss out.

Laughter, community, and social interaction are like essential nutrients. It's actually bad for your health to hole up in your kitchen with a 4-ounce chicken breast, wishing you were with everyone else. So throughout this book, I provide strategies for managing your eating so that you can be part of the group without going off the rails nutritionally. (See how I eat in restaurants on page 249.)

You can have fun with your friends. You can use systems to help in tempting times. You can even inspire others to follow your lead. Because you need your tribe—and the powerful medicinal tool of social connection—to be truly healthy.

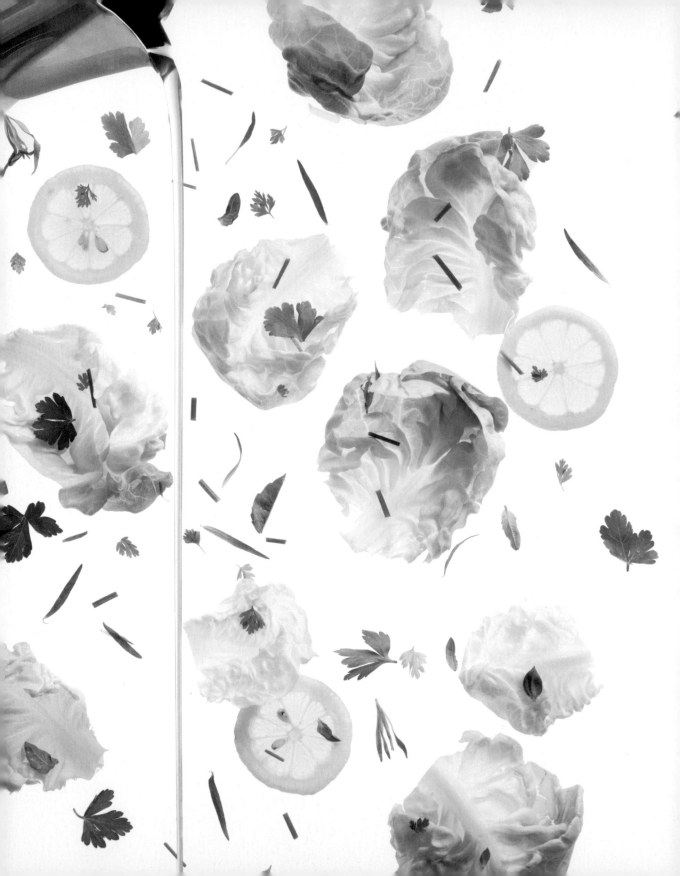

PART 2

FOOD FIXES

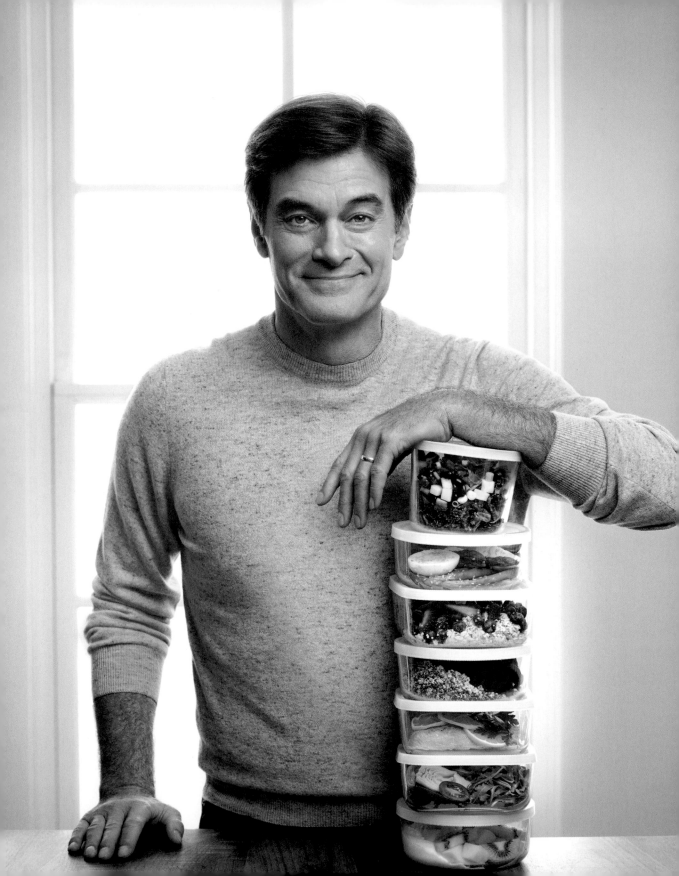

5

Food FIXES for Weight Loss

Three primary principles will normalize your weight for good.

There's a very good chance you're reading this book with one main goal: You, like 53 percent of Americans, want to lose weight.

You can envision the result. You want to be healthier, feel better, have more energy. You want to live happy and strong, not mopey and sluggish. You want a fix for the most prevalent health problem we face: We're too heavy.

So let's go ahead and acknowledge that this *is* a weight-loss book, but not in the traditional sense. Instead of losing weight any way you can to look great on the outside, you need to allow foods to fix your body from the inside. That, in turn, will *normalize* your weight, so that you can live in your body's comfort zone. After all, a healthy weight has a domino effect on many other facets of your life, improving your heart health, your inflammation level, your moods, and so many more measures of wellness. You'll lighten the load on your arteries, as well as your joints. You'll decrease your risk of developing diabetes, cancer, strokes, and most of the issues I cover in the chapters that follow this one. You'll lose weight, but more important, you'll gain a healthy future.

Every step along the way, FIXES foods will help you. Read on to find out how.

F (Fats with benefits): Omega-3s have been shown to reduce belly fat. According to one study in the *International Journal of Obesity*, people on a reduced-calorie diet who ate salmon (rich in omega-3s) three days a week lost significantly more fat from their middle than those who ate the same number of calories but didn't have fish. How do good fats help? By boosting metabolism and curbing hunger.

I (Ideal proteins): Lean proteins are key for keeping you full, and they're also the building blocks for your tissues. Plus, they're important for helping you lose weight. A New York University study, for instance, found that those who consumed recommended amounts of protein had lower amounts of excess body fat. Plus, protein is less efficient for your body to digest, which means you burn some of the calories you ingest as you're processing the food, essentially delivering a calorie discount—that is, you don't actually process all the calories that protein contains.

X (Xtra fruits and vegetables): Fiber keeps you full, so you're less likely to overeat, and fruits and vegetables are loaded with it. Get plenty of fiber in the morning with a produce-powered breakfast to help you through the day. Three recent studies showed that vegetarians lose more weight than meat eaters. (That doesn't mean meat is bad; it more likely indicates that vegetarians naturally tend to eat more vegetables.)

E (Energizing carbs): Complex carbs keep hunger at bay. In one recent study, people who ate a whole-grain-rich diet for six weeks burned an extra 92 calories a day compared to those who ate a refined-grain-based diet.

S (Special-occasion sugar): Careful here. Too many sweets and you'll jack up blood sugar and hunger levels, but used strategically, they can actually help. In one Italian study, those who ate dark chocolate (70% cacao) reduced their waist circumferences in just one week. Why? The darker stuff has anti-inflammatory properties and helps with

A PICKLE A DAY KEEPS THE DOCTOR AWAY

Vinegar with meals was used as a home remedy for diabetes before glucose-lowering drugs came around. The thought was that vinegar has acetic acid, which slows digestion and thus helps your body manage blood sugar. There might be something to it: Recent studies show that 1 to 2 tablespoons of vinegar when added to high glycemic foods can lower blood glucose and increase feelings of fullness. It's easy to put this idea into practice—just use vinegar with olive oil as your default salad dressing. And heck, help yourself to some pickles as a snack. If nothing else, they'll satisfy crunchy cravings.

THE FOOD THAT LOOKS LIKE A PILL (BUT WORKS EVEN BETTER)

I've got many secret weapons when it comes to weight loss, but one of my favorites is pulses (a term used by farmers long ago that's now coming back into fashion). They are plain and simple beans like cannellini and kidney, as well as peas, chickpeas, and lentils. (Green beans aren't technically a pulse.) A half cup of pulses (except for peas) has as much protein as three eggs, about a third of a day's worth of fiber, plus zinc, iron, and B vitamins. If you've been neglecting these superfoods, then add more of them to your diet. You'll also see plenty of them in my 21-Day Plan.

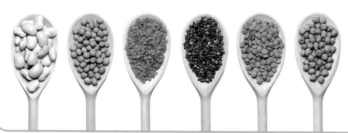

A few ways to get your pulse up: Puree them and spread on sandwiches, blend into dips, toss into salads for texture, or add to soups for extra heartiness.

insulin sensitivity, both of which influence how your body stores fat.

Think about eating for weight loss as a sort of quiet diet—not some strict plan that you're trying to follow for a certain number of days to achieve a certain number of pounds lost. Instead, eating the FIXES foods—and employing smart strategies—will become the automated vehicle by which you lose weight and get healthier. The approach will affect not just what you see on a scale, but what you see in a blood test—as well as how you feel.

One man in particular helped me understand the link between diet and health destiny. He came in to the hospital with chest pain and major clogs in his arteries. We determined that he needed heart bypass surgery. This man, who was in his fifties and weighed

about 450 pounds, needed to get into the OR as soon as possible.

The only problem? He weighed so much that we didn't have a table that could hold him for the necessary procedures. It's not a good feeling to tell someone that they should have surgery, but that you can't do it. He was left with just one shot: If he could lose enough weight so we could get him on the table, we could operate.

When you have only one chance, you take it, and that's what he did. He went on an aggressive diet—really focusing on vegetables, lean meats, and olive oil (sounds a lot like your FIXES, doesn't it?). He lost one hundred pounds in six months. Very dramatic results, but he was motivated. He didn't want to die, and that was his alternative. Now weighing 350 pounds, he was eligible for the operation.

You might assume that he came in, we operated, and he went on his way heart-healthily ever after.

That's not how this story ends.

Here's what happened: He came in to do the presurgery paperwork and I asked him about his symptoms. "Well," he said, "they sort of went away." The shortness of breath when he walked was gone. So were his other symptoms, including the chest pain. We did a full workup and determined that he had not only alleviated the symptoms associated with heart disease, but the clogging had cleared up enough that he no longer needed the surgery at all.

Amazing.

By switching to superfoods and losing weight, he reduced his risk of heart disease, and also a host of other problems. That's because extra fat triggers a cascade of chemical reactions

A FAST SOLUTION?

One of the more interesting trends in weight loss zeroes in on short windows of fasting (twelve hours). Many of us normally go without food for only six to eight hours a day, eating periodically throughout our sixteen to eighteen waking hours. More and more evidence is showing that regularly going longer periods without food is an effective strategy for losing weight.

In one study, subjects lost 10 percent of their weight in twelve weeks following a fasting principle. And some data shows subjects who use fasting methods had a reduction in total cholesterol (up to 21 percent) and triglyceride levels (up to 42 percent).

There are many variations of the fasting method—such as cutting back your calories by 25 percent a day or two a week. I don't want you to try this method during the 21-Day Plan. If you add fasting to your new eating approach, experiment with going for twelve-hour periods without food. For example, you could fast from seven P.M. to seven A.M. if you like an early breakfast to get you going, and don't mind an early dinner. You could also do midnight to noon if you find that you don't need breakfast first thing. You can still use my 21-Day Plan with the same meals and recipes. Try it a few days a week to see how you feel. At the very least, absorb this message: If you're a night eater, skipping that last snack will have some helpful weight-loss effects.

Researchers say it's not yet clear why fasting may be effective. It could increase the body's response to insulin or could change the way in which fat is utilized. Fat may be used for energy in the absence of immediately available food during fasting periods.

One note: Fasting doesn't give you license to eat like a *T. rex* the rest of the time. That is, if you fast for the twelve-hour window, but then gorge on junk, recalibrating your system won't work.

that wreak havoc on many aspects of your system. So if you're someone who needs or wants to lose weight—whether it's ten pounds or triple digits—think of this moment as your starting point. You are about to shift your dietary choices and habits in a direction that will make your body leaner and your internal systems stronger.

Everything in this book will help you lose the pounds. But I also want to share common strategies and ways of thinking among people who lose weight. My knowledge about this comes from working with and interviewing thousands of people who have gone through a successful body transformation.

PRINCIPLE 1: READINESS

It's the place where inspiration becomes action.

On the hundredth episode of *The Dr. Oz Show*, I brought in one hundred people who had lost one hundred pounds. While everyone who has struggled with weight can attest to the difficulty of losing it, there is quite a difference between dropping one hundred pounds and dropping, say, twenty. Losing triple-digits takes not only time, but also extra dedication and strategy.

When we invited those folks on the show, I expected a wide range of answers to the question "How did you lose the weight?" I thought people would say things like "forty-five minutes of cardio exercise a day" and

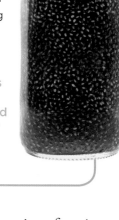

SNACK ON THIS

There are tons of healthy snack options out there, and you'll find a bunch in my plan on page 239. One of my favorites is plain Greek yogurt mixed with berries, nuts, or chia seeds. Research shows that an afternoon snack of plain Greek yogurt with a high protein content (24 grams) reduced hunger, increased fullness, and delayed subsequent eating compared with lower protein snacks or no snacks. And chia seeds may help regulate blood sugar, keeping your stomach happy for a long stretch of time.

Toss in Chia. Make your own chia-boosted drinks by adding a tablespoon of the seeds to juices and smoothies. Let stand for a few minutes until they plump up.

"egg-white omelets" and "no eating after six P.M." and "a picture of my skinny jeans hanging on the fridge door."

That's not what I got.

It turned out that the number one driver for losing weight was coming to the realization that losing weight mattered because *they* mattered. One man had his *aha* moment when his daughter told him she was upset because she didn't think he would be able to walk her down the aisle. A woman's husband confided in her that he was scared he'd have to live his later years without her because she was slowly killing herself. Seeing how much other people cared for them booted up their mental resolve to change their eating habits and related behaviors. Self-esteem ultimately triggered something that told them it was time to start—and finish—resetting their bodies and normalizing their weight.

Maybe just picking up this book is your ready point, or maybe there was some other trigger that inspired you to read this. Whatever it is, any *aha* moment requires more than just feeling ready—you need to be prepared to take action. After all, people don't plan to fail, but they do fail to plan.

Use your emotions as the engine that will help you develop the strategies I outline throughout the book and guide your choices going forward.

THE CALORIE CALCULATION

You're constantly burning calories in three different ways: **1.** You burn 60 to 75 percent just to fuel your organs. **2.** You burn another 15 to 30 percent through your activity and movement. **3.** You burn calories as you digest food. Foods that take more energy to digest work in your favor, because they burn themselves up with no extra work from you. Celery is the classic example, as digesting it actually burns more calories than those green stalks contain. Other foods burn a little extra as you digest, too, such as nuts, eggs, salmon, and certain other fruits and vegetables. Consider it a bit of a caloric discount. The calorie savings involving digestion is small, but hey, every bit counts.

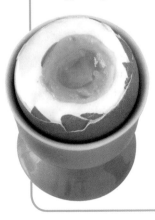

A whole egg has less than 100 calories. Try an egg or two soft-boiled for five minutes for a slightly runny yolk, a minute less if you like them runnier. For more on the health benefits of the incredible egg, see page 305.

PRINCIPLE 2: BALANCE

The big battle is won by addressing the double Q—quality and quantity.

If you follow my FIXES, you'll have the blueprint for what to eat, and those guidelines will help you naturally control your hunger, because you'll be eating satiating nutrients. But once you graduate from the 21-Day Plan, it's up to you to right-size portions. You *can* gain weight eating all healthy foods if you eat too much of them.

So there are two things to consider when following FIXES guidelines: 1) Know that choosing good foods will help regulate your diet. For example, fiber, fat, and protein all help stabilize your hunger so you're less likely to overeat. 2) None of that gives you license

EAT FAT, LOSE FAT

Here's a cool trick that some bodybuilders use: They eat sardines in olive oil—theoretically because the combo of protein and healthy fats in both the olive oil and the fish help keep them lean. That's not to say your goal is to look muscle-bound, but it does provide interesting insight based on a food choice made by people who are very concerned about how much body fat they carry. I love sardines, by the way. They get their name from Sardinia, where they used to be abundant. Give them a try—mash them up with olive oil and sliced scallions.

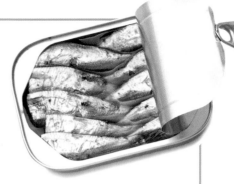

Sardines come with a bonus. You eat the soft, tiny bones along with the rest of the fish for a calcium boost.

to go berserk. Amounts do matter, so you should be aware of moderate portion sizes and finding the sweet spot between not eating enough and eating too much. My 21-Day Plan teaches lessons in quality and quantity—and will serve as a model for generous and satisfying portion sizes as you move to day twenty-two and beyond.

If you are trying to lose weight, you will automatically be cutting calories by following my plan (as compared to what you normally eat). That's a good thing. One study looked at factors contributing to weight loss. Those who had success decreased their intake by about 375 calories a day. That may not be the precise number you need to achieve, because there are so many other variables that go into weight loss. At the same time, the study's authors reported that increased consumption in fruits, vegetables, and low-fat dairy contributed to weight loss—suggesting the method people used to cut their calories. Veg-

etables are low-calorie, so you can eat more of them—and get more bang for your buck in terms of food volume.

FIXES foods generally mean fewer calories—and a smaller body in the long run.

PRINCIPLE 3: EMERGENCY PREPAREDNESS

Managing temptations is about controlling tough times.

If you've tried losing weight in the past, you already know: It's not easy. Sometimes, you get hungry. Sometimes, you get frustrated and want to vent via the vending machine. Sometimes, you are suddenly noshy when you smell food while walking through the mall. Temptation is all around us, and it makes the weight-loss struggle ever harder.

But here's the myth: Willpower alone can get you through. Many people argue that if you just "have the will" to resist, then you can be successful on any diet. I would counter that the various triggers that cajole us into eating are simply habits—that is, we've created our own Pavlovian responses. Turn on TV, open bag of chips. Strategies, like creating different eating environments so you don't always have to consciously engage your willpower, are what help win these battles. (I talked more about this in chapter 3.) Some research suggests that we may have a limited amount of willpower every day and we wear ourselves out if we constantly fight these tugs-of-war. When we run out of our decision-making *chi*, we start making poor decisions (often in the late afternoon, the witching hour for many people). But by making automatic decisions, we reduce temptation.

You may think that the story of hunger is all about the tongue or stomach, but it actually starts in the brain. There, the hypothalamus acts as a central hard drive for many bodily activities, including behaviors that key off of appetite and satiety. (By the way, that's not just for food and drink, but also the appetite you have for sleep and sex.) One of its jobs is to regulate how satisfied you feel and what actions you should take if you're not satisfied.

Two hormones, leptin and ghrelin, influence the hypothalamus. They work in relationship to each other to let you know whether you need food. In a perfect system, the two sides work together like salsa dance partners, moving gracefully with each other. Eat when you need calories to fuel your body; stop when you're energized so you don't store

LOW FAT ISN'T ALL THAT

What's the story with "diet" foods? Many of them are based more on marketing than sound nutrition. For example, "low-fat" may mean that a food is pumped with sugar or fake flavors. Take diet ice creams and fro-yo: They're touted as ways you can enjoy sinful sweetness without having to make any sacrifices. Sounds like a miracle, right? No sugar added! Well, they go heavy on the additives and artificial sweeteners. I once saw a diet ice cream sandwich that had fifty—yes, fifty!—ingredients. Oy. Pigs are actually fed artificially flavored food because it will make them fatter—not an example we humans want to follow. Better just to have a little bit of the real thing. That's the "S" in FIXES, after all.

too much fat. Your body, of course, wants this system to balance nicely. It doesn't want you to go hungry, and it doesn't want you to go haywire and overeat. It would prefer a perfect-ten dance, and that's where you come in.

Leptin is the satisfaction hormone (dancing around like a leprechaun). Keep those levels high, and you'll stay satisfied. Leptin shuts off your hunger and stimulates you to burn more calories. Ghrelin is the hunger hormone (angry like a gremlin). If ghrelin levels are really high, they'll make you want to motor through a box of Girl Scout cookies in three minutes flat.

LOVE YOUR LIVER

Fatty liver disease affects nearly one in three Americans. It happens when fat accumulates in the liver and damages it. You probably think of it as an alcohol-related disease, but fatty liver can also be caused by eating excess sugar and refined flour. How does it happen? The liver gets overwhelmed by the flood of extra sugar in your body and stores it as fatty deposits, which in turn triggers a damaging inflammatory response. The tough part is that there are no obvious symptoms of this liver damage, and it's dangerously related to heart disease and some forms of cancer. The way to help combat it: Eat FIXES foods, like omega-3s, and cut out all those added-sugar foods.

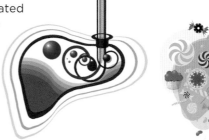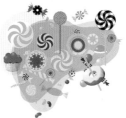

Scary Truth. If you put a liver that's been beaten up by too much fat and sugar next to one from a heavy drinker, they look nearly identical in terms of the damage to this important organ.

When your stomach gets empty at regular intervals throughout the day, it stimulates ghrelin production. You get little messages that you should eat, and some of those impulses are stronger than others. Those messages stop when you're satisfied.

How do you keep your leptin levels high and your ghrelin levels low? The most direct way is to eat the FIXES foods that promote satiety—that is, fats with benefits (F), ideal proteins (I), xtra fruits and veggies (X), and energizing carbs (E). They all take a long time to move through the digestive system, encouraging leptin levels to stay high, so that you feel satiated. But foods that go through digestion quickly—those pesky sugars and refined carbs—promote the production of ghrelin. That causes appetite to go up, so you eat more and create that vicious cycle of hunger.

So to avoid hunger extremes (feeling famished and feeling stuffed), you want the steady drip of FIXES foods, not the roller-coaster mayhem caused by processed and junky ones. There's no perfect formula—e.g., a rule that says eat three apples in the morning and you have the ideal leptin levels—so it takes some mindfulness on your part to thwart a hunger emergency before it unfolds. Focus on keeping your hunger levels even throughout the day and avoiding the peaks and valleys that cause overeating and weight gain.

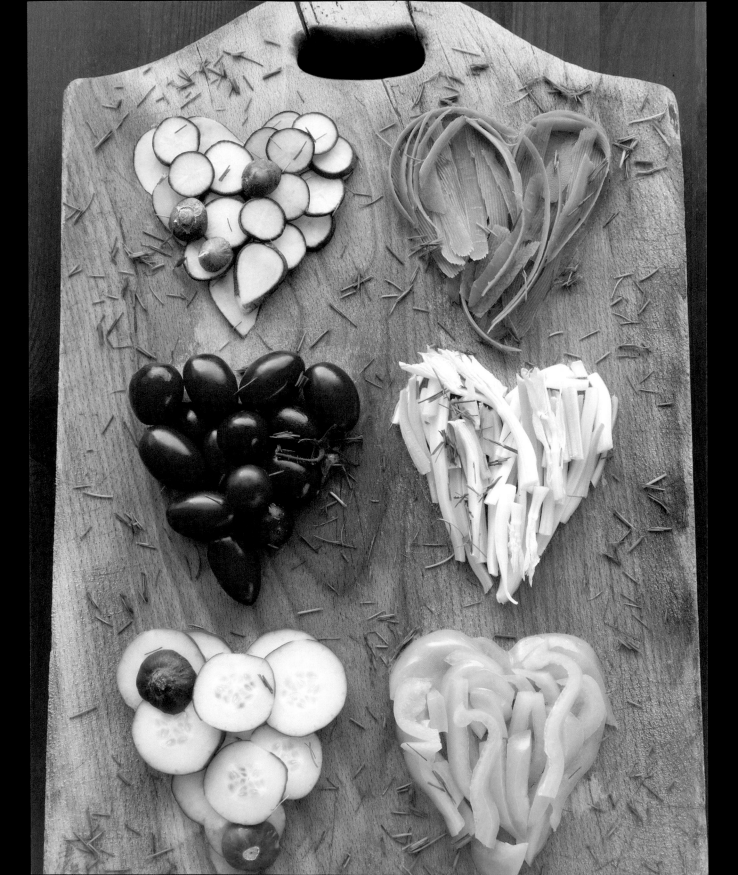

6.

Food FIXES
for the Heart

The natural way to keep your
arteries clear and your heart strong.

It's a sacred moment when I first see the heart in surgery. Cut the skin, split the ribs, open everything up—and there it is. As the heart beats, the muscle reminds me of the strength of a python. It's alive in its own way, somewhat reclusive as it cowers in the chest wall, unsure of what will happen next.

So the first thing I do to a damaged heart is caress it. I want to make peace with it and calm it. Amazingly, the heart does beat more slowly in response to a caring hand.

When we look inside, we know what to expect. All the diagnostics and assessments have told us why we're there and what we'll find.

I know there's a buildup of plaque if I see a substance that looks like dried icing or old French fries. Not coincidentally, the plaque resembles things that may have caused it.

If I feel the blood rumbling through an artery, like the turbulence in a hose, I know that the vessel is in trouble.

If there's a circular patch on the heart, like a black-and-blue bruise on a piece of fruit, that's the scar that shows the patient has had a heart attack.

If the patient has been a smoker, I can tell. How? A healthy heart has tissue like the finest linen. It's supple, soft, and easy to sew together. A heart damaged by smoking is more like cardboard. Connecting pieces together is more challenging.

Sometimes we see a heart that's enlarged and beating fast, like a scared bird fluttering in a cage. It's desperate to push blood forward to the rest of the body, but just can't find the power. We need to act fast in those cases.

Though there are many different surgeries to address various heart conditions, all of them share a similar mission: get the organ pumping strongly and efficiently and make sure that all pathways to and from this vital engine are cleared.

One of the reasons I fell in love with heart surgery is that it gives you immediate feedback. Either it works or it doesn't, right then and there. And I have spent many, many, many days of my career looking into the hearts of men and women whose life-thumpers were damaged by any number of things, including troubled genes, cigarettes, inactivity, and poor diet. We identified the problem, and we scheduled surgery to address it.

Whether you're at risk of heart disease (the country's number one killer) because of genetics or lifestyle, or you just want to make sure your heart keeps on working long and strong, you should take a keen interest in how food can help. Because frankly, I don't want to see you on that surgery table. I'd rather *you* take matters into your hands. Not with a scalpel, but with your fork and knife.

The primary way you do it? With the X in my FIXES foods—Xtra fruits and vegetables. The science is clear that a plant-based diet has an incredibly positive effect on the health of the heart. Fortify your plate with nature's best medicine, and you'll fortify your heart to carry you through life.

I can tell you the moment I knew we were in for a major change in our understanding about food and heart disease. It was 1989, and I was a young doctor attending a conference for the American Heart Association. Walking through the halls, I saw one room that was

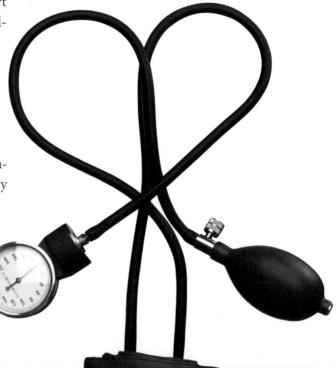

A CLOSER LOOK AT THE HEART

The aorta, the biggest blood vessel in the body, is about as wide as a garden hose.

Your heart has a built-in electrical system. Nodes—small masses of specialized muscle cells—send out electrical impulses that control the rhythm and speed of your heartbeats.

The tinier arteries don't accumulate plaque the same way large ones do. They still can cause heart attacks, however, by squeezing shut or opening up at the wrong times, especially in women.

Your heart isn't bright red! True color: a brownish-red with yellowish fatty streaks on it. (Some fat here is normal.)

Most common place for clogs: the left anterior descending artery, which supplies blood to large areas of the heart. Blockages there can be so deadly that docs call them widow-makers.

absolutely packed—everyone wanted to hear what the presenter was saying. This was the medical conference equivalent of fans jamming into a small club to get a glimpse of the Beatles.

The presenter was Dean Ornish, the founding father of a nutrition-based approach to heart disease. Dr. Ornish was really the first person to quantify the effect of a low-fat, plant-based diet on the reduction of heart disease. And other doctors were eating it up, so to speak.

His stats were staggering: 91 percent of the time, patients' symptoms of chest pain went away when they followed his program, which had a strong emphasis on eating the right foods. Remember, this presentation was given at a time when surgery and medication were the standard fix-its. And it wasn't too far removed from the era in which my father-in-law began his career as a heart surgeon. The protocol at the time? Patients were green-lighted to have cheeseburgers post-op and even given cigarettes at discharge to help them relax.

THE NO-EXCUSES SALAD

Maybe you've decided that packing a salad for lunch is a healthy eating solution. Yes—good answer! But it's not easy to transport a bowl of greens, veggies, and chicken without having it all become a soggy mess once you add dressing. Enter the mason jar salad. It's easy to fix and easy to carry, and you don't have to worry about any leaks or aggravations. Just construct it according to this formula and shake it up when you're ready to chow down. (My 21-Day Plan Salad in a Jar on page 198 will be your first of many.)

Bottom layer: Vinaigrette dressing made with olive oil (pour it in first so the rest of the ingredients don't get soggy)

Second layer: Crunchy vegetables

Next layer: Sturdy foods like hard-boiled eggs or chicken

Top layer: Greens (so they don't get crushed by the weight of the other add-ins)

Mix and match the ingredients as you like, then shake to coat with the dressing (or empty into a bowl) when you're ready to dive in.

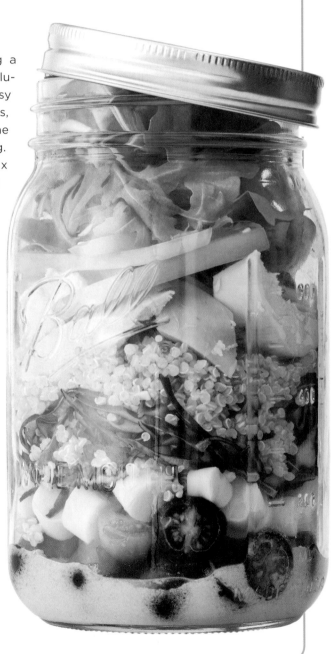

The doctors watching Dr. Ornish's presentation were thrilled to see his tangible, compelling data supporting the role of diet in health. In their heart of hearts, they knew that eating well was both healing and preventive—and now they had numbers to prove it and profess it.

I often saw anecdotal evidence in my practice. I remember a patient who was about fifty and in very good shape. He was actually more muscle-bound than paunchy (how you'd perhaps picture a typical heart patient). He wasn't overweight, he exercised every day, he didn't smoke, and he didn't have any typical markers that would indicate a problem (no high blood pressure, no diabetes). But he had advanced heart disease—likely caused by genetics since all the men in his family had heart problems by their forties. He was experiencing chest pain and, in fact, his coronary arteries were nearly blocked off.

Rather than schedule an immediate surgery, I put him on an aggressive diet plan in which he ate lots of vegetables and limited his saturated fats. What happened next was very interesting. The diet didn't cause the artery-clogging plaque buildup to disappear, but it did help his arteries to open up.

They dilated, which allowed blood to flow more freely. Think about it: If plaque is causing a 50 percent blockage in an artery, but then the artery opens up, the same plaque buildup may block only 25 percent of the artery. That's a viable path to healing heart disease. The

man's chest pain went away, and his risk of heart disease significantly lowered. In fact, I saw him recently, a decade removed from his chest pain, and he looked as vital as ever.

A surgical team didn't fix him. Food did.

This man's story and many, many like it offer good news for the rest of us, because they show that we don't always need invasive actions to fix problems. We each have more influence than we think over what happens within our heart and circulatory system.

Your heart works by pushing blood to and from it through your blood vessels. Blood, as you know from chapter 2, is a vital nutrient shuttle, moving everything you absorb through food to all your organs. The heart really works like the central hub. Every route, in some form or another, must come and go from there.

Trouble mostly happens in the arterial highways throughout the body rather than the heart itself.

Here's how it happens. The heart pulses out blood through the aortic valve into the aorta (that's the body's largest artery), and that's what sends blood out to all the rest of the organs. Tellingly, the first place the blood goes is to the surrounding coronary arteries, so the heart actually feeds itself before taking care of the rest of the body. (Side note: Doesn't that make the heart a great role model for all of us who devote ourselves to others? We need to prioritize our own health so we can help the people we love.)

With all that blood shuttling through the body, you can either have smooth traveling or twelve-vehicle pileups. Accidents come as a result of things that chip away at the arterial wall—high blood pressure, loads of excess sugar circulating in the bloodstream—both of which are linked to poor diet. Cracks are repaired with cholesterol, which is like the body's plaster. When the repair is done with lousy LDL cholesterol, it acts like cheap spackling and easily cracks with inflammation. This reveals underlying damage that can lead to sudden blood clots and closure of the artery.

A clog means that oxygen-and-nutrient-rich blood can't be delivered to your brain and other organs. It means that your heart has to work harder to push blood out and can't receive blood efficiently to do its job well. More clogs in more arteries equals more chances that you're going to have problems like high blood pressure, heart attack, and heart failure.

We can fix some of those issues with medication and surgery to clear clogs, no doubt. (That's what bypass surgery is. We're bypassing the damaged area and taking blood on a different route around the accident.)

However, if you're looking to strengthen your heart and even reverse damage before surgery or a life-threatening incident happens, you can use food to improve blood flow, quiet inflammation, and restore order on your arterial highways.

How? You eat foods that will minimize the chance that plaque will build up along the

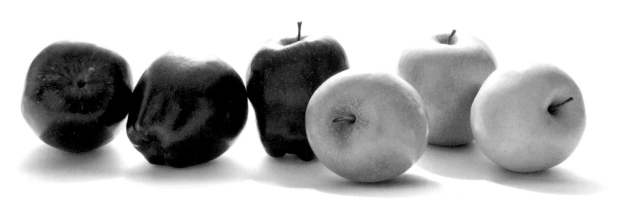

Fresh Apples. All apples have stores of potential disease fighters, with different kinds—Fuji, Red Delicious, Idared, Granny Smith, Jonagold, you name it—boasting various star compounds. Whether an apple's skin is ruby red, pale green, or yellow is less important than making sure you leave that natural wrapper on. It contains a good portion of the fruit's plant power and about half its fiber.

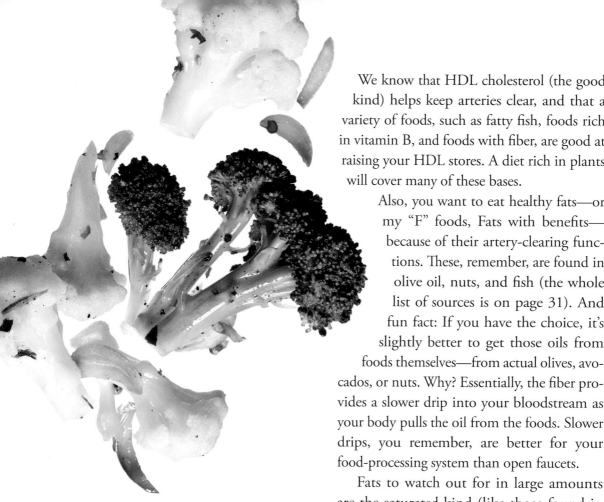

Try our Broccoli and Cauliflower Medley with garlic, lemon, and a pinch of red pepper flakes (see page 254).

We know that HDL cholesterol (the good kind) helps keep arteries clear, and that a variety of foods, such as fatty fish, foods rich in vitamin B, and foods with fiber, are good at raising your HDL stores. A diet rich in plants will cover many of these bases.

Also, you want to eat healthy fats—or my "F" foods, Fats with benefits—because of their artery-clearing functions. These, remember, are found in olive oil, nuts, and fish (the whole list of sources is on page 31). And fun fact: If you have the choice, it's slightly better to get those oils from foods themselves—from actual olives, avocados, or nuts. Why? Essentially, the fiber provides a slower drip into your bloodstream as your body pulls the oil from the foods. Slower drips, you remember, are better for your food-processing system than open faucets.

Fats to watch out for in large amounts are the saturated kind (like those found in red meat and dairy products). Those are the ones that jack up cholesterol, which can wind up as dangerous plaque on artery walls and trigger panicked 9-1-1 calls. While you don't have to eliminate red meat, I would recommend you severely restrict it if you have a significant risk of heart disease. (One of the first ways we learned about this was through studies of American soldiers killed in the Korean War. Their arteries were examined and high levels of plaque were discovered in previously healthy eighteen-year-old men who grew up on our typical red meat–rich diet.)

arterial walls and rupture. Remember, much of that damage is done by high blood pressure and excess sugar floating around in the blood—both usually caused by overeating in general, and piling on sugar and refined carbs in particular. Follow the FIXES approach, and you give your heart and arteries plenty of protection. You can also eat foods that will help stabilize existing jams so they don't hurt you.

THESE SEVEN INGREDIENTS ARE FULL OF HEALTHY FATS.

Here's how to add 'em to your plate.

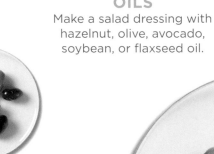

OILS
Make a salad dressing with hazelnut, olive, avocado, soybean, or flaxseed oil.

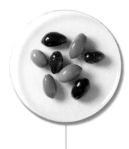

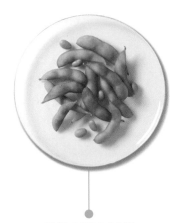

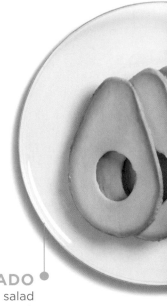

OLIVES
Snack on them straight up or add them to your favorite chicken dish.

EDAMAME
Scoop onto salads or toss with cooked quinoa.

AVOCADO
Savor in a salad or as a spread.

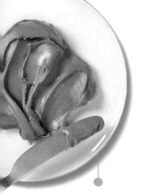

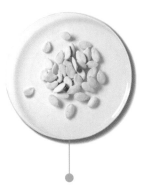

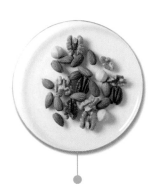

NUT AND SEED BUTTERS
Smear on sliced fruit and veggie sticks.

SEEDS
Pumpkin, sunflower, sesame, flax, hemp, and chia are all great sources of good fats. Sprinkle onto a salad, yogurt, or oatmeal.

NUTS
One of the healthiest noshes around. For extra flavor and no extra calories, try toasting them.

The fundamental difference between foods that help your heart and those that hurt it is what Dean Ornish tapped into way back at that early conference. Dr. Ornish and Dr. Caldwell Esselstyn, a leading heart doctor who was also a gold-medal Olympic rower in 1956, are two heroes in my book, for bridging nutrition and medicine.

Dr. Ornish released his first study linking dietary changes to heart disease in 1983. In this trial, he showed that the heart's ability to pump blood improves significantly after only twenty-four days of a dietary change, with a 91 percent reduction in the frequency of angina and about a 20 percent decrease in cholesterol levels, as well as a lower risk of cardiovascular problems. The magnitude of improvement was stunning and greater than many conventionally offered medications. Further studies by Dr. Ornish reinforced his initial findings. For example, in the 1990s, he found that even severe coronary artery blockages could be reversed in only one year when patients followed a heart-healthy eating plan (low-fat and plant-based). Total cholesterol dropped 24 percent and the bad LDL fell 37 percent—rates that were similar to those attributed to cholesterol-lowering drugs. And, not surprisingly, blockages dropped more significantly after five years than after one (moreover, those who didn't eat the heart-healthy diet had twice as many cardiac events as those who did).

Ornish's findings have been supported in a lot of research over the past couple of decades. For example, one major study of

I HEART DESSERTS

Limiting your sugar may make you think that your days of tiramisu are over. But don't worry. An occasional cupcake or treat isn't the problem; it's making sweets a habit over the long haul that is. The trick is managing "every once in a while." If you look at the recipes for Dark Chocolate and Beet Brownies and Banana "Ice Cream" on pages 327 and 329, you will see tempting and sweet desserts that are perfectly acceptable as special treats. The key revolves around ingredient-swapping and learning how to make healthy versions of unhealthy favorites.

Chocolate-Dipped Clementines are coated with pistachios for a touch of crunch (and protein). See page 329 for the recipe.

more than 126,000 people found that those with the highest intake of fruits and vegetables had a 20 percent lower risk of coronary heart disease. And a recent meta-analysis of twenty-three studies—involving nearly a million people—also demonstrated that a higher consumption of fruits and vegetables was associated with a lower risk of developing coronary heart disease.

Ultimately, this is one of the main reasons why my 21-Day Plan and FIXES approach emphasize produce so much. I want your plate to resemble a micro garden, with most foods reminding you of what they looked like when they were harvested (that doesn't mean you need to eat everything raw, just that the form of the food keeps its shape—hence, apples are better than apple juice and grilled eggplant is just fine, but when it's gooped up in batter and cheese, not so much). You'll be treated to lots of vegetables, as well as lean protein (like chicken, turkey, and fish). Some rice and grains are fine, too. Your goal is to avoid foods with lots of saturated fat and/or

THE BOTTOM LINE ON WINE

It's true that wine contains the heart-healthy antioxidants resveratrol and quercetin. A glass a day is A-OK (but wait until after you've finished the 21-Day Plan). One study in the *European Heart Journal* found that women in their forties, fifties, and sixties who drank seven servings of wine, beer, or liquor every week had a 16 percent lower risk of heart failure. But you can get those same disease-fighters in food, too. Resveratrol is found in blueberries, cranberries, grapes, peanuts, pistachios, and cocoa. And you'll tap into quercetin when you eat apples, blackberries, citrus fruits, dark cherries, grapes, onions, parsley, sage, and black tea and green tea.

Go smaller with your wineglasses and you may drink less. It's a trick of the eyes: Pour the same amount into small and large glasses, and it looks like less in the bigger ones—which leads people to sip faster and refill more. In fact, one study found that a pub served 9 percent more wine when it used 6-ounce glasses as opposed to 4-ounce ones. Keep it "pint-size" for fewer headaches.

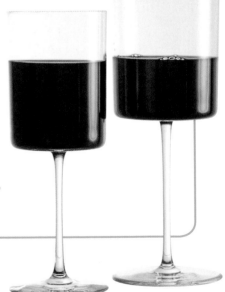

SHOULD YOU SHAKE OFF THE SALT?

Most Americans consume too much salt (high sodium is linked to heart trouble), but the majority of it comes from packaged, processed, and restaurant foods, not the shaker. Once you cut down on those, your sodium levels will plummet, which means if you want to sprinkle a little on your vegetables, go right ahead. If you're looking to lower your sodium intake, consider swapping out salt for citrus juice (such as lemon, lime, or even grapefruit). They have a similar tanginess.

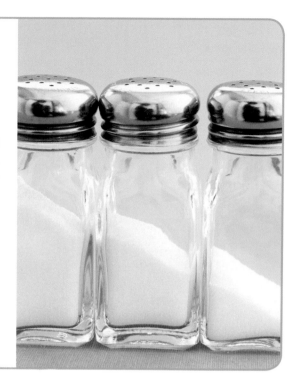

sugar, and anything processed. Eat this way and you prevent plaque from building up in the first place, keep the arteries clear, and minimize the risk of ruptures.

Not so excited by the idea of ramped-up veggie servings? Be brave with herbs and spices. You can season your vegetables with all kinds of combinations that keep things interesting. Slice cauliflower into "steaks" and roast them with Middle Eastern spices; add pow to a classic gazpacho recipe with minced jalapeños; sweeten carrots with cinnamon; charge up broccoli with turmeric. It's such a mistake to think that eating healthy must be boring, bland, and blah. Use your kitchen as a little lab to elevate everything you eat. Go there with flavor, knowing you're pleasing your tongue, and your ticker, too.

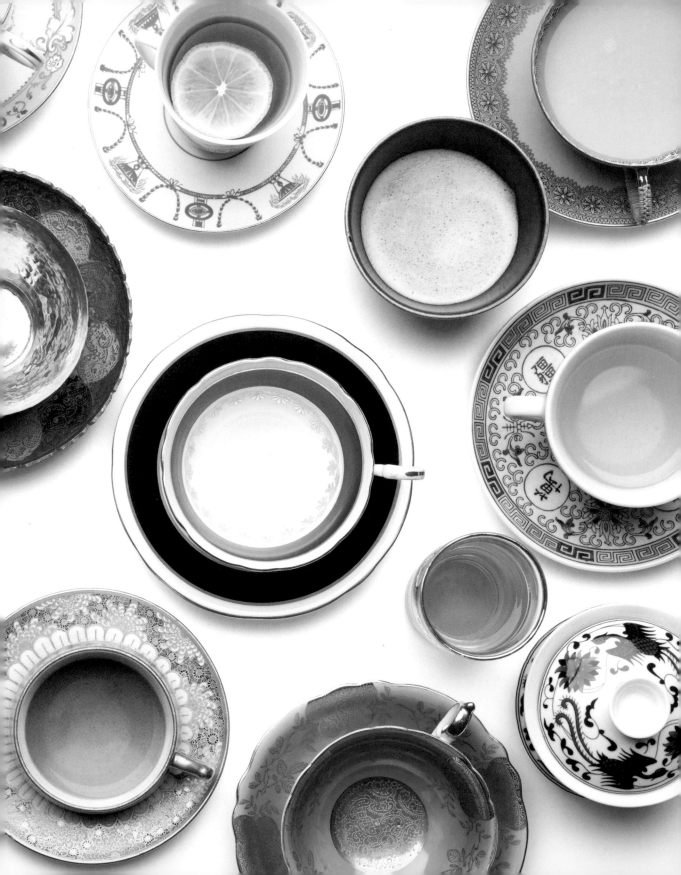

7

Food FIXES for Fatigue

Stick with the FIXES approach
for more zip, less zonk.

Start typing the words "why am I" in the Google search bar. The autofill that appears below could be *anything* from the philosophical—"Why am I alive?"—to the physical. You might expect the most popular question to focus on the health problem that plagues more than two-thirds of American adults: "Why am I overweight?"

The first thing that usually pops up: "Why am I always so tired?"

That's how big the issue of fatigue is. The almighty Google confirms it. And you confirmed it: In a reader poll for *Dr. Oz The Good Life* magazine, 74 percent of readers said they find themselves wishing for more energy every day, and 59 percent would rather have more energy than drop a dress size (nearly four in five also said they would rather have more energy than more sex).

So let's tackle this issue. Fatigue can be a mysterious and complicated ailment, because tangible data doesn't back it up the way, say, blood pressure indicates heart problems. You simply *feel* it. Maybe your body and mind just don't have the zip to get going in the morning. Maybe you feel that reach-for-sugar crash coming on every afternoon. Maybe you crash at the end of the day when the kids long for one last page of the book you're reading to them.

But you just can't. You're toast.

We all know what fatigue feels like, and we're all frustrated by it. We want more cheetah, less slug. We want to bounce through the day, not trudge through it.

I visualize fatigue like a ball of tangled yarn. The strands are influences—including sleep, nutrition, stress, activity, hormonal shifts, and a number of others—that jumble together in our anatomical energy center. You can't address fatigue without looking at all the strands, but nutrition? That's a big one.

Eating habits may be the cause of fatigue—or at the very least a contributing factor. (Fatigue can also be a sign of a number of problems, so if you feel out of sorts and don't improve with changes in nutrition and sleep habits, talk to your doctor.) The story of nutrition and fatigue starts with your basic bookends—what happens in the morning and before bed. But there's a whole lot that goes on in the middle, too. Let's examine how your body is fueled throughout the day and how your food choices inform your energy levels.

What You Eat

I felt the effects of profound exhaustion as a young doctor. One of my early responsibilities was in the ICU. The resident assigned to the ICU is never allowed to leave it, so you work through a thirty-hour shift—attending to any need that comes up throughout the day or night. This is one of the reasons why early career doctors run themselves into the

> ## EAT SMALLER TO LIVE LARGER
>
> One of the reasons you might be tired: Your meals are too big. When you eat a lot, quite a bit of blood has to rush to your digestive system to get those gastric processes going. The result? There's less blood flow to the rest of your body, which makes you feel more sluggish than a day-on-the-couch football fan. Try cutting portions back to where you're satisfied, not stuffed.

ground. (We've all watched TV hospital dramas, right? Burnout is a common storyline, because there's truth to the long hours and irregular sleeping and eating patterns.)

Because we couldn't leave the ICU, we were required to eat whatever we brought with us from home or whatever the hospital served to patients. Most residents didn't pack their meals, so they were subjected to meals such as a tasteless slab of meat loaf, thrice-boiled green beans, and whatever sort of potato concoction came alongside in those days.

When I started working there, I felt like a bug on the bottom of a shoe. Flattened. I had zero oomph.

Soon after, Lisa started packing my lunch. It often consisted of leftovers from a healthy dinner we'd had the night before, or she made me her tuna salad—tuna with garlic, celery, shallots, parsley, and other secret ingredients. Of course, I enjoyed it because it had more flavor than the factory food that came through the unit. More important, I noticed that my energy levels soared. I worked the same number of hours, but I felt great, I never got sick (despite working so close to sick people), and I chugged along throughout the day. (My high-octane MO became a bit notorious. In a *New York Times* story about me some time later, the author said that energy levels should be measured in a "full Mehmet unit.")

I take pride in my ability to seize as much of the day as I can, but it has nothing to do with some special genetic makeup and everything to do with the fuel I use. My FIXES foods, in the right proportions of carbs, protein, and fats, provide a steady drip of nourishment that keeps your energy account in perfect balance.

What does the FIXES approach avoid? This classic vicious cycle: You're tired, sluggish, need a jolt. When you hit that slump—through the coaxing of convincing gremlins

disguised as brain hormones—you reach for the one thing that can make you feel better instantly: quick-acting carbohydrates that will FedEx sugar to your brain and other organs for immediate energy. The only problem with quick-acting carbs? They disappear as fast as they show up. So the temporary pop you feel is just that—and you crash as quickly as you soar. Then you reach for more carbs to make you feel better, and the cycle starts over again. Moreover, the flood of those fast carbs is exactly what leads to weight gain and other health problems.

Food FIXES work the exact opposite way: They provide long-lasting energy because they keep you satiated without immediate rises and falls. Energy comes in the form of those healthy fats (why nuts are a good snack), satiating protein (chicken or fish at lunch), and slow-digesting carbohydrates (why crunchy carrots are a better snack than anything that's been living for months in a vending machine). They give you sustained energy levels and ultimately will help

THE SIDE DISH FOR DROWSINESS

To help improve sleepiness after a day of overdoing coffee, have a serving of cauliflower, Brussels sprouts, kale, or broccoli at dinner. Studies show that these cruciferous vegetables can break down caffeine faster, which may help you reduce sleep disturbances.

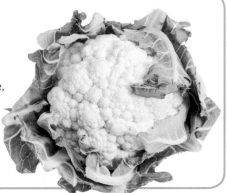

3 WAYS TO BUZZ UP YOUR BREW

Got a love affair going with coffee? So many of us do. I'm not trying to get between you and your best caffeinated friend. If you like it, drink it in moderation and don't gunk it up with a lot of sugary extras. The big thing is just to get out of the habit of thinking that you need a cup with you at all times. It's more likely you're just in the habit of sipping something while you're working, driving, or watching the kids, and you automatically assume it has to be coffee. Try alternating drinks—a cup of coffee, then fruit-infused ice water—and see if that doesn't support your energy levels without going cold turkey on your favorite warm drink. Or try some other options as well:

Use hemp milk or almond milk: They're both flavorful and are better alternatives than junking up your coffee with syrups and such. Add a dash of cinnamon for flavor without sugar.

Make bulletproof coffee: Instead of cream and sugar, add a dollop of butter and coconut oil. The short-chain fatty acids slow the absorption of caffeine, which will help stretch the energy you feel over a longer time period. And the addition of fat will also help you curb hunger. Lisa blends ours for a few seconds for better emulsion; otherwise, the coconut oil floats on top.

Try hot water and lemon: This has been trendy in the last few years, and I'm a fan because the citrus helps get the gastric juices flowing. It gives you something to sip on (your coffee addiction may be more of a behavioral habit than a need for caffeine) and has a nice, quiet taste.

you sleep better at night. That's why a steady consumption of FIXES foods—in the morning, during the day, and at night—is the main way to keep energy levels consistent throughout the day.

What You Drink

Coffee has become the ubiquitous American symbol of the energy boost. You know how it was discovered? The legend goes that an Ethiopian goatherd noticed that his goats stayed up all night when they ate certain berries. The herder, named Kaldi, took the berries to a monastery, and they, too, noticed the pep-in-the-step qualities of the berries, so one monk dried them and started using them to brew up a beverage. That monk experienced the same bounce that the goats did, and coffee was born.

Now we get can't enough of our favorite go-go-go beverage. All because of some zippy goats.

I'm not an especially big coffee drinker (as a surgeon who once did operations that lasted into the double-digit hours, I couldn't run off to the toilet because of the digestive prodding that follows a cup of joe). I do like to drink green tea or black tea, with just a tiny bit of sugar. (Tea's origin story? It is believed to have been discovered thousands of years ago by a Chinese emperor when tea leaves blew into a pot of boiling water.) Whatever type of tea you favor, from Earl Grey to jasmine green, tea is one of the world's great health drinks. It contains compounds that are linked to all kinds of health benefits, such as reducing risk of heart disease and cancer. As long as you don't sweeten it up with a truckload of sugar, it's a wonderful alternative to the high-calorie drinks you may rely on. But there's nothing wrong with having a cup of coffee in the morning if you like it.

In fact, you'll be slurping up health benefits; that's because coffee (caffeinated or decaffeinated) does come with disease-fighting properties. Daily coffee drinkers have a lower risk of dying from diabetes or developing heart and neurological diseases than non–coffee drinkers, according to a major Harvard University study. Other research has shown decreased rates of certain cancers among those who drink caffeinated coffee (three to five cups per day seemed to have the best rates). And it has also been linked to better moods and improved memory. The power comes from beneficial compounds called polyphenols, many of which have antioxidant properties. And then, of course, there's the real reason so many of us drink coffee: the caffeine jolt, which can release adrenaline and mood-boosting dopamine to make you feel good, as well as sharpening concentration and even improving workout performance. Caffeine's energizing effects peak forty-five minutes after the first sip (you do get rid of about half the caffeine through pee, by the way).

But I have two questions I want you to ask yourself about what you drink, whether it's as a morning boost or an afternoon pick-me-up: One, what's in your coffee? If your mug is

KNOW YOUR LABELS: DECIPHER THE COFFEE CODE

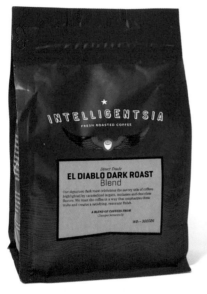

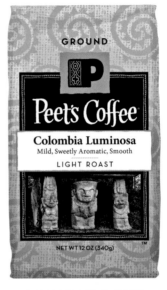

DARK ROAST

The more time in the roaster, the darker the beans. That means they're also more bitter.

LIGHT ROAST

Lighter beans hang on to their original flavor and caffeine better, so they taste fruitier and may give you a bigger jolt.

SHADE GROWN

Farmers grow beans under or around the natural forest canopy, forgoing excess fertilizer and pesticides.

FAIR TRADE CERTIFIED

It suggests growers got a fair price for their beans.

ORGANIC

It means different things in different countries, but the USDA stamp signifies that the beans were grown and roasted with few to zero synthetic pesticides.

pumped with sugar, syrups, and whipped this or that, then the benefits you get energywise just aren't worth it. All of those add-ins can contribute to weight gain, mood swings, and energy dips. Two, how much do you rely on caffeine as a get-you-through-the-day crutch?

Whether in the form of coffee, sodas, or well-marketed energy drinks, there's a problem with perpetually pumping caffeine into your system. Our bodies only have so much energy throughout the day, and we're designed to use that energy at a steady pace until bedtime, at which point a restorative rest reboots our system so we can do it all over again. So ingesting caffeine doesn't allow you to tap into a secret reserve of energy that you'd otherwise never feel; it's more like taking a withdrawal out on your day's allotment. The more you divest from it early, the less you'll have available later.

When we try to pull a fast one on our energy system—say, by flooding our bodies with a gas silo's worth of coffee in the morning—we leave less for later. Instead of having steady

4 WAYS TO MAKE YOUR COFFEE TASTE EVEN BETTER—WITHOUT THE SUGAR!

- Grinding your own beans won't change the health benefits, but it may make for a better-tasting cup. The best container for locking in the bean's flavor is the bean itself.

- Keep coffee stored in a vacuum-sealed pouch to minimize exposure to oxygen, which is what degrades the taste. It'll stay reasonably fresh for about one month after opening. The freezer is fine (if beans are in a zip-top freezer bag, they'll keep for up to six months), but the fridge is a no-go because moisture can get inside the container.

- Brewed coffee is up to 98 percent water, so if your tap water tastes like a steel pipe, so will your coffee. Use bottled or filtered water to improve taste.

- Use the industry-standard ratio of 6 ounces of water for every 2 tablespoons of ground coffee.

Rev Your Workout. Drinking a cup of coffee fifteen to sixty minutes pregym can make your workout feel easier, research has found. It can also slightly increase performance.

energy levels available, we take out a big amount early, and that's when we find ourselves craving those carbs and sugar and, you guessed it, more caffeine throughout the day.

The goal shouldn't be to avoid caffeine altogether (there's nothing inherently wrong with it, unless you are a person who experiences unwanted side effects—which is my issue). But be strategic. Do you really need a cup first thing in the morning, or do you make it because that's your habit, just as my childhood candy drawer was mine? Would it help you more at eleven in the morning, when energy naturally begins to dip? It's something to consider, so that you rely less on caffeine as your be-all and end-all, but perhaps as more of a supplement or a kickstarter when you need it.

I also think that if you eat the FIXES foods and drink water consistently throughout the day, you'll find that your energy levels will be higher and you're less likely to experience the highs and lows you might get relying on quick-fix beverages.

Before You Sleep

More than half of the people polled in our magazine survey say they tend to eat more when they're low on energy and nearly 30 percent eat sweets when they hit that slump. We're pretty quick to self-medicate when it comes to fatigue; we instinctually know that food can help us, even if we don't always choose the best thing. But the core of fixing fatigue is fixing your sleep, and it turns out that the right food can help you here, too.

Lack of sleep may well be one of the most far-reaching problems we have, as it's linked to heart problems, obesity, depression, memory issues, and more. The time of day when you sleep seems to play a role as well. That is, all hours are not created equal. Some data is showing that the hours you sleep before midnight are more important than those that you sleep after. Practically, sleeping from ten P.M. to six A.M. is better for your body than sleeping from midnight to eight A.M. Needless to say, there are many reasons why we don't

YOUR HEADED-TO-BED SNACK

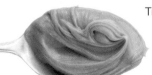

Try a tablespoon of peanut butter and a small banana a few hours before bed. Peanuts and bananas contain the amino acid L-tryptophan, which the body converts to melatonin. It also provides a boost of serotonin that helps relax you.

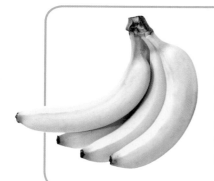

TRY THIS, CONK OUT

One of my new favorite teas is banana peel tea from sleep doctor Michael Breus, Ph.D. It's got magnesium, which is soothing, and potassium, a muscle relaxant. To make it, cut off the ends of a banana, slice it into three pieces—with the peel on—boil for ten minutes, strain, and serve. Breus recommends having it an hour before bed.

always hit the hay before midnight (work schedules, getting caught up on your favorite celeb's Instagram posts, etc.), but once there, you want to nod off fast and stay conked.

While there's no magic potion that will automatically induce sleepiness, you can eat and drink to help lull your body into lights-out mode. The food fix you can use to help involves melatonin, a hormone released by the pineal gland in the brain, which is the first signal to your body that it's time to sleep. One of my favorite sources of melatonin is tart cherry juice (my father grew up on a tart cherry farm and the whole family slept like babies). You don't need a lot—maybe four ounces at dinnertime so the melatonin has time to act. I like cutting it with sparkling water because the juice is too sweet for me; that way you get a bit of a sweet spritz, which actually makes for a nice, healthy dessert as well. While the data is limited, small studies show that tart cherry juice helps

reduce insomnia and increase total sleep time.

Other things my family likes to use to help improve sleep: lemon balm tea and turmeric milk (half a teaspoon of the spice added to a cup of warm milk with a little honey). Both seem to bring on drowsiness. One of the reasons to use milk is that it aids the absorption of magnesium, which helps muscles relax. Being tense and being in pain are two main causes for insomnia and sleep-quality issues, so the natural muscle relaxant can aid in both of those areas. (As an alternative, see a cool idea for magnesium-rich banana peel tea, above.)

Oftentimes, energy—or lack of it—is representative of what we eat and drink. Eat high-quality foods, and you'll have the same kind of chutzpah; go with the junk, and you'll feel like that, too. Your goal is to supply your body with energy-giving nutrients that help keep you up when you're up, as well as shut you down when it's time to rest, restore, and recharge.

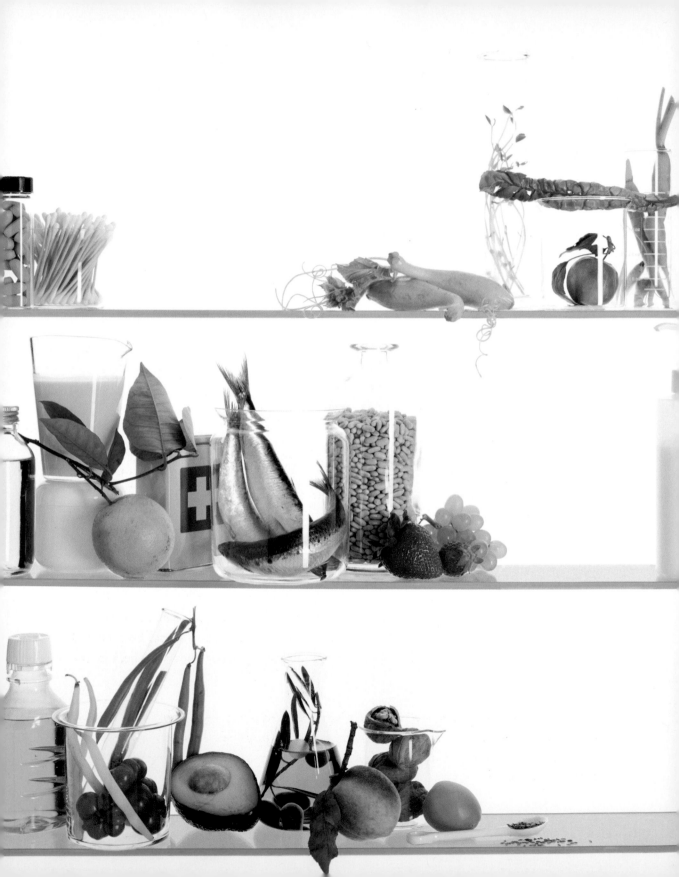

8

Food FIXES for Pain

Pain is one of medicine's most complicated challenges, but the right food can help you feel better.

The worst pain I ever felt happened some ten years ago when I broke a tooth. I was flying to do an appearance on Oprah's show, and we experienced some bad turbulence. Just as I bit down on a nut (healthy stress reliever!), we hit an air pocket. I felt my tooth snap as we dropped a hundred feet. Hour by hour, the pain just kept getting worse. Turned out I'd cracked the root, and it was getting infected and inflamed. I did the show, probably looking like a cross between a chipmunk and an Ultimate Fighter, then flew home.

When you fly, any air trapped in your body expands. You don't normally feel it except in your ears, unless you, say, have an abscess like I did. The pain was off the charts. I would have gladly replaced Dustin Hoffman with the crazy dentist in *Marathon Man* just to get relief. Using words that I could never print or say on TV, I went straight to my local hospital and saw a dental surgeon, who drained the abscess without bothering to use anesthesia because the pressure was so high.

Felt. So. Good.

Yes, the pain was bad enough that a surgeon jamming a needle into my gums came as heavenly relief. But even in horrible moments like my plane ride from hell, it's important to realize that the biological purpose of pain isn't sinister. It's actually intended to help, not hurt. Pain is a message to take action.

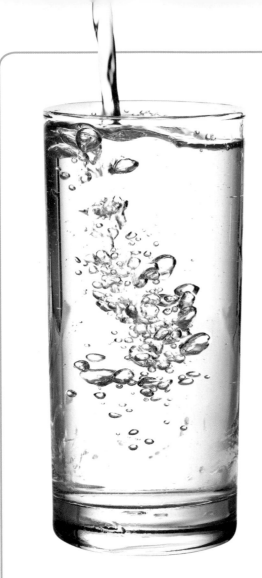

THE 10-SECOND HEADACHE RELIEVER

Being even a little bit dehydrated can cause a headache. In one study, 47 percent of people found that swigging six extra glasses of water a day helped relieve chronic headache pain.

Let's say you touch a hot pan handle. The burn you feel on the tips of your fingers triggers a message from your nerve endings that instantly instructs your body to remove your hand before you scorch it black.

Without that signal, there's no way for your body to protect you from dangerous situations. This is why people with diabetes who have nerve damage in their feet sometimes must have limbs amputated. They develop infections, but they have no pain signals to tell them something is wrong. And if they can't see or feel the infection on the bottom of their feet, it spreads so badly and for so long that the only method of treatment is to amputate.

So we have to appreciate that pain is nature's way of alerting your brain to something wrong in your body. Your body senses pain through two sets of nerve endings—one that operates slowly and one that operates quickly. The fast ones are surrounded by what's called a myelin sheath, which is a fatty protective layer that speeds the pain sensation's transmission to your spinal cord and brain so you can react quickly (dropping the hot pan, for example). The slower kind of nerve endings don't have that sheath, so what you feel is more of a deep pain rather than a stabbing one. That's often the way people describe chronic pain—the kind that radiates through the body day after day.

Like every family, the Oz squad has experienced its share. Lisa has felt aches in her lower back and my dad has dealt with lots of knee pain. From many years of operating, I've had quite a bit of back trouble as well (standing with your head bent over looking into a chest cavity isn't exactly perfect posture).

It's important for me to say that with any chronic pain issues, you should be working with your doctor, because your goal shouldn't be just to erase or mask the pain, but also to find and treat the root cause. Even if there's nothing serious behind how your feel, pain will weaken other aspects of your health. When you can't sleep, you're less healthy. When you're bound to the couch or bed, you're less healthy. When you use brownie bites to counteract pain with a little pleasure, you're less healthy.

IS FOOD RESPONSIBLE FOR YOUR HEADACHE?

There are lots of reasons why your head may be pounding like a jackhammer, but dietary culprits are worth investigating.

Caffeine withdrawal: If you skipped your usual morning coffee, it can lead to a headache. That's because the blood vessels in your brain are used to the constriction that caffeine produces. When you don't give them the daily fix, blood rushes through at full throttle. To manage the overflow, the blood vessels swell, which creates the pain.

Skipping meals: Your brain needs a steady dose of blood sugar to operate. Missing lunch may mean that your brain is on empty, so a headache is a way of calling out that it needs fuel. Stick to snacks and meals made up of FIXES foods that don't produce extreme sugar highs and lows.

Diet drinks: Almost all diet sodas contain different levels of aspartame (an artificial sweetener found in more than six thousand food items). Research shows that aspartame in diet sodas may be a dietary trigger of headache in some people. And research also shows that the additive may inhibit levels of feel-good chemicals like serotonin, which could trigger migraines.

Something new: Lots of foods can trigger headaches—most notably chocolate, nitrate-containing meats, MSG, and foods that contain the amino acid tyramine (which is in red wine, aged cheese, smoked fish, and figs). If you've added something new recently and you've started to experience more headaches, try scaling back on one particular food at a time to see if you can ID the bad guy.

Chronic pain continually influences your emotional state, your work, your sleep, your play, your relationships, everything.

The solution usually involves a multitactic approach. The first step is to figure out the acute issue and work on preventing or healing it. For example, one of the root causes of low back pain can be tight muscles in the hamstrings, hips, and other areas. Or it could be that you have a herniated disc that is bulging into the nerves in your spine. So if you can't eliminate the cause, you won't get very far in managing the pain over the long haul. For headaches, which can be caused by so many factors, the trigger may be food or hormones or something environmental. And when you start to delve into problems where people experience chronic pain—as is the case with ailments such as fibromyalgia and arthritis—the treatments are varied, nuanced, and complex, involving medications, exercise, and sometimes more advanced medical options.

Easing Aches with Food

No matter what hurts and why, you can complement your main treatment plan by addressing pain with nutrition.

Before modern medical developments, ancient cultures often used food and herbs as modes of pain relief. There are many examples that were chronicled in writings and oral histories. Sage was used by Native Americans to relieve a variety of hurts, and the ancient Greeks are believed to have used barley soup with vinegar and honey to help with diseases of the chest. The Egyptians had their laborers eat a diet featuring radishes, garlic, and onion, which they believed would stave off diseases. (In fact, these foods do contain compounds that have been shown to have a protective effect.) Nutrition wasn't their only method, but in the absence of pills and procedures, they chose food, spices, and herbs to do their healing. The ancient Ayurvedic traditions of the East offer numerous solutions that have passed scientific muster centuries later.

Our modern storehouse of knowledge about nutrition and the body lets us target pain more accurately. Why do these foods help? I'll back up to explain: If you remember the tale of inflammation (described on page 19), it's your body's response to some kind of injury. This is a good thing, because it's an attempt to send helpers to your broken or damaged body part or tissue.

You can see how that works for something like a twisted ankle: Trip on the sidewalk and your ankle might swell up to the size of a cantaloupe. Inflammation happens there, and you feel pain because your body sends signals up to your brain that you shouldn't go skipping through the park anytime soon. The nerves play a major role, communicating what is hurt to your brain, which is actually the place where we evaluate the damage.

Inflammation makes the danger detectors in your brain more sensitive, so when you're injured, your brain is very aware of it—and attempts to protect you from further injuring yourself. Your swollen ankle is incredibly sensitive when you walk, even though you may not actually hurt the tissues by walking. Those "ouch!" messages are a protective mechanism—sort of like a biological harness to keep you from making a bad thing worse.

So now take the same principle and apply it to something that you may not see on the surface, like joint pain. Through years of natural wear and tear, the cartilage cushion between your joints decreases and you can wind up with bone-on-bone rubbing. When that happens, it triggers an inflammatory response in an attempt to heal the area. This is a good thing, because the intent of the immune system is to repair. But the inflammation (think of the red swollen twisted ankle, but all of that happening inside your body) can irritate the nerves around the injured spot, and that's what fires those pain signals to make you feel horrible.

Food won't do much for a twisted ankle (you'll need rest, ice, compression, and elevation for that), but it may help in the case of something more chronic, like joint pain.

Because if you eat to settle down the inflammation, you will quiet the signals that cause pain. That doesn't mean you'll fix the structural damage that you may have, but you can make it feel better—and when it comes to pain, that's one of the main goals, right? The other problem occurs because inflammation—when your immune system is in overdrive to fight off a problem—causes your body to churn out chemicals that can actually damage tissues. So you're getting walloped from all directions with damaged tissue from the injury as well as collateral damage from inflammation.

Inflammation is one of the reasons controlling your weight is so important. Fat cells don't just sit there in the body; they're active—meaning that they spit out compounds that actually increase inflammation, which then triggers a higher immune response and, in turn, more inflammation. One of the ways to combat that is by getting the right fats in your diet—because the combo of omega-3s (from fatty fish and walnuts), for example, and omega-6s (from seeds, nuts, and the oils derived from them) regulates your immune response to calm down inflammation. Most

I'LL DRINK TO THAT

Want a one-two anti-inflammatory punch? Try stirring ground cinnamon into your coffee. Both have compounds that have been shown to reduce inflammation. And the cinnamon adds a fancy coffeehouse flavor!

people get enough of the omega-6s; it's the omega-3s we need to bump up. This helps control your weight, and, in the process, eases chronic pain.

We had a babysitter who had debilitating arthritis. It was so bad that she couldn't hold pots and pans, or even stir food, which was sad, because she loved, loved, *loved* to cook. One of the things she did to address her pain was up the amount of fish in her diet, because strong evidence suggests that omega-3s lubricate joints better (more on that in a minute). The change helped her enough that she was able to go back to doing what she enjoyed the most.

Delicious Pain Relief

As you pull back on certain inflammatory foods and ingredients (processed stuff and simple sugars), you should replace them with superfoods that have restorative powers. The FIXES foods should be your go-tos, and the meals in the 21-Day Plan will get you started.

The ultimate anti-inflammatory pain reduction plate? Mine would include salmon, salad with extra-virgin olive oil, and a glass of wine. Here's why:

The fish: As I've said, the strongest research about pain centers around omega-3 fatty acids, the fat found in some fish like salmon and mackerel. Many studies have shown that regular dietary consumption of fatty fish may help to prevent the development of inflammatory diseases. It's difficult to make sweeping statements about pain and diet, because the research typically centers around a specific ailment rather than a far-reaching issue like pain. But you can take cues from their findings. And these omega-3s are important because of the way they regulate the immune response by telling immune soldiers to pull back and not constantly fight. In a study of people who consumed fish oil for neck or back pain, 60 percent stated that their overall pain was improved, and 60 percent stated that their joint pain had improved. Another

A LITTLE SQUEEZE WILL DO YOU

Ever wonder why lemon is traditionally served with fish? Yes, it tastes good. Yes, it's better for you than goopy tartar sauce. But the practice seems to stem from the Middle Ages, when people believed that the fruit's juice would dissolve any bones that were accidentally swallowed.

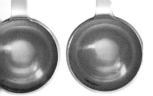

Aim for 2 teaspoons of extra-virgin olive oil per serving of dressing.

example: A recent analysis of eighteen studies found that the fats in fish and fish oils lowered the levels of an inflammatory substance by 17 percent in people with rheumatoid arthritis.

The salad: Top off your superpower veggies with extra-virgin olive oil, which has been shown to have anti-inflammatory properties. One study looking at a substance derived from virgin olive oil called oleocanthal found that it can reduce arthritic pain. Another German study found that olive oil may lessen pain because it contains a number of components that have anti-inflammatory potential, such as polyphenols and plant sterols. This research further underscores that you don't have to fear fats; instead, embrace the healthy ones. And veggies are always good choices, as many of their vitamins have been linked to decreasing various kinds of pain.

The wine: Nope, I'm not suggesting that you fill your glass to mask the pain. Uncork a bottle because wine is rich in a substance called resveratrol, which also has antiaging properties. (We talked about other foods high in resveratrol on page 102.) While most studies on resveratrol and pain mainly use animal models (so actual wine isn't used), some research does link the substance with decreased pain in people. For example, one study found that the addition of resveratrol resulted in a reduced pain score—and four of five patients with endometriosis pain reported complete reduction of pelvic pain after two months of adding resveratrol. Another study, while not directly looking at pain, did show that resveratrol was associated with an increase in a hormone called adiponectin, which has been shown to have anti-inflammatory effects. I'm not suggesting a glass of wine will cure pain, but if it gives a little boost of anti-inflammatory powers, that's not a bad thing.

Above all, following the 21-Day Plan will be your antipain starter kit, getting you used to the foods that will help. While you may need reinforcements in other nonfood forms depending on your problem and its severity, you can be sure that one of your most important weapons is eating to bolster your body, not break it down.

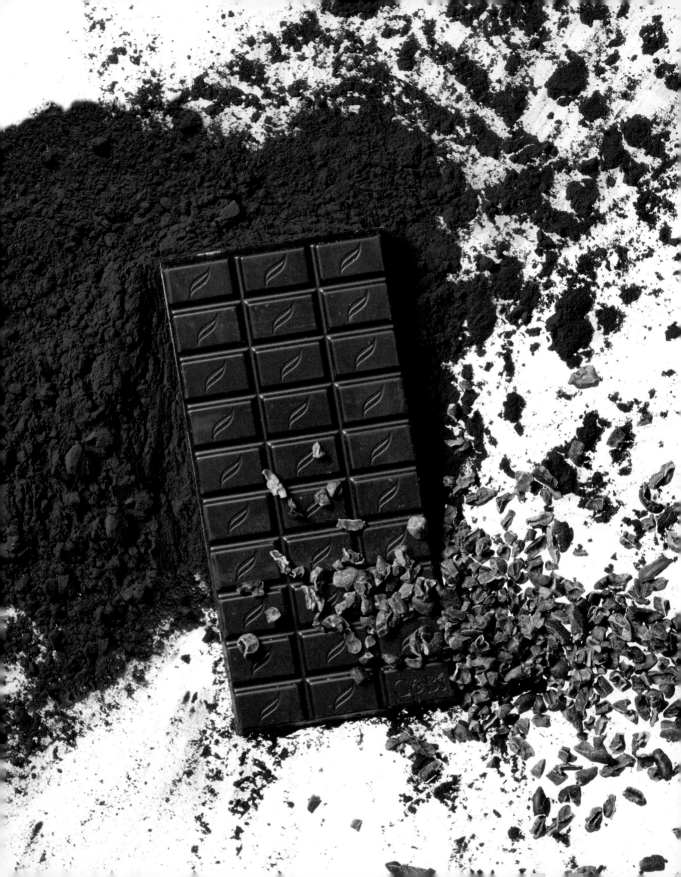

9

Food FIXES
for Brain Power

Food can improve your memory, sharpen your mind, and keep your brain firing for life.

We've all done it at some time or another. You can't remember where you parked the car or the last of the four things you needed at the store or the command that undoes what you just did on your computer. You blank on the name of your friend's husband. You space on the day of the week and plenty of other stuff that should be easy to recall. (Garlic! That's the fourth item!)

Don't panic: It's a natural part of aging. Your memory declines just like your eyesight, muscle tone, and bone density does, often in ways that don't seem to make sense. Why in the world can you recall the name of your third-grade teacher but space about whether you unplugged the curling iron three minutes ago now that you're out the door? Again, we all experience slight overall brain drain as we get older; your IQ drops five points per decade after the age of thirty. Here's a fact that may surprise you: Memory loss starts at age sixteen (and you thought it was Snapchat that made your teenager's mind mush). The decline is so minimal that you don't even recognize it, but by age forty, you might start to notice the effects.

We can't entirely brush off these quick "senior moments." Many of us take a second to pause and think something along the lines of, "I hope it doesn't get much worse." That's because we harbor a deep fear of memory loss; in fact, several surveys, including one of my own, have shown that this scares people more than cancer, heart attacks, and accidents. Maybe you're afraid because you've watched loved ones struggle through Alzheimer's or dementia, or you've heard the stories about the pain people experience with those diseases. I saw it firsthand with my grandmother, who had dementia in her nineties. She was always a strict and old-fashioned grandmother, but when her mind changed, she became combative, angry, and frustrated, and when she spoke, the words were intelligible but the phrases didn't make sense. She had a paranoid fear that people were talking about her. We were doing that, yes, but not in the mean way she imagined—we were just commiserating about how we hated watching her slip away. Absolutely, it was sad to see someone I loved not even know what she didn't know.

But here's the thing: Alzheimer's, dementia, or memory-related problems are not necessarily inescapable. You can prevent some of these issues, slow their progression, and, in some cases, even reverse them.

Exercise has been shown to be the most effective brain defender. According to a review of sixteen studies, people who are physically active on a regular basis reduce their risk of Alzheimer's by 45 percent. What's regular? It's not complicated: 150 minutes a week of moderately intense aerobic exercise, meaning that you're working hard enough for your heart to beat fast, but not so hard that you're

too breathless to talk. This simple prescription helps to promote new networks of small blood vessels, which allow more glucose and nutrients to reach more brain regions.

And then there are brain exercises, another key to lowering your risk of cognitive decline. Exercising your noggin helps to keep it plastic and strong. (*Plastic*, by the way, is the word scientists use to describe the brain's ability to continually learn and develop.) It's the old "use it or lose it" mantra—you want to continually challenge your brain to help it perform well. "Using it" is what builds the hard wires and connections that fend off neurological deterioration.

A final tactic centers around food: feeding your brain the nutrients it needs to optimally function. But before we get into the food specifics, let's peek inside that machine so you know what you're tinkering with every time you eat and drink.

Your Brain's Inner Workings

The best way to think about the brain is to visualize a cell phone network. Your brain's nerve cells, called neurons, are like individual callers. They send and receive messages to and from each other. When this information goes from one neuron to another, you've had a successful call, and that neuron stores away the information. This is how memory is built: neurons talking to each other, transmitting messages, and filing them away for future use.

In our cell phone analogy, it's not only the neurons that need to be working well to

Turmeric has played a starring role in both tasty curries and holistic medicine for ages, with research pointing to the health perks of an antioxidant it contains, including a possible impact on your brain. Now the peppery spice is going mainstream. You'll see it popping up as the star ingredient in everything from tea to snacks, but bring it to the front row of your spice rack, too. Sprinkle turmeric on eggs, lentils, roasted veggies, rice, and whatever else you've got cooking tonight.

successfully store memories—the network must be fully functional, too. We've all been in plenty of places with "no bars," no connection, no signal. It's not that your phone is on the fritz. It's that the connection fails. Here's how that happens in your brain. The space between neurons is called the synapse, and neurotransmitters are chemicals that bring info back and forth across it. The most common one is called acetylcholine. A shortage of it can be what causes those "dropped calls."

Other things can mess up this transmission between neurons. For example, if you don't use the network often, that synapse will weaken. Makes sense, right? If you're learning piano or a foreign language, you're more likely to remember it the more you practice. If you skip lessons for a few months, you'll forget plenty. We strengthen our synapses the more we use them, creating a stronger and stronger signal. Information can flow because that signal is ultra-high-speed. The mantra "it's like riding a bike" might work for, well, riding a bike. But it's a bit of a misnomer because memory relies on repeated use for you to retrieve bits of information.

The other signal disrupter comes in the form of a protein fragment in your brain called beta amyloid. This is a substance that cuts off signals (like tree branches falling on power lines) and is considered one of the likely causes of Alzheimer's. Related to that, fibers may build up inside of neurons, tangling them and causing a disruption of information exchange and memory.

Your genetic inheritance largely dictates how much of that gunk-inducing beta amyloid you have, but you can limit the damage. How? Your body produces a protein (it's called APOE) that sweeps away the gunk, and some research has shown that you can influence how much of it you have. Getting regular exercise helps you here, too. There's also a food influencer: The spice turmeric, which is found in Indian foods and many of my FIXES recipes, can help increase levels of that brain-sweeping protein.

Other things that can cause cognitive problems: a drop in the neurotransmitter acetylcholine and a decrease in a substance called BDNF (brain-derived neurotrophic growth factor, if you want the mouthful name). I compare BDNF to Miracle-Gro for the brain, because it supports nerves that allow us to learn. Unfortunately, it decreases as we age; inflammation and stress can also deplete your supply. Unsurprisingly, eating saturated fat and refined sugar might also make your BDNF levels fall because of the inflammation that they trigger. So cutting back on these the FIXES way will help to safeguard your natural brain fertilizer.

Keep-Sharp Foods

Of course it's not just what you don't eat, but what you *do* eat. Here's how to maximize your Fix-It plan to help slow brain drain.

First order of business: The "F" in FIXES—fats with benefits. Because your brain is the fattiest organ, healthy dietary fats are essential to protect against memory-related diseases. Why? Saturated fats are rigid molecules, while omega-3 fats are flexible. When our brain is repairing itself and making neurons, it prefers flexible cells rather than rigid ones that don't adapt as quickly to new influences. You can help by feeding it the right building blocks for your neurons. Fish is a fantastic source of omega-3s, and plenty of research connects eating more of it with brain health. A *Journal of the American Medical Association* study showed that people with the highest levels of DHA (the fats found in fish) had a 47 percent reduction in risk of developing dementia. And an *American Journal of Clinical Nutrition* review of twenty-one studies found that just one serving of fish a week was associated with lower risks of dementia and Alzheimer's disease.

The second must-eat category to keep your brain kicking also keeps your heart ticking:

lots of fruits and vegetables. I can't overstate the importance of a plant-based diet when it comes to your brain health. For example, a recent study in the journal *Alzheimer's & Dementia* looked at a Mediterranean-based diet (which my FIXES approach follows). Researchers found that a high consumption of vegetables (especially leafy greens) was beneficial to brain health.

But the positive effects didn't stop with veggies. These researchers also found that people who reported a higher consumption of one specific fruit—berries—had a slower rate of cognitive decline.

It's also a good idea to add seeds to your diet (heck, just lump them together all at once and have a salmon salad topped with berries and seeds). A 2015 *British Journal of Nutrition* study looked at the diet habits and cognitive function of more than 2,500 people; they found that a higher intake of lignan, a chemical compound found in sesame seeds, flaxseed, and pumpkin seeds, was associated with less decline in cognitive function, memory, and information processing. The people who had the lowest lignan intake? They had a 3.5 times greater decline in cognitive function and a 6 times greater decline in memory. But forget their brain powers—seeds are crunchy-good eating (get started with the recipes on pages 240 and 241).

Finally, embrace that special-occasion sugar in the form of dark chocolate. Research is showing that flavanols—phytonutrients found in foods such as chocolate, tea, red wine, and blueberries—help facilitate brain connections. They may also protect brain cells from toxins and the negative effects of inflammation. A small study looked at older people whose memories were in good shape for their ages. Three groups of people drank a brew containing different amounts of cocoa flavanols. The greatest improvement in mental tests came from the high flavanol group. (Side benefit: the cocoa flavanols also reduced blood pressure and improved insulin resistance.)

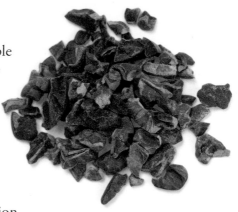

Cacao Nibs. Because these roasted and cracked cocoa beans are 100% cacao, they're especially high in flavanols. They're crunchy and unsweetened, with a raw chocolate taste. Try them on yogurt or in a smoothie.

Isn't it nice to know there's a food formula to keep your body's most complex organ working like a well-oiled machine? By following my FIXES approach to eating, you'll be doing what you can to make your brain steely and strong—and that will help you remember all kinds of important info. Quick! Which foods contain lignan?

LOSE THE WEIGHT, HANG ON TO YOUR MIND

Being overweight will slow down your mind as well as your movement. A recent University of Arizona study of more than 21,000 people found that those who are heavier run a higher risk of cognitive decline later in life. Why? Overweight people tend to have higher levels of inflammation, which is also associated with memory problems.

OKAY, BUT WHAT ABOUT MERCURY?

I eat a lot of fish, for reasons you see throughout this book. It's good for your brain, it's good for weight control, it's good for your heart. One of the potential drawbacks, however, is that fish can contain the toxin mercury. Recently, I found out that my levels were higher than they should be, and there is some evidence that mercury can have a *negative* effect on your brain function. I had to cut back on my consumption of larger fish, which have higher mercury levels because they've lived longer and eaten more, since they are

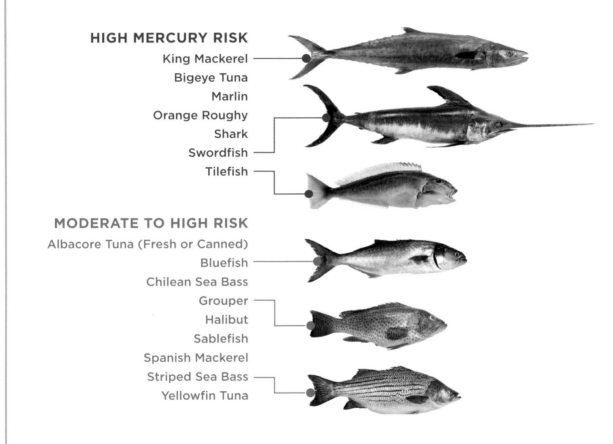

HIGH MERCURY RISK

King Mackerel
Bigeye Tuna
Marlin
Orange Roughy
Shark
Swordfish
Tilefish

MODERATE TO HIGH RISK

Albacore Tuna (Fresh or Canned)
Bluefish
Chilean Sea Bass
Grouper
Halibut
Sablefish
Spanish Mackerel
Striped Sea Bass
Yellowfin Tuna

higher on the food chain. While the risk isn't totally understood, you likely don't need to reduce your fish intake, since most of us don't currently eat enough. If you get fish into your diet several times a week, the benefits outweigh the potential risk. Overdoing it would likely only happen if you became an everyday fish-eater, and mostly downed the kinds that have high levels of mercury. Smaller species are safer since they don't gobble up lots of other fish and so don't accumulate high mercury levels. Now I eat low-risk and moderate-risk fish and seafood three or four times a week and rarely eat the ones at the top of the list.

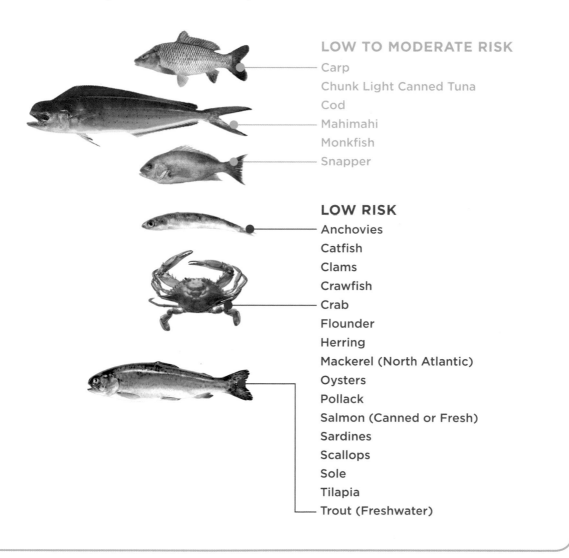

LOW TO MODERATE RISK

Carp

Chunk Light Canned Tuna

Cod

Mahimahi

Monkfish

Snapper

LOW RISK

Anchovies

Catfish

Clams

Crawfish

Crab

Flounder

Herring

Mackerel (North Atlantic)

Oysters

Pollack

Salmon (Canned or Fresh)

Sardines

Scallops

Sole

Tilapia

Trout (Freshwater)

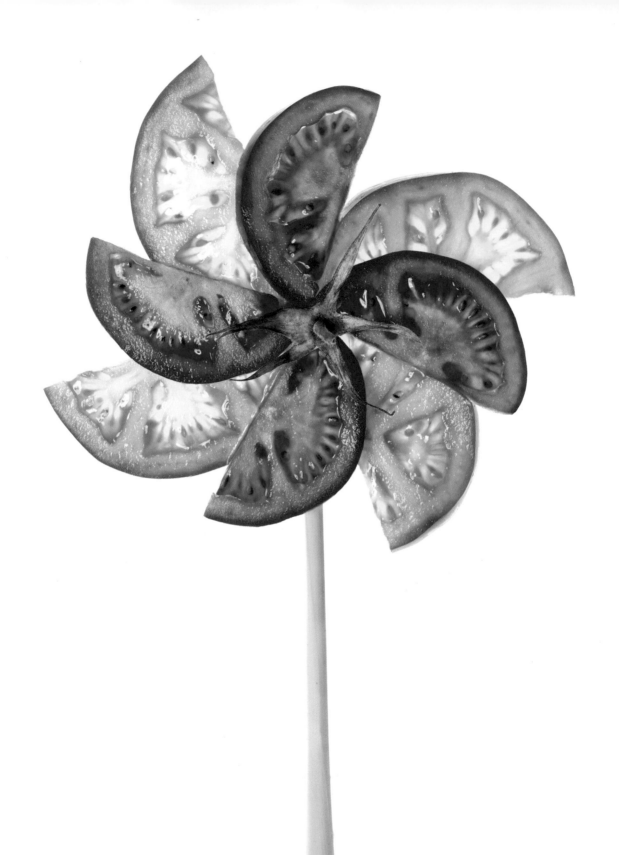

10

Food FIXES
for Bad Moods

Feeling a little cranky, moody . . . off?
Choose foods that will turn your well-being back *on*.

In medicine, we often think of formulas: x symptom + y symptom = z condition. The answer to that equation dictates the treatment options. Some conditions, however, don't have clear formulas. Some are nuanced in their appearance, which makes them trickier to treat. Some diagnoses are more art than science.

That's certainly the case when it comes to mood issues—a kitchen-sink category that contains stress, anxiety, or just feeling down. You can't simply take an X-ray, MRI, blood test, or other diagnostic that shows something's not right. There's no biomarker that can tell us, hey, your mood has a reading of thirty-two tears per minute so you should be treated with two tablespoons of whatevericillin.

Like any health issue, mood problems have a wide spectrum of severity—some are episodic and minor, while others can be chronic and life-threatening. Important note: Major mental illness requires professional help, so please don't rely on this chapter to magically resolve it. If you have any doubt about whether what you are feeling is serious enough to warrant a doctor's visit, it likely is.

Here, I'm addressing the common and normal fluctuations of emotions including frustration, anxiety, and blues that many of us experience as we cycle through our lives. People with minor mood issues—the kind we will deal with in the next few pages—can have difficulty describing their state of mind. Perhaps artists capture this kind of trouble better than anyone; think of a painting from Picasso's blue period or a piece of classical music or a poignant lyric from a pop song that nails the sense of something wrong instead of right with the world.

But even if you can't quite put your finger on the origin of your mood, you may instinctively put your fingers on something else: food.

When we feel off, we self-medicate, and many times, food is the drug of choice. I'm lumping several "problems" into one category—feeling down, anxious, angry, etc.—but there is a common thread. They all make us more prone to emotional eating.

The instinct to eat isn't always bad, however. In fact, used in the right way, food can actually change your brain chemistry to balance the hormones that influence your emotional state. Unfortunately, most of us prescribe ourselves the wrong kind of medicine. Sometimes it's half a jar of peanut butter or a mega bowl of ice cream. Sometimes it's too much alcohol. These kinds of OTKC (over-the-kitchen-counter) medications have real dangers—including the possibility of addiction. Let's take a look at the emotional dynamics.

Different forces are in charge when you make decisions. The executive function—located in the cerebral cortex—gives you the ability to see a problem, analyze it, make a choice, and find a solution. It's how we get things done from day to day. It's the part of the brain that has helped us survive, thrive, and continue to extend our lives as individuals and as a species. Executive function allows you to read this book, make decisions about food, and be smart about how you fill your plate.

Other decisions are more emotional and/or instinctual; you're reacting rather than thinking. These responses are associated with a part of the brain called the amygdala, which helps regulate fear, love, temptation, and anxiety. It impels you to gobble down a cake pop at the mall because you saw a kid eating one and it looked darn good. It has you reaching for a bag of chips when a relative sends you a super-annoying text. It makes choices about food without consulting your master eating plan, just by reacting.

Often the two functions work together. For example, your emotions may tell you that you're attracted to someone, and the executive function allows you to cook up the best way to ask that person on a date. But here's the interesting thing: The amygdala is darn persuasive, which is why emotion can override logic and reason. In the thick of things, emotional impulses can shove the executive aside, so self-control does take some work and strategy.

Without that, we can fall prey to feelings and impulses, rather than knowledge-based decisions, as humans did when our only big decision was whether to fight an enemy or flee from one. There was no time to carve a pro/con list on the wall of your cave. There was no need for twenty-one-day plans because you didn't even know whether you'd make it through the next twenty-one minutes. Instinctual responses gave you the best chance of staying alive.

Now consider how emotions and impulses apply to modern-day food choices. What happens when you're tired or cranky or have low energy? Your body knows it needs a boost and that the quickest way to spark up is to flood your system with sugar. That's why, at tough moments, you crave fast-acting sugars and carbs. Even if logic tells us that a candy

SUSTAINABLE ENERGY SOURCES: SNACK EDITION

It would be nice to have a stress-bypass operation that could cure bodies of life's mental clogs and the cravings that come with them. No such luck, so you need foods that satisfy hankerings without the body damage of classic fast-grab snacks. Be prepared with a satisfying alternative that will help you maintain energy levels. Some ideas for when a mood strikes (see more snack ideas in chapter 3):

Cheesy: Popcorn tossed with nutritional yeast. It hits the spot for fewer calories than a block of cheddar (or a box of highlighter-orange crackers).

Creamy: Plain Greek yogurt with a drop of vanilla extract and some blueberries on top. Simple and rich-tasting.

Crunchy: Roasted chickpeas. (You can make them yourself or buy them prepackaged at the grocery store.) They're high in protein, and a smart substitute when you're jonesing for chips.

Salty: Edamame, either sprinkled with flaky salt or drizzled with low-sodium soy sauce.

Spicy: Hummus with a swirl of sriracha sauce. Dunk your favorite snacking veggies.

Sweet: Fruit with peanut butter. The nut butter brings extra satiation power and slows down the absorption of sugar.

bar isn't the best choice, the urge to get more energy and the "up" feeling that comes with it can send us on a vending machine run.

The problem: That treatment works like a shot of nutritional novocaine. It's only going to mask your low mood temporarily. The candy bar may numb what hurts or stresses you for a bit, but it doesn't do anything to help the long term. And the pain continues when the anesthetic wears off. But smart food strategies can help you thwart these low, frazzled, or furious moments.

Two common issues involving mood—high stress and feelings of sadness—deserve special attention.

Stress: Whatever trigger has you on edge, the process is the same. Nerve signals send messages to the brain to let you know you'd better do something to calm the agitation. Once the amygdala receives the signal, it tells another part of your brain to produce some helpful hormones. One is adrenaline, which made sense for ancient times. You needed that boost to prepare you for fight or flight. Another is the stress hormone cortisol, which can be helpful, because it enters your bloodstream and triggers a surge of blood sugar. It does this by tapping into stores and also tampering with insulin so that more blood sugar is available for energy. How is that good? It provides you with energy, which works well when you need to flee the beast or meet the deadline. But when you have chronic stress, that increase in blood sugar—as you remember from

chapter 2—is no good for your circulatory system. You don't use it up in the moment of fight or flight. It's just *there*, nicking up your arteries, for one. And it also creates a vicious cycle, where blood sugar spikes, then plummets, and you wind up once again reaching for those simple sugars. Your body jumps onto the merry-go-round that doesn't stop: messed-up hormones, messed-up hunger, messed-up eating, messed-up body.

Blue Moods: Research suggests that two key hormones—serotonin and dopamine—play roles in your mood. When dopamine and serotonin are high, you feel good. And when you feel good, you want to keep doing the thing that feeds that dopamine and serotonin rush. Take one guess as to something that creates a rush of those feel-good hormones. Yep, sugar. The sweet stuff stimulates dopamine in the rewards center of the brain (just like other things do, including social stimulation, sex, drugs, etc.), as well as indirectly boosting serotonin. So when you feel down, it's not uncommon to want to reach for something that will make you feel up, aka sugary treats.

Eating sugar regularly may temporarily mask the down moments, but over time, the same cascade of problems happens: higher blood sugar, more collateral damage to your arteries, more weight gain, and so on.

So what's the solution?

I absolutely want you to use food as a mood-lifter, but not in the typical way. How do you eat to treat the problem, not the symptom? How do you use food as a long-term prescription to make you feel better daily, to help quell stress, to be happier? By now, it won't surprise you that my Rx for matters of the mind involves FIXES foods. Ideally, eating protein with slowly-absorbed carbs (like sweet potatoes, nuts, and brown rice) will calm those sugar-seeking moments.

Upping your fruits and veggies is part of the mood-boosting arsenal, too, as we see in a recent study of fourteen thousand people done by University of Warwick Medical School researchers. In that research, about one-third of people who scored high in mental well-being tests reported having five or more portions of produce a day, compared with just 7 percent who ate less than one serving. The thought is that some fruits and vegetables contain antioxidants that could influence parts of the brain associated with optimism.

But eating for a great mood goes beyond the X in FIXES. My entire approach—emphasizing healthy oils, beans, and plants—serves as the baseline for a healthier, happier brain. In a study of 3,500 older adults, greater consumption of a Mediterranean-based diet was significantly associated with lowering the risk of symptoms tied to mood issues. Researchers suspected that B vitamins, antioxidant nutrients, and healthy fats (all part of your FIXES) made the difference.

It's especially important to focus on omega-3 fatty acids, like the ones found in salmon, walnuts, and seeds. A 2015 review of research on the benefits of omega-3s found that they protect against mood and anxiety

SHOULD YOU "B" WORRIED?

More than 30 percent of people over the age of fifty have a B12 deficiency. As we age, we don't absorb B12 as well, so we get less of it through our food sources. The trouble with that? B12 helps your nerve cells communicate with one another. When you have low levels, it's difficult for your cells to send and receive messages, making you more prone to worry and anxiety. Since B12 is only found in animal-based products, including fish and shellfish, some meat, eggs, and dairy (all on the 21-Day Plan), it's especially important for vegetarians and vegans to think about alternative sources. Those include fortified products like soy and cereal.

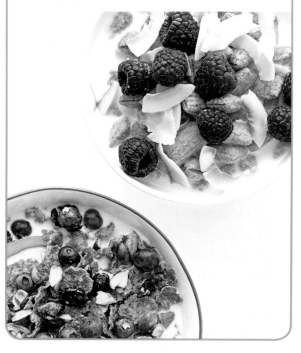

disorders because they improve brain function. And a 2016 meta-analysis of thirteen studies found that omega-3s had a beneficial effect on symptoms associated with depression. Why? Still unclear, but it's likely because of the anti-inflammatory powers of these healthy fats. (Inflammation is thought to disrupt signals in the brain, which can be related to depression and mood.) Healthy fats also help brain cell membranes to become flexible so they can rapidly create new connections and adapt to stress.

Remember the story of Luigi and the Blue Zones? Well, there are also blue zones for actual blues. Psychologist Stephen Scott Ilardi looked at several cultures that had nonexistent rates of depression. One of the groups was the Kaluli people of the Highlands of Papua New Guinea. He pointed to research showing that of two thousand Kaluli people interviewed, there was only one marginal case of depression. That's an extraordinary finding when you consider that the Kaluli lead hard lives. Ilardi noted their high rates of violent deaths, infant mortality, and infections. So why didn't they experience depression?

THERE MAY BE PLENTY OF FISH IN THE SEA, BUT SALMON IS ONE OF THE HEALTHIEST

Salmon is packed with omega-3 fatty acids, which are big-time heart helpers as well as mood improvers. They may keep your cholesterol in check, protect your blood vessels, and drive down your blood pressure.

Bake it all-in-one. Stack thinly sliced veggies, a salmon fillet, and lemon slices on parchment paper. Fold paper over, then pinch the edges to make a packet. Bake at 400°F until cooked through (about 15 minutes).

Healthy hack your bagel craving. Spread some cottage cheese on a slice of whole-grain toast. Top with smoked salmon, a slice of tomato, carrot and cucumber shavings, and red onion slices.

Make salmon salad. With a fork, mash canned salmon, a dollop of plain Greek yogurt, and a splash of lemon or lime. Fold in diced avocado, if you like. Load up a sandwich, or serve with crackers and crudités.

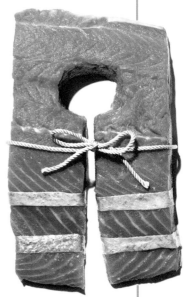

Ilardi pointed to six lifestyle markers, including exercise, social connections, and of course, food: The Kaluli diet had the right balance of omega-3s and omega-6s. He argues that the modern American diet has too many omega-6s, which can be inflammatory (and thus can be related to depression), and not enough omega-3s (found in fish and other sources), which are anti-inflammatory. The Kaluli eat lots of fish, so their omega-3s were in balance—an important factor for mood control.

The massive benefit of omega-3s is just one reason fish is such a big part of my 21-Day Plan and a foundation for the way you'll eat for the rest of your life. Fish contains nutrients that feed your brain—not just so you're sharper, but so you feel better. Will you never have sugar cravings again? Of course not, and there's nothing wrong with special-occasion sugar—if you go for it *occasionally*. As for everyday hankerings? Handle those by creating the environments I talked about in chapter 3. If you strategize and prepare to manage hunger and temptation by having healthy foods near you, you'll reach for them, rather than junk. (See the box on page 77 for my ways to satisfy any in-the-moment craving.) Executive brain, you've got this.

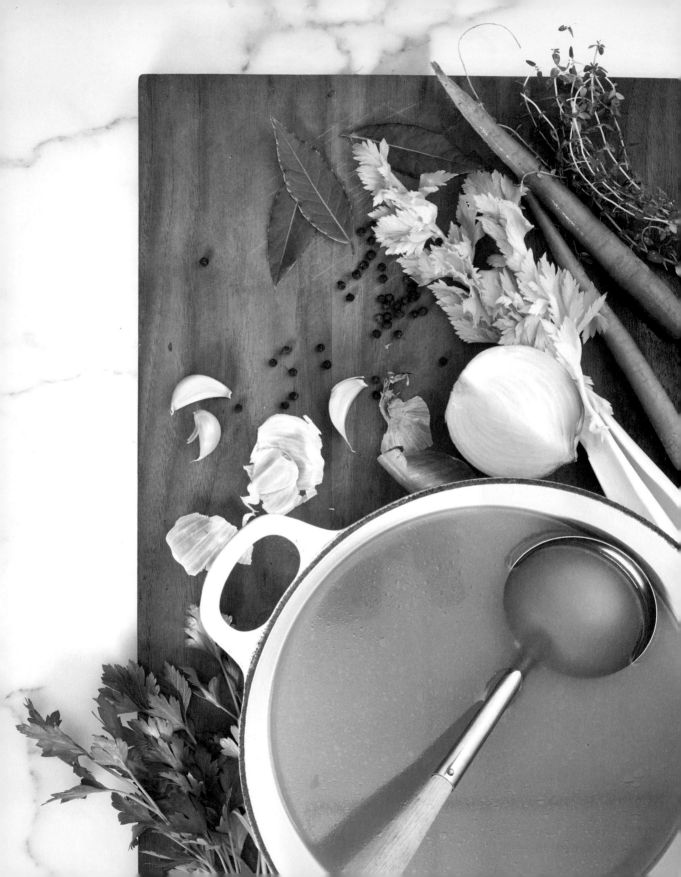

11.

Food FIXES for Immunity

To protect against sniffles, the flu, and more serious bodily invaders, you need to feed the troops.

Have you ever wondered this: *How did Grandma know?*

How did she know that the minute you got sick, you should be pumped up with orange juice and chicken soup? Our grandmothers—and their grandmothers and theirs—always had a food fix. They knew that good eats could make you well before science caught up. Maybe it was instinct. Maybe it was trial and error. Maybe it was wisdom passed down the family tree right along with holiday rituals and wedding rings.

Or maybe our elders were up on their history of Moses Maimonides. The twelfth-century Jewish physician and philosopher is said to have been the first to write about the medicinal benefits of hen and rooster eaten in their own broth. He wrote that this concoction "neutralizes the bodily constitution," which, really, is just a twelfth-century way of saying "food fixes." (And then he went a little off the deep end, claiming that eating the testicles of any living creature could increase libido!)

Chicken soup is actually more of a proxy for two other things that are happening—hydration and warmth, both of which can help thin the mucus of a nasty cold and open things up, so you feel better when you're sick. In addition, chicken soup usually has a lot of sodium, so it encourages you to drink fluids, always a good thing. Other research even suggests that it works by changing the function of your immune cells so they're better able to move around and help fortify you. (These reasons are good enough to freeze some homemade broth and have it ready to go for when you need it.)

While Grandma probably didn't know all that, she always seemed to have a good sense of which kitchen concoction could cure your cold—or prevent you from getting one in the first place.

The last time I was *really* sick? It was a bout of food poisoning from what I suspect was either bad fish or bad sauce (or a bad sauce on top of bad fish). My body rebelled fiercely—from both the north and the south. I was so cleaned out that, heck, I could have had a colonoscopy the next day. It was horrible. But besides that memorable-for-all-the-wrong-reasons day, I don't have a long illness history, because I just don't get sick. In the last decade, I have never missed a day of work because of illness; I may get stuffy or deal with a sore throat once or twice a year, but nothing more than that.

The funny thing is, I *should* get sick more than I do. It's common for

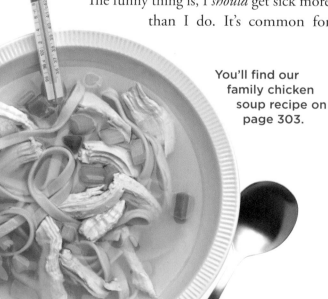

You'll find our family chicken soup recipe on page 303.

THE QUICK TRICK TO FEND OFF COLDS

Gargle with tap water for a minute or so. Researchers in Japan found that people who did this three times a day or more caught fewer colds—and if they did come down with something, some symptoms were milder than in those who didn't gargle.

me to shake a hundred hands a day, which is a leading cause of sickness, as bacteria and viruses jump from person to person. I've spent much of my career in a hospital, aka ground zero for germ transmission. Even if my whole family is sick, I know I likely won't come down with anything. And no, I don't wear rubber gloves and surgical masks wherever I go.

My diet (and my sleep) protects me. Because I follow the FIXES principles, my immune defense system is fortified to handle the invaders that enter my body. And a strong immune system does more than just fend off minor illness; it helps settle down inflammation, which, as you've seen, is the root of so many medical issues.

The food answer for strengthening your immune system revolves around making sure you get plenty of vitamins and minerals, which are most often found in those omnipotent fruits and vegetables. The current thinking is that micronutrients (vitamin A, D, C, E, B6, folate, B12, zinc, selenium, iron, and copper) are most responsible for boosting the immune system.

That's because they fortify the immunity soldiers in your body. If you think about your immune system as an army of fighters ready to fend off attacks, then of course you want to provide it with foods that will strengthen it to stand up to the most powerful invaders. After all, you wouldn't want your country's army fueled on sugary

4 IMPORTANT LITTLE MINERALS (AND WHERE TO FIND THEM)

Minerals of all kinds help your body function; it's why you need balance in your diet and another reason it makes sense to take a daily multivitamin. Be sure to get these four:

Copper: You only need a little, and your multivitamin delivers. So do oysters, cashews, kale, mushrooms, and clams.

Iron: After age fifty, women need less iron, and multis for this age group reflect that. But you don't have to stay away from iron-rich foods like tofu, spinach, and lentils.

Selenium: Most Americans get adequate amounts of this mineral from food. Brazil nuts are brimming with it (eat no more than three a day to avoid overload), and it's also found in cod, shrimp, tuna, and salmon.

Zinc: Get it from oysters, beef, sesame seeds, cashews, pumpkin seeds, spinach, and chickpeas. Extra zinc can be helpful when fighting a cold, but too much of it can work against you and may eventually create a copper deficiency. If you take a multi with zinc, stick to one zinc lozenge every two to three hours at the onset of cold symptoms. A bonus: This mineral is needed to help us taste, so I often administer it to surgery patients who say they've lost their sense of taste.

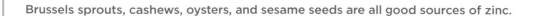

Brussels sprouts, cashews, oysters, and sesame seeds are all good sources of zinc.

cereals and nachos. You want it powered with foods that will sustain its energy to fight the good fight whenever necessary. That's exactly what you do with your internal soldiers. You feed them the good stuff.

Eating the FIXES way will do that, because of the diversity of vitamins and minerals you'll down every day. These nutrients bolster the function of your body-protecting immune cells—helping them not just fight attackers, but also identify them better to

HIT YOUR C NOTE

You think of orange juice when you think of vitamin C, but you can get a nice surge of immunity protection from strawberries. Not only are they full of fiber, folate, and potassium, but they're also a major source of C. It only takes ten of them to fulfill your daily needs. Put them in smoothies or yogurt, have them as dessert, or create a healthy and satisfying PB&"J"—spread no-sugar-added nut butter on whole wheat bread, and layer with sliced strawberries.

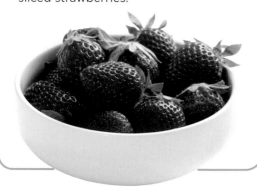

stop them in their tracks before they wreak havoc on your body.

This is how it all works:

Imagine your body as an airport. Nobody gets into the terminal without passing through multiple layers of security. Part of your immune system works as the TSA screening agents, who will put things through a few checkpoints to see if they're safe or need to be sent away and destroyed. Sometimes invaders slip by the TSA agents, and that can be what causes harm.

At the cellular level, it all starts with communication. Cells called macrophages are always on alert, patrolling the body for trouble, like security cameras or drug-sniffing dogs. They try to get the lay of the land for the entire body. All the while, they gobble up and destroy run-of-the-mill germs, but if they spot major trouble, they call in reinforcements. These are defense cells called T cells and B cells.

Your immune system can recognize whether something's foreign, because just like the people standing in that TSA line, every cell needs to have some kind of identification. If your immune system recognizes cells that don't have the proper ID for your body, that's when it gets to work to kill off the offenders.

Some cells simply attack and kill invaders, whether they're germs, bacteria, viruses, or other things that your immune system is unfamiliar with. Sometimes, they overreact to those foreign invaders, which creates a major inflammatory response (allergy symptoms are

3 COOL WAYS TO EAT AN APPLE

One large apple has 5 grams of fiber and 14 percent of your daily vitamin C—important for your immunity and for keeping weight off. Go ahead and chomp on an apple as a snack or dessert, but if you're looking to spruce things up, try these methods:

Make crispy apple chips: Thinly slice an apple, sprinkle on some cinnamon, and bake at 225°F for about 45 minutes.

Sauté apple wedges in olive oil with fresh thyme and lemon juice. Top them off with a splash of balsamic vinegar.

Cut them up and mix them with cabbage and grated carrots to create a coleslaw. For dressing, try plain Greek yogurt, lemon juice, and just a touch of maple syrup.

an inflammatory response that shows your immune system is trying to get rid of a specific allergen, for instance). They may even attack your own body, thinking that healthy cells are foreign, such as with autoimmune diseases. Those are a bit like friendly fire, if you will. Food is a vital defense, because various nutrients can have a positive effect on the functioning of your immune cells, so that they work well in the capacities they need to—whether it's ID'ing foreign invaders, destroying them, or overall protection against the many microscopic skirmishes going on inside your body.

Now, let's say the fight takes place in the form of a run-of-the-mill infection. Your immune cells come in full force and overwhelm it. The result: An inflammatory response that causes the symptoms you feel, be it a runny nose or sore throat or sudden middle-of-the-night bathroom drama.

As we age, we lose a bit of our ability to produce some immune cells, so we may have a tougher time repelling infections when they come up. Food can help—by bulking up and strengthening the defense force.

In order to best strengthen your immune system through your diet, you want a balanced mix of vitamins and minerals, so that means paying special attention to the "X" in my FIXES foods—in the form of Xtra fruits

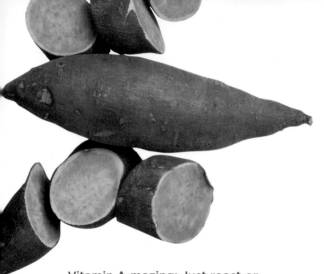

Vitamin A-mazing: Just roast or microwave a sweet potato and dress it up a little—consider pumpkin or sesame seeds or Parmesan cheese and greens.

Garlic: It's antibacterial, antiviral, and antifungal. No wonder garlic is one of the foods on my unlimited list, and I recommend you eat it as often as you can. Roast it with veggies, mince it and add it to salad dressing, or use it as part of a rub when roasting chicken or other meat. Other benefits, by the way: Garlic has been shown to lower LDL cholesterol, lower total cholesterol, lower blood pressure, and reduce your risk of blood clots and stroke.

By all means, make a great chicken soup when you're under the weather. And while you're at it, toss lots of veggies in there—because that may very well prevent you from getting sick the next time.

and veggies. A colorful plate—mixing up the fruits and vegetables you have every day—is one of the best things you can do to improve your immune system, because the whole swath of compounds in the plant kingdom will fortify your body.

To zero in a little, research does suggest that vitamin A has the most firepower and that vitamin A deficiencies are linked to higher rates of infections and lower immune function. How does vitamin A help? By pitching in to create the immune cells that fight off pathogens. So for the maximum boost, focus on things like sweet potatoes, carrots, squash, and leafy greens.

In addition to foods with vitamin A, several other eats have been found to have special immune-boosting power, such as:

Mushrooms: They contain powerful compounds called beta-glucans, which have been long known for their immune-enhancing properties. They stimulate your immune system by binding to macrophages and other scavenger white blood cells, activating their anti-infection functions.

HOW TO FEED A COLD

I vote for chicken soup because it helps calm irritated nasal passages and airways. And don't believe the myth that it's good to starve a fever. When you're weak, your body does need nutrients—and plenty of water. So eating when you're sick is smart. Some other nutritional tricks:

Green tea and honey. Nutrients in green tea help prevent viruses from infiltrating your body, and the honey can coat your throat and keep coughing to a minimum.

Frozen grapes. Sucking on these will numb a sore throat; plus, grapes offer a boost of vitamin C, one of the key nutrients for immunity.

Vegetable juice can help you get much-needed nutrients when you don't feel like eating.

Yogurt or kefir: The good bacteria (probiotics) in these can give your immunity a powerful leg up. In fact, in one study, when people with colds took probiotic supplements, they recovered faster than those on a placebo and said their symptoms were 34 percent less severe. Check the labels for products that contain *Lactobacillus* and *Bifidobacterium* (also called *Bifidus*) strains.

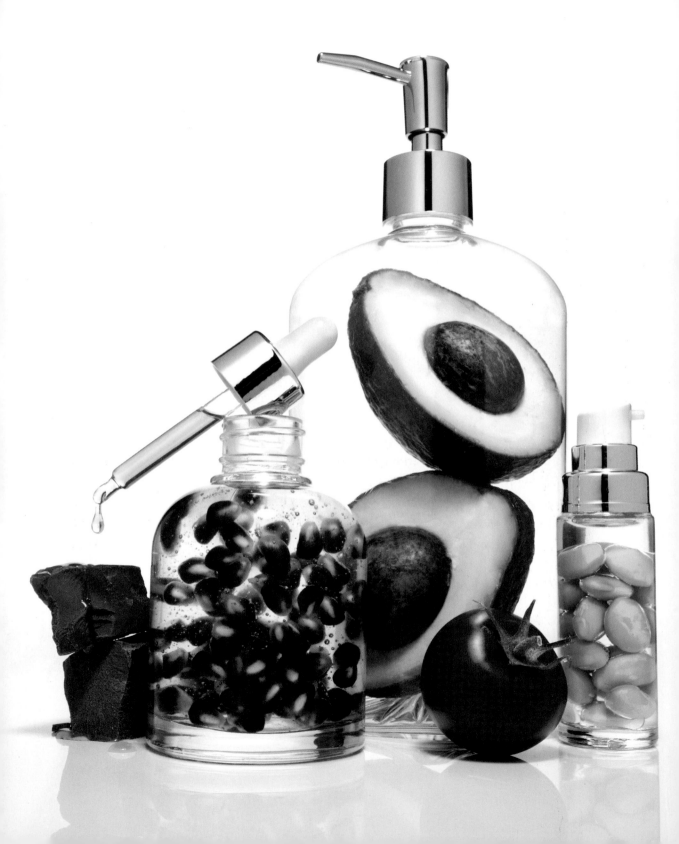

12

Food FIXES
for Skin and Hair

Looking good on the outside starts
with what happens on the inside.

I like to joke that Lisa and I had an arranged marriage because our fathers were friends for years before we ever met.

I got to know Lisa's dad, Gerry, when he came to Turkey as a visiting professor and I offered to show him around. But I had never met any of his children. Then one night when I was a med student, my parents were meeting Lisa's parents for dinner in Philadelphia, and I came along. Lisa joined the party, too.

The first time I saw her, she looked like a dove. Glowing, pure, radiant.

She thought I was the maître d'.

Our story is just a variation on the one many couples tell, about how two people (or at least one) tingled when they saw each other for the first time.

For me, the love-at-first-sight cliché was true: Lisa was as stunning as could be, and our initial physical attraction ignited a lifelong spiritual and soul-filling bond. That spark led to a journey that has produced the next two generations of our families. Which is a somewhat long way to say, how you look matters. Not in the superficial way, but in a deeper, more evolutionary way. Attractiveness is really a proxy for good health, and we assess, deep inside our subconscious brains, someone's longevity and compatibility through how they look.

I also have to say this: Lisa's *entire family* looked good. They had clear, luminous skin. They had full hair. They practically oozed good health. Heck, even their cats, dogs, and horses were poster pets for well-being.

There's no doubt in my mind that it all stemmed from the way they ate. As I mentioned in my introduction, they grew vegetables in their garden, they minimized sugary foods, and even their pets ate kibble that wasn't mega-processed.

I want to briefly look at two things that may seem like they don't matter much when compared to major diseases and conditions: your skin and hair. These are important for two reasons. First, skin and hair problems may indicate other systemic issues. Second, there's a relationship between how you look and how you function.

Outer appearance is a barometer of inner health. When we look strong and vibrant, most likely, we feel that way, too. And what we do in the kitchen is as important as what we do in front of the bathroom mirror. That's because both skin and hair are nourished by vitamins and nutrients that keep them strong and vibrant. It's no surprise that antioxidants and vitamins are key ingredients in many topical skin and hair products, since these nutrients help feed the supporting structures that build your hair and skin.

As you've probably figured out, I love stories about how ancient cultures used food to improve their health. They also knew how food and appearance were linked. The ancient Aztecs were believed to eat avocados not just because of the flavor, but because the oil helped rehydrate their skin in harshly windy climates. Far Eastern cultures have long used various herbs as topical ingredients to revitalize skin. The ancient Egyptians used

PREP SCHOOL

Make the most of skin-friendly foods: The antioxidants in tomatoes and carrots—lycopene and beta-carotene—are more potent when you cook them in a healthy fat, like olive oil. Foods with the antioxidant vitamin C (peppers, broccoli, kale) are best eaten raw or stir-fried just enough to heat them without sapping their color or crunch. By the way, the average American eats twenty-two pounds of tomatoes a year. A full 59 percent of those are canned, and pizza is a major delivery system. Then there are the sugar-laden ketchups and sauces—processed forms, rather than the real thing. Eat them the way nature intended.

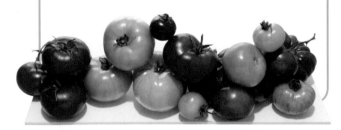

YOU'VE GOT FOOD ON YOUR FACE

You can make your own exfoliating scrub with food sources and use it to gently slough away dead cells for a fresher complexion. Do it once or twice a week at night and before you wash your face. Mix and match the ingredients below (one from each column) to create your own skin-saving concoctions.

Exfoliant (4 TABLESPOONS)	Binder (4 TABLESPOONS)	Oil (A FEW DROPS, OPTIONAL, FOR SCENT)	Booster (2 TEASPOONS)

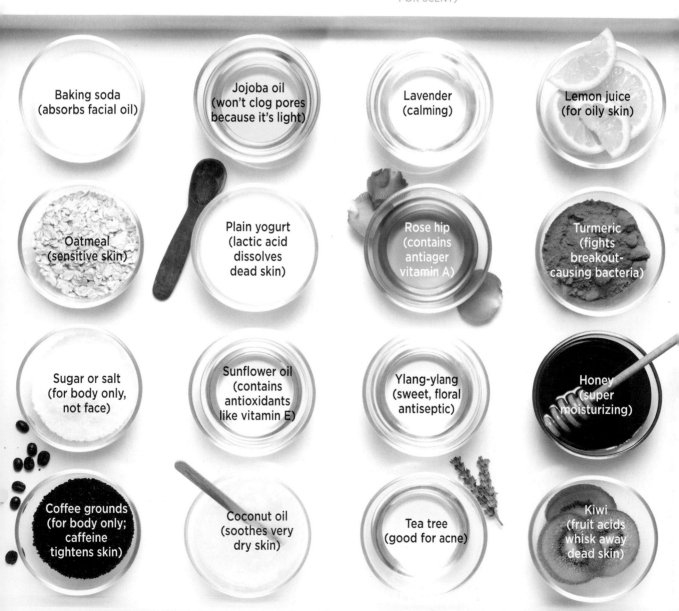

Exfoliant

Baking soda (absorbs facial oil)

Oatmeal (sensitive skin)

Sugar or salt (for body only, not face)

Coffee grounds (for body only; caffeine tightens skin)

Binder

Jojoba oil (won't clog pores because it's light)

Plain yogurt (lactic acid dissolves dead skin)

Sunflower oil (contains antioxidants like vitamin E)

Coconut oil (soothes very dry skin)

Oil

Lavender (calming)

Rose hip (contains antiager vitamin A)

Ylang-ylang (sweet, floral antiseptic)

Tea tree (good for acne)

Booster

Lemon juice (for oily skin)

Turmeric (fights breakout-causing bacteria)

Honey (super moisturizing)

Kiwi (fruit acids whisk away dead skin)

oils like sesame to make skin look soft and youthful; they produced soap using olive oil; and Cleopatra was thought to take milk baths as a way to exfoliate and soothe her skin.

These cultures intuitively experimented with food to fortify and beautify their bodies. They stuck with what they found effective. We do that, today. When my daughter Arabella was going through some periods of dry and dull skin, we suggested she boost her diet with omega-3 fatty acids because of the oil's healthy properties. (We actually tried this on our pets first, and when their coats improved dramatically, we moved on to experimenting with Arabella. This was my mother-in-law's idea, so I would have blamed her if it had failed!) The change worked, likely because omega-3s are rich in two compounds (DHA and EPA) linked to improved skin. (Though

IS YOUR HAIR HUNGRY FOR THESE?

Your hair can look and be healthier when you use certain foodie ingredients as part of your cleansing process (once a week or so is fine for these).

Argan oil: An oil that comes from the nut of a tree in Morocco, it contains antioxidants and vitamin E. Argan oil helps prevent hair from breaking and makes it feel smooth and soft. Rub a dime-sized drop into wet hair. Comb it in to distribute evenly, then style your hair as you normally would.

Brown sugar: A natural exfoliant. It can remove dead cells on your scalp. Combine it with avocado oil (filled with vitamins and antioxidants). Mix one part avocado oil and two parts brown sugar. Wet your hair and rub the mixture into your scalp for a few minutes. Rinse, then shampoo and condition as you normally would.

Espresso: You can put a shot in your conditioner to help give your brown hair a color refresh, making it look deep and rich. Those with blond hair can use chamomile tea, and redheads can use one part carrot juice and one part beet juice. Mix the ingredients into the conditioner and work the mixture through wet hair. Let it sit for fifteen minutes, then rinse thoroughly. Reapply conditioner (without the added ingredients) and rinse again.

ARGANÖL

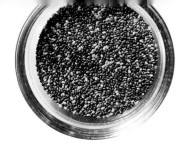

There are so many ways to use omega-3 stars; here's just one: Soak 1 tablespoon of chia seeds in 1 tablespoon of water to plump them, then stir them into salad dressing.

FACE FACT

If your skin is pink from the inflammatory conditions rosacea or acne, there could be trouble in your gut. Foods like kale that have prebiotics (a type of fiber that feeds the good bacteria in your digestive system) may help. Walnuts have lots of omega-3 fats, which can also calm skin breakouts.

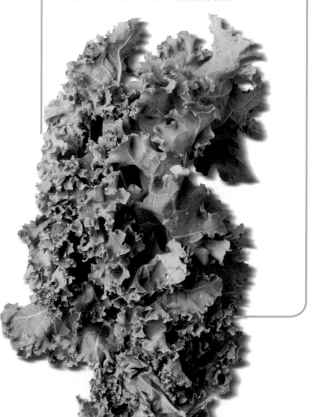

Arabella's problem wasn't acne, the fats have been shown to alleviate that condition as well.) As you remember, these fats are found in cold-water fish, including salmon, tuna, and sardines, but you can also get them in walnuts, chia seeds, or flaxseed.

The lesson? What's good for the body on the inside is also good for the body on the outside. If you try the 21-Day Plan and follow the FIXES formula going forward, you will not only tap into ingredients that benefit your skin and hair, you'll also weed out some of the culprits that can steal your glow. Not surprisingly, one of the worst things for your skin is sugar (and refined carbohydrates). Why? You guessed it: inflammation. When you eat sweetened foods, it causes your blood sugar to spike for about fifteen minutes. In response, your body churns out a type of protein that triggers inflammation. Anecdotally, some people report skin issues after eating sweet foods, and this might be one of the reasons. In addition, higher blood sugar can stiffen up collagen fibers, which may make the skin less springy. Sugar also sticks to proteins and makes your skin sallow. This is why diabetics may have a discolored complexion.

Your skin is your anatomical wrapping paper. Most of us only care about it when it burns, wrinkles, or breaks out in unidentified thingamajigs (are those ant bites, pimples, or some kind of fungus?), but we ought to show our skin a bit more appreciation, considering its genius structure. Containing 70 percent water, 25 percent protein, and 5 percent fat, your skin is your body's largest organ, and it makes up 15 percent of your body weight. Skin acts as a barrier to the outside environment, but it's also an absorber. For example, there are thousands of chemicals in our modern world that can be readily absorbed by our skin. You want to feed your wrapper with nutrients that will strengthen not just its appearance, but also fortify its underlying structures, to help keep irritating chemicals out of the body.

Your epidermis—the outside layer—is the part of the skin that we all see. Because dead cells slough off approximately every thirty days, it's a self-rejuvenating layer. The innermost layer, called the subcutaneous tissue, is made up of fat and helps insulate your body.

The real action happens in the dermis, the middle layer of your skin. This is where you find the hair follicles and sweat glands, plus tiny blood vessels (they feed your skin nutrients) and lymph nodes to help fend off toxins.

WASH YOUR SKIN FROM THE INSIDE

Part of the reason skin gets damaged is lack of moisture. Drinking plenty of water every day (there's no magic number, but eight glasses is a nice goal to shoot for) will help produce a Broadway spotlight glow. Many fresh foods are mostly water (cucumbers are 96 percent water and tomatoes are 94 percent water). Munch a piece of watermelon, too, because its high water content makes it great at hydrating the skin. Other fruits with the same effect are cantaloupe, honeydew, and strawberries.

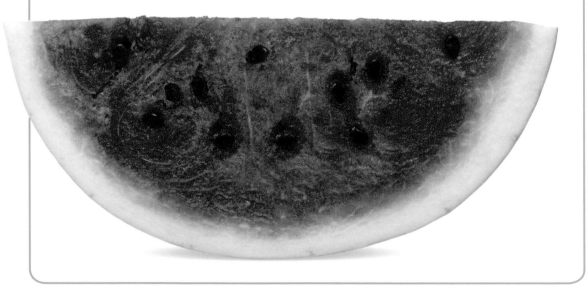

The dermis is made up of cells called fibroblasts. These are your workhorse cells, because they make collagen and elastin—proteins that give skin its strength, suppleness, and resilience.

One of the main reasons skin ages or loses its glow is the gradual weakening of collagen and elastin. When they get damaged (from aging, sun exposure, toxins, and poor diet), skin loses its ability to stretch. It gets rigid, sags, and splits.

Because your skin is attached to muscle, creases can form when you move your face and body. Over time, that area forms a groove. It's sort of like a stress fracture; repeated movement over time wears skin down, which creates inflammation and damages the collagen. Years pass and the process causes the groove to deepen: That's a wrinkle.

So if you want to minimize damage that comes in the form of wrinkles and overall dullness, you need to protect your skin from outside assaults (by regularly using sunscreen), and also nourish it with a variety of foods that keep elastin and collagen strong.

Now, a quick look at your hair: The average person's head has up to 150,000 hair follicles. That number stays consistent over time; what changes is the thickness and condition of the strands, and if they actually stay on your head. Perhaps the most interesting thing to know about hair health is that each strand has its own blood supply—blood from the body feeds into the tiny blood vessels in the hair follicle. That's the living part—the bulb at the base of the strand. The actual strand we see above the skin is the dead part, though it is made up of proteins that influence how your hair looks. The right foods help nourish the cells that make hair grow lush, and improve the quality of oils that lubricate each strand to give it a shiny appearance.

My plan and FIXES foods are loaded with nutrients that will improve the skin on your face, your scalp, and all over your body. Want to *really* focus on skin health? Kick off every day with a breakfast specifically designed to get you glowing. Try these suggestions:

EVERYONE'S FAVORITE SUPERFOOD

High-quality chocolate has flavonoids shown to boost blood flow to the top layer of the skin by up to 100 percent, delivering oxygen, vitamins, and minerals to the epidermis so it can build new cells, one study found. My three favorite kinds of chocolate? Dark chocolate with 70% cacao or more, cacao nibs, and unsweetened dark cocoa powder.

Drink up: Start with a cup of green tea. Women who drank it regularly for three months experienced 25 percent less damage when exposed to UV rays, according to a study in the *Journal of Nutrition*. Green tea contains a catechin called EGCG, an antioxidant believed to promote good skin health by protecting against sun damage (but you still need sunscreen). Also, make sure to drink water throughout the day.

Eat one of these:

Option 1: Veggie omelet. Eggs contain lysine and proline, which are amino acids that help form collagen. Don't be yolk-shy: They have vitamin B12, which may fight against dark spots, plus hydrating nutrients like lutein and zeaxanthin. Add any veggies you like, and be sure to include some spinach. (See the recipe on page 310.) Dark leafy greens are full of phytonutrients called carotenoids, which help keep skin taut. Yellow peppers, carrots, and squash are good choices as well, because of their carotenoids. One study by British researchers found that women with a higher intake of them had fewer crow's-feet. Add some shiitake mushrooms, which are a good source of zinc, a mineral that's been shown to improve skin's ability to heal itself; they also have copper, which your body needs to build collagen.

Option 2: Oatmeal with add-ons/Smoothie with add-ins. Whether you choose oatmeal or a smoothie, include one or more of these ingredients:

Chia seeds, which have 5,000 milligrams of omega-3 fatty acids per 2 tablespoons. Omega-3s help prevent the loss of moisture in the skin, thus slowing down the formation of wrinkles. Eating omega-3s may also help fend off melanoma.

GRAY ANATOMY

A deficiency in vitamin B9 (folic acid) or B12 can lead to prematurely gray hair. These vitamins help with the production of DNA and RNA and help produce methionine, an amino acid connected to hair color. Foods rich in folate, the natural form of folic acid, include asparagus, chickpeas, lentils, lima beans, spinach, and cooked rice and pasta. Adults should get 400 micrograms of folate a day (600 micrograms for pregnant women and 500 micrograms for women who are breastfeeding).

Pomegranate seeds, for their antioxidants and vitamin C, which helps stimulate new skin cells. One study found that those whose diets were high in vitamin C were less likely to have a dry, wrinkly complexion.

Raspberries, because they contain the antioxidant ellagic acid, which protects against collagen-sapping sun damage.

Unsweetened coconut, which is high in an anti-inflammatory fat. By keeping inflammation low, it helps prevent the breakdown of collagen.

Option 3: The grab-and-go. Need a breakfast that's quick, but also skin-friendly? Try a piece of whole-grain toast with almond butter, banana slices, and a squirt of honey. Two tablespoons of almond butter give you 50 percent of your daily vitamin E needs, an antioxidant that fends off free radical damage that can lead to premature aging and skin cancer. It also has unsaturated fatty acids, which combat dryness and soften wrinkles. Honey has trace minerals like manganese and selenium to fight free radicals, and it's less likely than white sugar to cause the blood sugar spikes linked to skin aging.

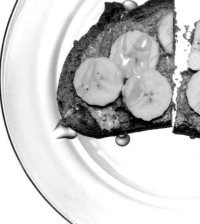

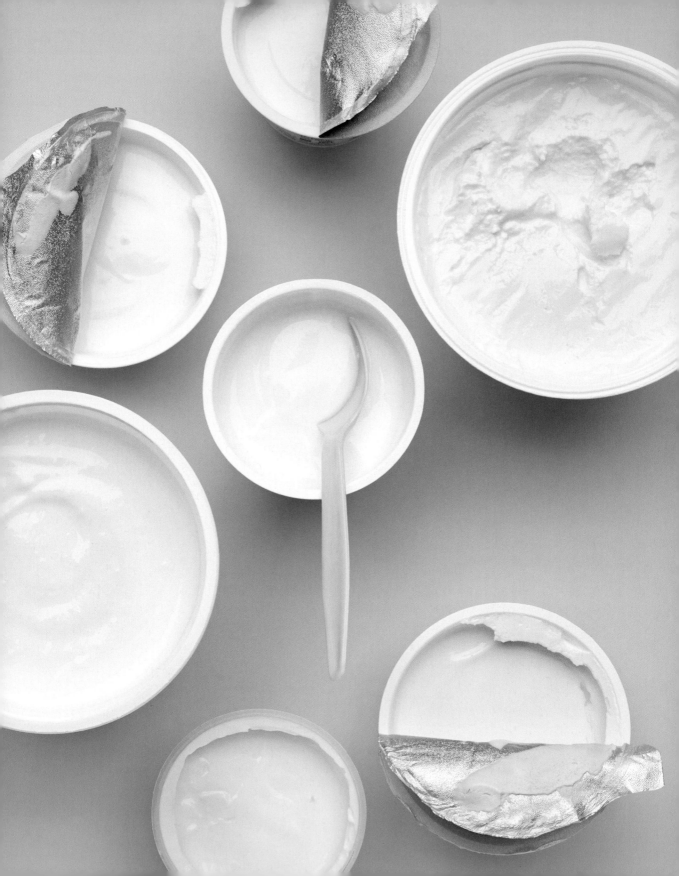

13.

Food FIXES
for a Healthy Gut

The digestive system is one of your body's command centers. Keep it happy and you'll do more than settle your belly— you'll improve your overall health.

When most people think about the gut, their minds go to a couple of places. Possibly first: *Why is mine so big?* And second: *Why do I have bloating, gas, constipation, or an overall yucky feeling?*

No matter what you're thinking right now, I want you to hang on one second and consider this: Your gut—the intricate system of organs involved in the digestive process—is really your second brain, because it plays a major role in your moods, your immunity, and many other aspects of your general health. So before I get into the common tummy ailments, it's important for everyone—whether you suffer from bellyaches or not—to understand one of your body's main control centers.

Like your brain, your stomach, colon, and small intestines pilot so much of what you do, how you feel, your behaviors, and your health outcomes. These organs even share hormones in common with your brain. For example, the feel-good hormone serotonin is in large abundance in your gut. Let's look at how it all works together and why this chapter is about more than just constipation and bloating.

You have 100 trillion or so bacteria living in your body—this world is referred to as the microbiome. Different types of bacteria perform different functions, and they come in the classic good versus evil variety. Some can help your health, and some can hurt it. Your goal isn't to eradicate the bad ones; the key is to establish an equilibrium. Some researchers like to equate the system to a rain forest, because you need a wide variety to allow the ecosystem to flourish. The good kind, unsurprisingly, make your system thrive. The bad guys can cause trouble when there's too many of them, and can become toxic to the body.

A thriving rain forest is diverse, and the same can be said about the microbiome. The more types of beneficial bugs you house, the healthier you're likely to be. There's a lot to be discovered about these microbes, but we do know that the gut holds the richest diversity of them in the body—more than a thousand species. Many experts believe that your gut health may have as much effect on your overall health as your genes. For example, it seems that bacteria in your gut influence a number of things, such as:

Inflammation: Some of your bugs take nutrients from your diet and do good with them. When you eat right, these bugs help your body make vitamins and turn food into other nutrients, like short-chain fatty acids—which are some of the most powerful anti-inflammatory agents in the body. But when you eat unhealthy fats and starches, your bad bacteria are more likely to secrete a substance called endotoxin that sparks your immune system to go on the defensive, triggering inflammation.

Appetite: Scientists have observed that slim people have a diverse population of bacteria, while overweight people have less variety. One form of bacteria seems to have an influ-

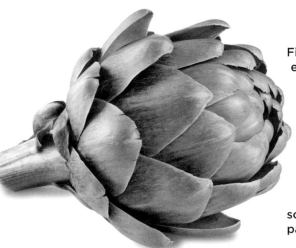

Fiber-rich artichokes are an adventure to eat and easier to prepare than you might think. Just cut off and discard the tough outer leaves and trim the sharp points off the remaining leaves. Boil water with a squirt of lemon juice and add the chokes. Lower the heat, cover, and simmer for thirty to forty minutes. Serve with a squeeze of lemon juice and a little salt. To eat, peel off the leaves and pull off the delicious soft flesh with your teeth. Messy and tasty! When you reach the fuzzy protective layer over the artichoke heart, scrape it away. The soft heart underneath is sweet, tender, and the best part of all.

ence on levels of the hormone ghrelin, which controls your appetite. Your food choices can have an impact on these bugs; for example, nondigestible compounds in apples promote the growth of friendly gut bacteria, which stabilize metabolism and help you feel full.

Immunity: Nearly three-quarters of your fighter immune cells live in your gut. So your immune system and gut communicate with each other, making decisions about what to attack. Researchers believe that the more diverse your gut bacteria, the more finely tuned your immune system will be.

Mood: Because of the abundance of serotonin in the gut, your intestines influence your emotional state, too. Having a diverse gut microbiome seems to help lower depressive symptoms.

Perhaps best of all, good bacteria can play a role in helping you eat more of the FIXES foods by stopping your cravings for junk. When you eat good foods, the bacteria in your gut ferments them and produces gas and short-chain fatty acids—that's what signals your brain to stop eating foods that can have harmful effects.

You don't have to do anything exotic or complicated to improve the ecosystem inside you. No point in obsessing about which strains of "good" bacteria you're getting, because scientists say there's not enough research yet to pinpoint the key players in big issues like obesity, heart disease, or brain health. For now, a healthy diet is the number one way to create a robust microbiome. Once you start making changes, your bugs respond rapidly and the composition of your gut bacteria can change within hours.

Your primary goal is to eat plenty of fiber, which is guaranteed on the FIXES plan. Fiber is your microbiome's favorite food. While your bugs eat all the same nutrients you do, it's fiber that feeds the "good" bugs. The big problem with most simple starches and low-fiber foods is that few actually make it to your colon, where the vast majority of your bugs live. Simple carbohydrates and sugar are immediately absorbed through the small intestine and move on to various body parts to be used as energy or turned into fat. Anything that's not used keeps traveling through your system. On the flip side, foods rich in fiber don't get digested in the stomach or absorbed in the small intestine, which means they get to keep traveling until they reach the colon, where they become food for the healthy bacteria there. A few fiber superstars to look for: almonds, artichokes, barley, beans, jicama, and oats. Some of these foods—artichokes and oats, for example—are prebiotics, meaning they help improve the function of the good bacteria already in your gut.

In addition, if you embrace experimentation with your produce, you can help diversify your gut's ecosystem. So don't just rely on two or three vegetables you like; take a chance on a new fruit or veggie every time you shop. It could solve dinner boredom along with a host of body issues.

Now for your next question: What about probiotics? They've been touted as the key to repopulating your gut with good bacteria, and they come in a variety of fermented food forms (yogurt, sauerkraut, and kefir products all contain organisms purported to improve gut health). In terms of microbiome health—that is, diversity of bacterial population—there's no way to know whether a particular strain in a particular food is the one you need to diversify your own personal gut population. So healthy fermented foods are good, but don't pour money into iffy supplements. Instead, emphasize generally fiber-rich foods, as well as a wide range of fruits and vegetables.

Bellyaches

Now you know the global view of the gut and how you can influence it to shore up

Good bacteria turn cabbage into sauerkraut. Not a fan? Try miso, soy sauce, kefir, yogurt, kimchi, or fermented pickles.

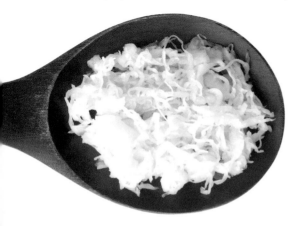

your overall health. But what's happening when you're bothered by GI issues? We're talking about a wide variety of complaints from going to the bathroom too much or not enough, bloating, certain foods disagreeing with you, or just overall stormy feelings brewing in your center.

I remember one woman from an early episode of my show. Her bothersome symptom: She would poop only once a week. Once a week? Heck, I knew people who seemed to go once when the sun rose, once when the sun set, and twice in between. But I had never known anyone who flushed her digestive system only one time every 168 hours. She felt frustrated and uncomfortable, as if her belly were loaded with bricks. Even worse, she was sure there was nothing she could do about the problem.

I gave her a simple fix: more fiber in her diet. Since the average person only gets about 16 grams of it a day and she was well below that, we gradually increased her to 25 grams a day, using more fruits and vegetables and fiber heroes like beans. (We did it slowly because if you increase fiber all at once, it comes with a side order of a lot of extra gas.) Her story had a happy ending: She quickly got "regular" and relieved the symptoms she had been experiencing.

For people dealing with a tumultuous gut, I recommend using food to help calm the turmoil. And you can tweak the Rx depending on your problem.

Overall belly discomfort: Even if you're not diagnosed with something specific like celiac disease (in which gluten damages the small intestine), you might have an intolerance to certain foods or nutrients. In these cases, you may want to eliminate foods on a rotating basis to see if you can identify the troublemaker.

The most common way people do this is by eliminating wheat products from their diet. You stop eating all forms of wheat, even the good whole-grain kinds, to see if it's the source of your pain and discomfort. Many people find that they can settle their stomachs this way.

You can try this with other food groups as well—for example, with dairy products or meat. Mind you, those groups aren't *bad*; it just goes back to what I said early in this book. We're all made differently, and how our bodies react to certain foods differs from person to person. Experimentation can go a long way in pinpointing the source of your tummy ruckus.

To do an elimination diet, remove just one group of foods at a time (do more than that, and you won't know what the trigger is if you start to feel better). Go for a week or two, and if you don't feel any better, add back what you just eliminated, and try cutting out a different food group.

Constipation: As I told the woman on my show, it's all about fiber, fiber, fiber. We simply don't get enough, and fiber helps move

YES TO YOGURT

Yogurt—milk fermented with bacteria—can help your digestive health because its beneficial bacteria can ease some symptoms associated with a cranky bowel. I like old-world yogurt—Greek yogurt—because it is strained to remove the whey, which makes it thicker and protein-rich. But don't just eat it because it'll help your gut. Yogurt helps improve blood pressure because of its potassium content (there's more in a cup of yogurt than in a banana). It strengthens bones with its calcium; some yogurts are also fortified with vitamin D, which helps you absorb the calcium. And it lowers your risk of developing type 2 diabetes. According to a Harvard University study, one serving of yogurt a day lowered the chance of getting the disease by 18 percent, possibly because its probiotics quiet inflammation and balance blood sugar levels. A super way to eat yogurt: Add chia seeds. Chia absorbs twenty-seven times its weight in water, forming a thick gel that slows digestion and can help regulate blood sugar.

things through the gut. When combined with water, it forms a gel-like substance that expands in your digestive tract so you are no longer trying to push what feels like toothpaste through five feet of colon. Fiber also decreases appetite, as it takes up more volume in your digestive tract, which dials down the hormones that increase appetite and keeps you feeling satisfied longer.

Diarrhea: Though probiotics won't necessarily repopulate your microbiome, there is some evidence to suggest that they can help with diarrhea. For example, studies have shown that two strains of beneficial bacteria (*Lactobacillus GG* and *Saccharomyces*) can shorten a bout of diarrhea when it's related to taking antibiotics or a dangerous colon bug called *Clostridium difficile*. (That bacteria can be deadly. Make sure you see your doctor to establish the cause for any extended bout of diarrhea.) And in several studies, probiotics (*B. infantis*) can help calm some symptoms of irritable bowel syndrome (like abdominal pain and bloating).

Bloating: Several foods may help you feel less like a parade float and more like yourself. For example:

Asparagus has a natural diuretic effect that helps flush excess water from your body. (Cabbage and cauliflower, on the other hand, make you gassy.)

Fennel or fennel seeds can reduce gas and that puffy feeling.

Ginger can help you expel some gas that may be contributing to your pain.

Papaya contains a substance called papain that helps your body break down hard-to-digest foods. It can act as a laxative to help move the bowels and ease the constipation that may be causing gas and bloating.

Pumpkin can act as a mild diuretic to help you get rid of excess water.

I want to tell one more story to emphasize the important role your digestive system plays in other systems in your body. When my daughter Zoe was seventeen, her thyroid levels were so out of whack that her doctor recommended medication to regulate them. But like most teenagers, she didn't want to be stuck on medication, which would disrupt her thyroid function and be hard to wean off of. So we experimented with diet. She eliminated wheat, dairy, and red meat. And she didn't just eliminate, she also added powerful FIXES foods to her plate. Her thyroid levels

COOL CARB-TERNATIVES

One of the most common ways to settle down a cranky digestive system is to get rid of refined carbs and sugars. But cheer up—that doesn't immediately translate to "no more pasta." There are plenty of less-processed pasta alternatives that contain more useful nutrients and taste great. Here's what you get in a 1 cup serving of these options:

Brown rice noodles: 4 grams of fiber; 4 grams of protein

Chickpea pasta: 8 grams of fiber; 14 grams of protein

Quinoa pasta: 4 grams of fiber; 4 grams of protein

Soba noodles: 3 grams of fiber; 6 grams of protein. These are made from nutty buckwheat. Some early studies show that buckwheat's compounds, flavonoids like quercetin, might help cognition and memory. Buckwheat is also a good source of vitamin B and magnesium.

If you do eat regular pasta, quell the effect of refined carbs by bringing in fiber and healthy fats (think sautéed tomatoes and olive oil). Cook pasta until it is just al dente to lower its glycemic index.

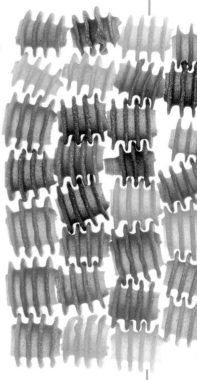

went back to normal without meds, and more than five years later, she hasn't had a problem since. She is still off bread and red meat, but has reintegrated dairy, and her thyroid is doing great.

While Zoe doesn't have celiac disease, it is interesting to note the connection between the gut and hormonal issues. There is evidence to suggest a link between celiac disease and auto-immune issues involving the thyroid, but it's not clear whether one causes the other or if there might be a genetic disposition.

Whatever the reason, Zoe's recovery underscores the importance of working the nutrition angle to help cure what ails you. Turn to the next chapter to meet your army of superfoods, and start nourishing your "second brain" along with every other part of you.

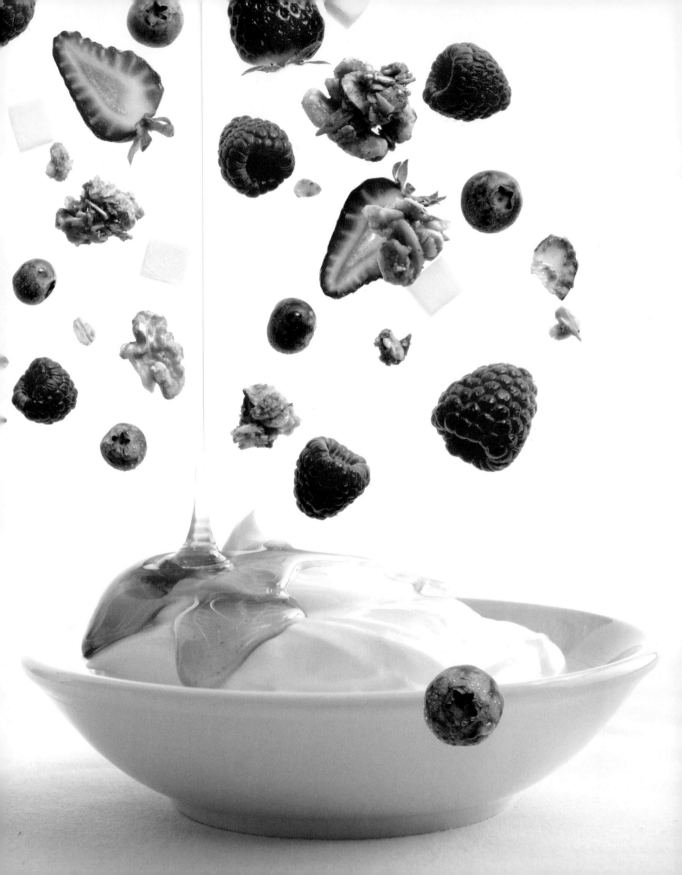

PART 3

EAT IT, LOVE IT, LIVE IT

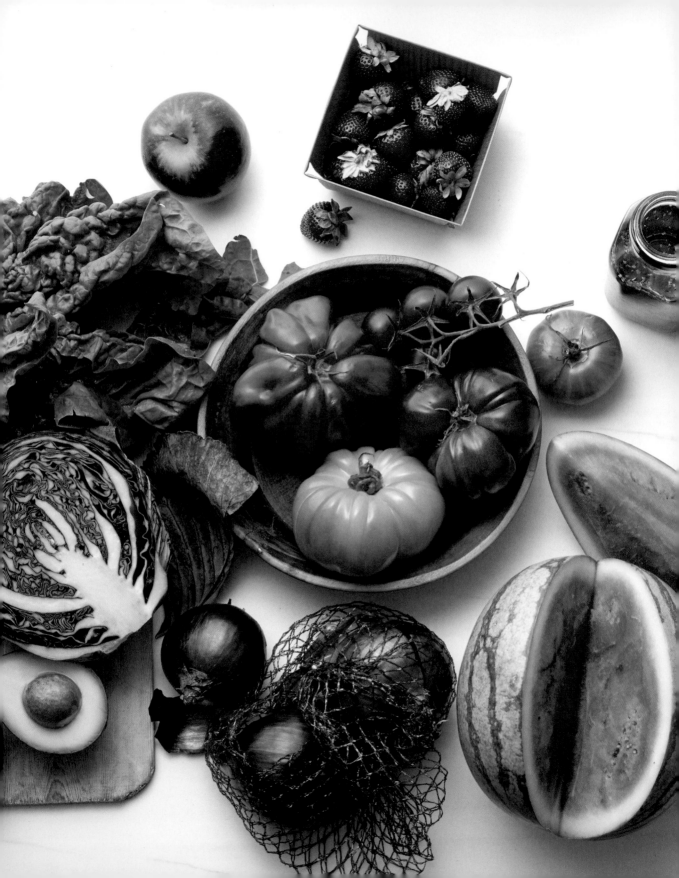

14

The *Food Can Fix It* 21-Day Plan

To a child, three weeks before a birthday seems like a lifetime away. To an adult, three weeks to get a major project finished whizzes by. It's all about your perspective. When you're looking at the entire spectrum of your life, twenty-one days is a blip—just a small moment among many.

So here's what I ask of you. Give me one of your blips.

Stay with me for three weeks. That will give you the time to:

- Retrain your palate
- Begin to experiment in the kitchen
- Automate new healthy habits that will swallow up old, unhealthy ones
- Shed a little weight—if you're looking to lose extra pounds
- Teach your body how good it feels to eat foods that heal

I want to be clear. I'm not hawking a "lose twenty-one pounds in twenty-one days" crash diet. And I'm not at all implying that you can switch up your eating for a few weeks and erase heart disease or reverse diabetes.

This is a sensible, well-paced plan. It won't make you feel deprived or hangry, or fill your brain with visions of cheeseburgers. Follow it faithfully and you could lose three to four pounds in the first week—mostly water weight, but it feels great!—and one to two pounds a week afterward, most likely shedding seven to eight pounds by the end of week three, since the menu is full of satiating meals that help your body feel full on less. Not bad for a blip of your time. (If weight loss isn't one of your goals, no problem. An online calorie intake calculator, such as the My Weight Manager at www.supertracker.usda.gov, can help you figure out how much you should be eating to maintain your current weight. Once you know, you can play around with portion sizes and additional snacks.)

Think of this program as a great first date that will lead to a new relationship between you and food—an invigorating, delicious, lifelong bond. You'll fall in love with foods that satisfy and energize while you leave behind calorie-dense junk that packs on weight, hurts your health, and generally makes you feel lousy. In the end, this way of eating—started now and continued for good (see chapter 16 for day twenty-two and beyond)—will help you normalize your weight and recalibrate many of your body's systems.

This is the way to let food fix it.

Why twenty-one days? That timing gained some traction in the world of behavioral science starting in the 1960s, and it has remained a commonly accepted period for making changes and ingraining them as habits. Because we can't just get rid of bad old ways; they need to be replaced by good new ways, and rewiring your neurons takes a few weeks.

Here's what you can expect from these three weeks: You'll eat way more vegetables than ever before and make friends with all the FIXES foods from chapter 2—several per meal, in fact.

You'll eat foods that have been shown to reduce cravings on a chemical level. (Remember page 159, where you learned about fatty acids that signal to your brain to quell can't-stop-eating urges? Those show up here.)

You'll pull way back on added sugar and retrain your palate so you don't even miss it. You'll replace guilty pleasures with foods you feel good about (no need for those little sugar-plus-fat bombs that drop out of the vending machine at three P.M.). You'll eat healthy fats—more than you thought were "allowed" and enough to keep you happily satiated.

You'll also cook more from scratch, and find it surprisingly easy. You'll discover flavor-boosting kitchen tricks that prove vegetables can dazzle your taste buds *without* being deep-fried, coated in goopy sauce, or otherwise stripped of their nutritional value. (See the next chapter for the delicious recipes.)

My plan brings whole foods to the forefront, because they're more of a home game to the body. Remember the big lesson from chapter 2: Your cells and organs immediately recognize and understand what they're dealing with. Unlike highly processed food, your body knows exactly where to direct the nutrients in whole foods to promote your overall well-being. Plus, they're more filling, more flavorful, and less padded with the junky stuff that puts weight on your body.

With more than thirty delicious, filling,

and easy meals to choose from (all with super-food ingredients), you will not only find recipes you like, but you'll also redefine culinary pleasure for yourself. Most important, you'll start reversing any damage caused by your old, less-than-ideal ways of eating.

If you're the kind of person who does better sticking to a detailed outline, then by all means, follow the 21-Day Plan to a T and use it as your nutritional road map. But you can also swap meals to address your personal health concerns or to accommodate your lifestyle. Mix and match breakfasts, lunches, dinners, and snacks to your heart's content (literally). Above all, I want this plan to be easy. To that end, I've calculated all the calorie counts for you—breakfast clocks in under 420 calories per serving, lunch at 430 or fewer calories, snacks at under 400 calories total per day, and dinner at 520 or fewer calories—so you don't have to worry about tallying. I'm also including a shopping list (see page 181) to make stocking up a cinch.

You're three weeks away from feeling slimmer, healthier, happier—and understanding how you want to eat for the rest of your life. Let's get started.

The 21-Day Plan: Basics

Every day, for three weeks, you'll eat three meals a day and two snacks. You can follow the schedule I've laid out for you, or you can choose from five breakfast recipes, seven lunches, twenty-one dinners, and twenty-one

snacks. If you decide to make your own schedule, just hold to these five simple rules:

1. Eat fish at *least* twice a week. As we've seen in previous chapters, fish has been linked to heart health, brain health, and overall longevity. Leftovers are your best friend here—you can make a salmon entrée for dinner one night and use a leftover fillet as a salad protein for lunch the next day. (See my take on mercury on page 128.)

2. Treat red meat like a treat. Red meats like beef and pork aren't as good for you as the leaner kinds of protein (like poultry, fish, and veggie-based proteins). It's not entirely off the table, but you shouldn't have it every night, either. That goes double if you're watching your cholesterol levels. So I've only included one red meat recipe on my plan—a salad with skirt steak—and you should make it no more than twice during these twenty-one days. (Red meat FYIs: In general, it's best to stick to cuts of beef that are at least 90% lean. Choose grass-fed meats over grain-fed when you can.

3. Lean into beans. Research increasingly suggests that your body benefits from plant-based proteins. At least once a week, try to have a plant-centric dinner, with beans, legumes, or tofu playing the starring role on your plate.

4. Hydrate. Often your brain confuses thirst for hunger, leading you to overeat when all you really needed was to chug some water, so aim for eight or more glasses a day. Do whatever it

TRY NEW FOODS—LIKE THESE!

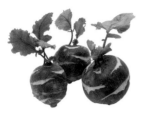

Kohlrabi: Related to cabbage, very tasty raw or cooked, roasted, or tossed into soup.

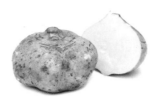

Jicama: Crunchy and delicious sliced into chunks in a salad.

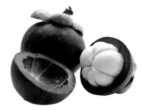

Mangosteen: Sweet and a good source of vitamin C.

takes to make that happen—whether it's buying bottles of the sparkling, unsweetened kind, jazzing it up with squeezes of fresh citrus juice, or setting a phone alarm to remind you to sip.

5. Be food-brave. If you come across an unfamiliar ingredient, like the three you see above, try it. If you encounter a food you're *meh* about, give it a second chance. Quite possibly it was prepped badly when you were a kid, or canned instead of fresh, or your palate just wasn't primed for it then (but will be soon). In other words, don't let a memory of bland tofu or a soggy heap of greens keep you from experiencing a perfectly seasoned tofu steak or our crunchy rainbow salad with buttermilk dressing. Prepare to be converted.

Here's what this plan serves up:

A dose of protein with every meal. This macronutrient's satiating powers are unparalleled. You'll get a hit at breakfast, lunch, and dinner to help you feel full and *stay* that way longer.

At least two servings of complex carbohydrates every day. Bring on the brown rice, beans, and whole grains. (Whole wheat pasta? A-OK. Whole-grain bread? Go right ahead.) They're excellent sources of fiber, which, like protein, helps you feel full. Fiber also aids digestion, helps to lower "bad" LDL cholesterol, and is less likely to spike your blood sugar levels than simple carbs—things like white bread, white pasta, cookies, cake— that yo-yo your energy.

As many nonstarchy vegetables as your heart desires. Any veggie listed on page 172 is fair game. I'll shout out tips for how to snack on them or add them to recipes, but feel free to pile them sky-high onto whatever you're eating. (Noshing on veggies between meals and snacks works, too.)

Just the right amount of fruit. That's one to two servings a day. Not all fruits are created equal. Some fruits—like apples, berries, cherries, pears, grapefruits, plums, and peaches— are less likely to spike your blood sugar and

THE FITNESS FACTOR

This meal plan is geared for the needs of a moderately active person—meaning someone who gets in 2½ hours of moderate aerobic exercise every week. There are plenty of ways to hit that mark. A two-hour hike on a Saturday and a midweek workout class will get you there. So will taking three brisk, ten-minute walks every day but weekends. Alternatively, you could take an hour-long water aerobics class, play a few sets of doubles tennis, and take a thirty-minute powerwalk. Or you could really cobble it together with four 15-minute brisk walks, a half hour jog after work one day, thirty minutes of yardwork on a weekend, and two 15-minute stints of body weight exercises, like push-ups, wall sits, and lunges. The possibilities are endless.

What this means for the diet: If you're less active than the above, you might only need one snack instead of two. If weight loss is an important goal for you, try skipping one snack a few days a week. On the other hand, if you're *more* than moderately active—meaning that you either work in three-plus hours of moderate exercise every week *or* that you opt for more intense exercise (like running, swimming laps, or interval training), you may want to add another snack before workouts.

spark cravings than other fruits (such as pineapple and watermelon). But that doesn't mean you can't have other kinds. You just have to pair them with the right stuff. In my plan, fruits are always paired with a protein-rich food (such as nuts or yogurt) that help to balance out their natural sugar content and avoid those side effects. (And if you've never tried watermelon pizza, you've got to—just top watermelon wedges with a little feta, some fresh mint, and a pinch of coarse salt.) You'll get a serving of fruit nearly every morning with breakfast, and if you're craving something sweet later in the day, you can have a fruity snack.

A healthier approach to fats. New research increasingly shows that the best kinds of fats—the monounsaturated kind—raise your "good" HDL cholesterol to keep your blood

levels in check. And you've heard how they benefit the brain, blood flow, digestion, inflammation, and more. Accordingly, you'll be having up to 2 tablespoons olive or canola oil per day on this plan. You'll also eat healthy fats in their whole-food form in fish, avocados, nuts, seeds, and more.

One thing missing from the plan? Added sugars. You won't find any extra sweet stuff in these recipes. For just these three weeks, I'm going to ask you to limit your added sugars to no more than 3 teaspoons a day. (Extra credit for swearing off completely—but if you think you'll feel deprived and depressed without a spoonful of sugar in your coffee or a drizzle of honey on your yogurt, it's not worth making yourself crazy.) When I say sugar, I'm talking about sugar in all forms: the

THE **ARTICHOKES**-TO-**ZUCCHINI** UNLIMITED VEGGIE LIST

All vegetables are good vegetables, but these nonstarchy picks do the best job at filling you up for very few calories. Eat as many as you want, whenever you want 'em. You can snack on them raw, with a splash of vinegar (such as balsamic) or lemon juice for flavor. You can also steam them and add them to any meal to plump it out. If you come across one of these veggies in a recipe, feel free to add more than what the recipe calls for. (This works especially well with leafy greens—they cook down nicely into just about anything.) I've noted some tasty ways to snack on these and to add them to meals throughout, but be creative—the veggie sky's the limit.

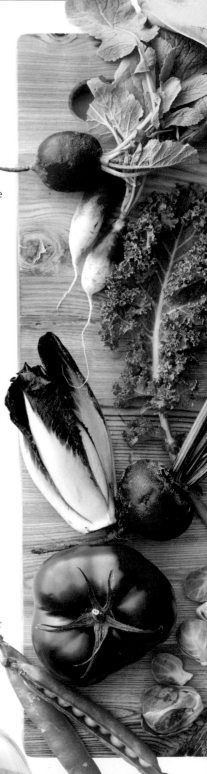

Artichokes Simple prep instructions are on page 158. Or use canned if they are packed in water.

Asparagus

Bamboo shoots, canned. Add to a pot of brown rice for flavor, toss into a stir-fry, or slice thin and add to a salad for crunch.

Beets

Broccoli If you buy a head of broccoli, you can spiralize the stem and add it to a pasta dish to bulk it up. Throw the broccoli "noodles" into the pot with the pasta a few minutes before it's done cooking.

Brussels sprouts

Cabbage

Cauliflower

Celery

Cucumber

Daikon radish Steam and top with a squeeze of lemon, or use as a snacking veggie— they're great sliced and dipped in peanut butter.

Eggplant Try slicing it thin, then steaming it for 15 minutes. Then add it to a saucy dish, like a stir-fry or pasta.

Greens collard greens, kale, romaine, spinach, Swiss chard, etc.

Hearts of palm, canned. Use as a salad topper, mince and add to tomato sauce, or steam, blend, and add to broth for a creamier soup.

Leeks Cut raw leeks into thin slices and add them to salads.

Mushrooms

Okra Halve raw okra and top with a little salt and pepper.

Onions

Peppers

Radishes Slice thin and use on anything that needs a bit of texture: tacos, sandwiches, grain dishes.

Rutabaga Peel, boil, and mash for a creamy side dish.

Snow peas

Sprouts alfalfa, bean, pea, soybean, etc.

Sugar snap peas

Tomatoes Canned are fine, too.

Turnips Try them boiled and mashed with a little salt and pepper.

Water chestnuts, canned. Slice this crunch star thin and use it in soups, salads, and stir-fries.

Zucchini

usual white kind, honey, maple syrup, agave syrup, turbinado sugar, brown rice syrup, and convenience foods with sugar on their ingredients lists. It tends to sneak into foods you might not think of as sweet—check the label on products like tomato sauce, yogurt, even salsa. (Starting in July 2018, food companies will be required to list added sugars on their labels, but until then, you need to read the ingredients list to be sure. And remember that sugar sometimes disguises itself on food labels—look out for syrups; words that end in "-ose" like maltose, dextrose, sucrose; the word "cane"; and fruit juice. The complete list of names is on page 53.) Cutting back and paying attention to sneaky sugar sources will help you unlearn the craving and retrain your taste buds. By the end of the process, you may be surprised to discover that foods that you once found delicious now seem overly sweet.

But a slice of perfectly ripe mango? Sublime.

I'd also prefer that you avoid artificial sugar entirely, if you can—remember, this plan is about real, whole foods, and those yellow, pink, blue, and green packets shouldn't be an exception, nor should the added artificial sweeteners found in many store-bought foods and drinks. (Some experts even think that artificial sweeteners may cause changes in your microbiome that make you less sensitive to sweetness so you need more to feel satisfied. Boom—weight gain.)

As for beverages, stick to the basics, please: water, coffee, and tea. When it comes to add-ins, just trust your common sense. A splash of milk in your coffee is fine; flavored syrups are not. Sparkling water with a squeeze of citrus: Oz-approved. Soda, diet or regular: Nope. And same goes for sugary juices, like orange or apple juice.

HEY, DUDES! MEN SHOULD DO THE PLAN, TOO.

These meal plans are geared to accommodate both men and women, but because men tend to be taller and heavier than women—and therefore need more calories for basic body maintenance—guys may need to eat a little bit more than what's outlined in the plan. That online calorie intake calculator I mentioned earlier on page 168 (or a conversation with your doctor) will help you set your calorie goal. Once you know how much higher your intake should be, you can decide how you want to make up those extra calories: maybe with a double serving of brown rice at dinner, an extra ounce of nuts with your afternoon snack, a large portion of chicken breast at dinner, or a bit more cheese sprinkled on your salad.

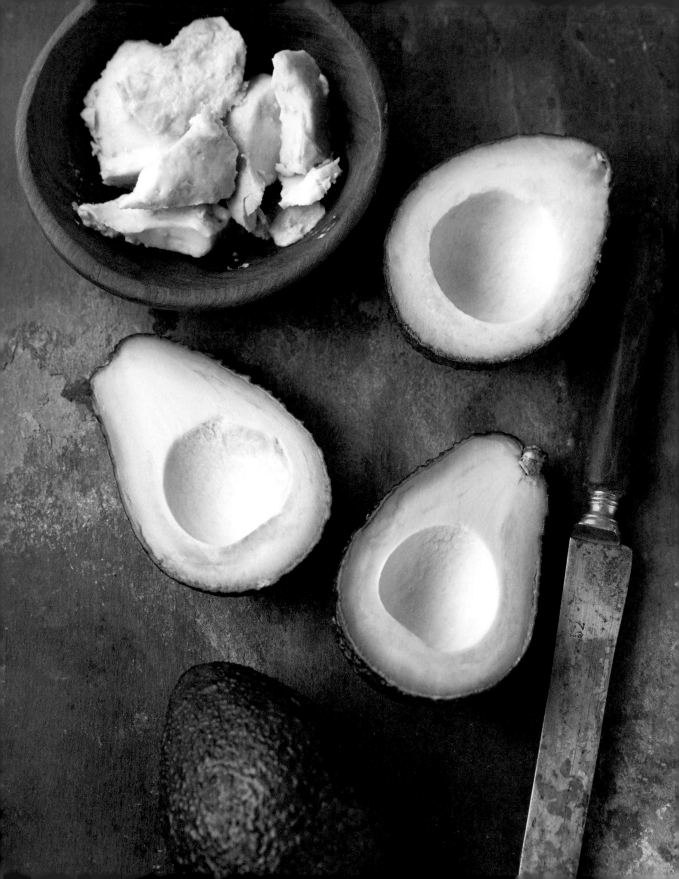

The 21-Day Plan

Reminder: Feel free to follow this exactly or to mix and match breakfasts, lunches, snacks, and dinners as you please.

WEEK 1

	DAY 1	DAY 2	DAY 3	DAY 4	DAY 5	DAY 6	DAY 7
Breakfast	Greek yogurt with berries	Eggs with salsa and beans	Blueberry-oat parfait	Greek yogurt with berries	Peach smoothie	Peanut butter–banana overnight oats	Eggs with salsa and beans
Snack	Apple with nut butter	Greek yogurt with nuts or berries	String cheese and crackers	Hard-boiled egg and crackers	Veggies and string cheese	Veggies and nut butter	Fruit and nuts
Lunch	Open-faced veggie sandwich	Rainbow salad with mixed greens, chicken, and buttermilk dressing	Supergreen salad with chicken and Parmesan	Wild rice bowl with egg	Salmon power bowl	Salad in a jar	Open-faced Italian turkey sandwich
Snack	Smoky hummus with veggies	Old Bay popcorn with super seeds	Smoky hummus with veggies	Veggie rolls with nut butter	Sweet potato strips	Frozen grapes with Greek yogurt	Sweet potato strips
Dinner	Lemony salmon with broccoli and tomatoes	Whole wheat penne with chicken	Spiced lentils with roasted green beans and quinoa	Spicy shrimp and quinoa bowl	Cauliflower Pizza Margherita	Mustard and quinoa–crusted salmon with cauliflower rice	Salsa turkey burger with baked sweet potato fries

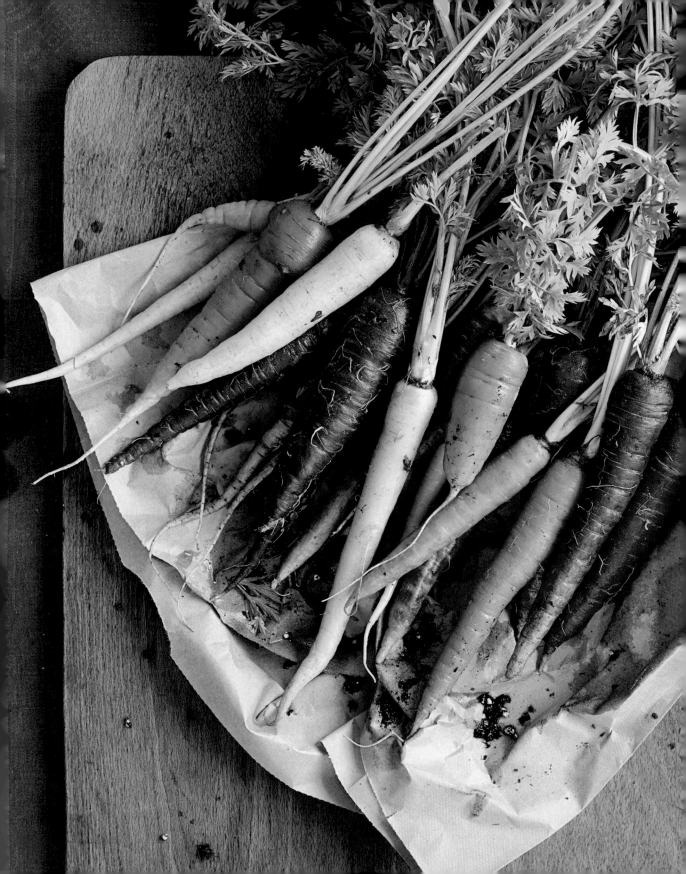

WEEK 2

	DAY 1	DAY 2	DAY 3	DAY 4	DAY 5	DAY 6	DAY 7
Breakfast	Greek yogurt with berries	Eggs with salsa and beans	Blueberry-oat parfait	Greek yogurt with berries	Peach smoothie	Peanut butter–banana overnight oats	Eggs with salsa and beans
Snack	Apple with nut butter	Greek yogurt with nuts or berries	String cheese and crackers	Hard-boiled egg and crackers	Veggies and string cheese	Veggies and nut butter	Fruit and nuts
Lunch	Salad in a jar	Salmon power bowl	Supergreen salad with chicken and Parmesan	Open-faced Italian turkey sandwich	Rainbow salad with mixed greens, chicken, and buttermilk dressing	Open-faced veggie sandwich	Wild rice bowl with egg
Snack	Veggies and artichoke dip	Paprika-almond popcorn	Veggies and artichoke dip	Curried carrot sticks	Chili-spiced pumpkin seeds	Veggies and avocado dip	Chili-spiced pumpkin seeds
Dinner	Salmon hash with sunny-side-up eggs	Black bean bowl (with grilled chicken, optional)	Pasta salad with shrimp and herbs	Mediter-ranean chickpea burger	Whole wheat panko and herb-crusted chicken	Steak night salad with couscous	Blackened tilapia tacos

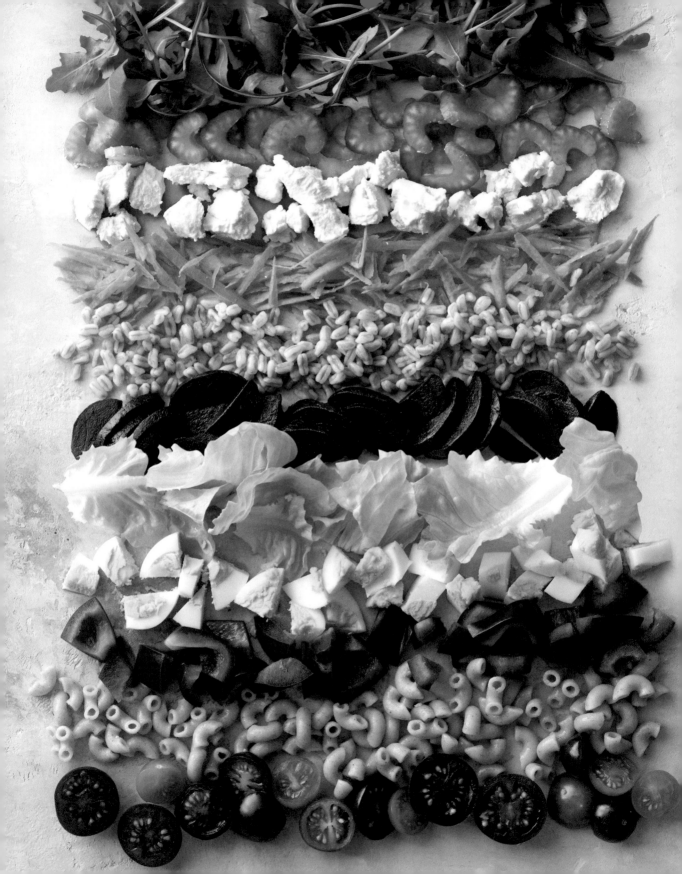

WEEK 3

	DAY 1	DAY 2	DAY 3	DAY 4	DAY 5	DAY 6	DAY 7
Breakfast	Greek yogurt with berries	Eggs with salsa and beans	Blueberry-oat parfait	Greek yogurt with berries	Peach smoothie	Peanut butter–banana overnight oats	Eggs with salsa and beans
Snack	Apple with nut butter	Greek yogurt with nuts or berries	String cheese and crackers	Hard-boiled egg and veggies	Crackers and string cheese	Veggies and nut butter	Fruit and nuts
Lunch	Salmon power bowl	Open-faced Italian turkey sandwich	Supergreen salad with chicken and Parmesan	Salad in a jar	Rainbow salad with mixed greens, chicken, and buttermilk dressing	Wild rice bowl with egg	Open-faced veggie sandwich
Snack	Veggies with edamame pesto dip	Old Bay popcorn	Veggies with edamame pesto dip	Brussels sprout chips	Roasted chickpeas	Tomato "pizzas"	Roasted chickpeas
Dinner	Quick chicken fried rice	Asian tofu steak with noodles	Quick whole wheat pasta with broccoli sauce	Arugula salad with fried eggs and asparagus	Balsamic-glazed chicken with Brussels sprouts and brown rice	Quick tuna puttanesca	Baked eggs with Swiss chard

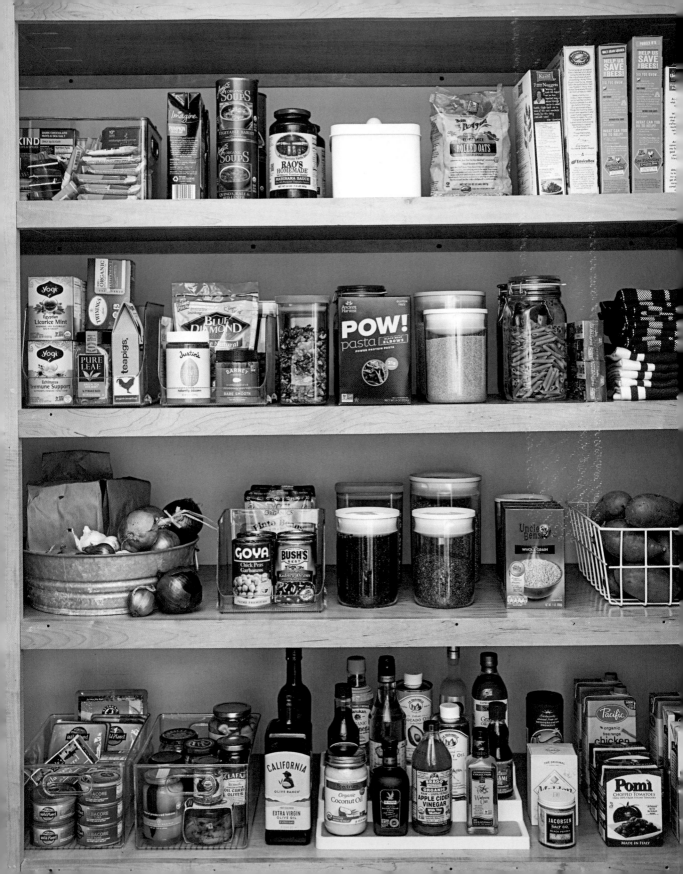

Shopping List for the Basics

Start with the following staples that will be used for the 21-Day Plan. (The recipes start on page 186.) In addition, you'll pick up perishables once a week for the duration of the plan.

PANTRY

Artichoke hearts, water-packed (3 [14-ounce] cans or jars)
Black beans (4 [15-ounce] cans)
Brown rice (large box)
Bulgur (small box)
Capers
Chia seeds
Chickpeas (3 [15-ounce] cans)
Diced tomatoes (28-ounce can)
Flaxseed, ground
Healthy crackers: whole-grain, seed-based (such as Mary's Gone Crackers), or nut-based (such as Blue Diamond)
Hearts of palm, canned
Lemon juice
Lentils, dried green
Mustard seeds
Nut butters: peanut, almond

Nuts: slivered almonds (small bag), plus any nuts of your choosing for snacking
Oil-packed tuna (5-ounce can)
Olives, Kalamata (large jar)
Pasta: whole wheat penne (2 boxes), whole wheat spaghetti (1 box), whole wheat rigatoni (1 box)
Popcorn kernels
Quinoa (large box)
Roasted red peppers (16-ounce jar)
Rolled oats
Salsa (you can also make it yourself. If purchasing, 3 jars, no added sugar)
Sesame seeds, white
Sunflower seeds, shelled
Tomato sauce, no added sugar (1 [24-ounce] jar)

Vanilla extract, pure
Vegetable broth (low-sodium), homemade (page 302), or store-bought
Whole-grain bread (look for 100%)
Whole wheat couscous (small box)
Whole wheat panko (small container)
Wild rice (small box)

HERBS AND SPICES

Basil
Black pepper
Blackened spice rub
Chili powder
Cinnamon, ground
Coriander, ground
Cumin, ground
Curry powder
Garlic powder
Old Bay seasoning
Onion powder
Oregano
Paprika

Paprika, smoked
Red pepper flakes
Rosemary
Salt
Salt, coarse
Thyme
Turmeric, ground

OIL AND VINEGAR

Balsamic vinegar
Canola oil
Canola oil cooking spray
Extra-virgin olive oil
Olive oil
Red wine vinegar
Sherry vinegar
White wine vinegar or white balsamic vinegar

CONDIMENTS

Dijon mustard
Dijon mustard (coarse-grain)
Soy sauce, low-sodium
Sriracha sauce

Now you're all set to get going. Remember, one of the keys to success is to set up your environment to make it easier to eat well. So the last thing I'll say is this: Before you start the plan, rid your pantry, refrigerator, and freezer of any tempting junk. When you start with a clean slate in your home, it will give you the best chance to do the same for your body.

I hope you enjoy the next twenty-one days (your recipes are coming up in the next chapter). After you're done, let me know how it went, how you felt, and how your body changed. Just post your message on my Facebook page (Dr. Mehmet Oz) along with the tag #foodcanfixit. *Bon appétit!*

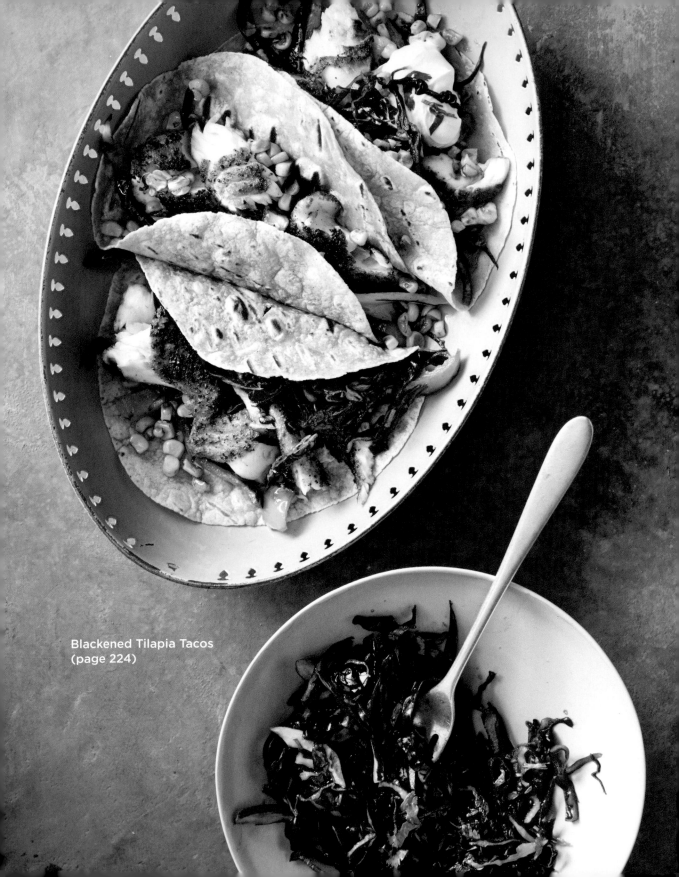

Blackened Tilapia Tacos
(page 224)

15

The Fix-It Recipes

These recipes—designed for you to use in the 21-Day Plan and beyond—will do more than deliver optimum nutritional balance. They'll tune you in to the joy of preparing healthy and delicious dishes. They're all uncomplicated, because cooking shouldn't feel like putting together an IKEA cabinet. For me, there's no joy in *that*. You'll find short ingredients lists and simple steps throughout. That said, you'll also learn some nice new skills in the kitchen, and meet plenty of unexpected flavors. So let's get started with some of my favorite meals, all integral parts of the 21-Day Plan.

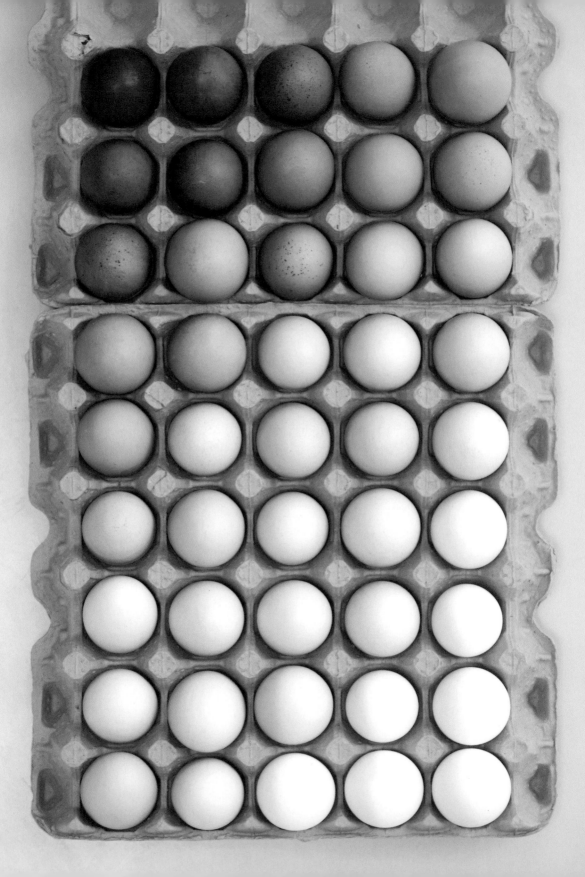

BREAKFAST

Start the day strong with a powerful hit of
protein, satisfying fiber, and wake-you-up flavor.

All breakfasts serve one.

Greek Yogurt with Berries

SERVES 1

1 cup plain 2% Greek yogurt

½ cup berries
(fresh or frozen)

In a small bowl, combine the yogurt with the berries. (If you're struggling with the tart yogurt taste, stir in a drop of pure vanilla extract or pulse the yogurt with the berries in the blender to distribute their sweetness throughout.)

Note: If you're feeling berried out, mix things up with nuts or fresh herbs.

---

192 CAL, 5 G FAT (3 G SATURATED), 20 G PROTEIN, 18 G CARB, 16 G SUGAR, 2 G FIBER, 76 MG SODIUM

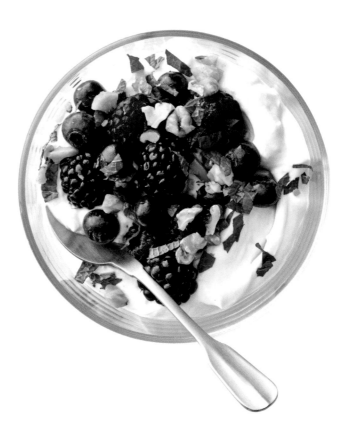

Eggs with Salsa and Beans

Whip up this quick homemade salsa, or substitute up to 1/3 cup jarred salsa (just make sure it has no added sugar). You can make a double or triple batch of this low-calorie flavor-booster and save it for future meals—and veggie-dunking needs.

To make the salsa: In a small bowl, combine the tomato, shallot, cilantro, and jalapeño. Stir in a squeeze of lime juice and add a pinch of salt.

To make the eggs: Heat a medium skillet over medium heat. Coat the skillet with cooking spray, add the eggs, and cook, stirring to scramble, until set, about 4 minutes. While the eggs are cooking, zap the beans in a microwave on high for 2 minutes. Plate the eggs; top with the beans and salsa.

---

196 CAL, 10 G FAT (3 G SATURATED), 15 G PROTEIN, 12 G CARB, 3 G SUGAR, 3 G FIBER, 428 MG SODIUM

EXTRA VEGGIE POWER! Toss mushrooms into the skillet after adding the cooking spray; sauté for 5 minutes, then add the eggs. Or serve the eggs over a bed of spinach.

For the salsa

⅓ cup chopped tomato

1 tablespoon chopped shallot

1 tablespoon chopped fresh cilantro

½ teaspoon diced jalapeño

Lime

Coarse salt

For the eggs

Canola oil cooking spray

2 large eggs

2 tablespoons canned black beans, rinsed and drained

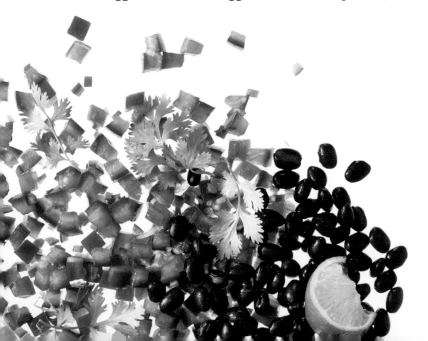

Blueberry-Oat Parfait

SERVES 1

¼ cup rolled oats

1 cup plain 2% Greek yogurt

1 cup blueberries (fresh or frozen)

1 tablespoon chia seeds

¼ teaspoon ground cinnamon

In a jar or bowl, layer the oats, yogurt, blueberries, chia seeds, and cinnamon. Stir before eating to mix in the oats. (If you like your oats a little softer, you can throw this together the evening before and refrigerate it overnight.)

_____

362 CAL, 5 G FAT (4 G SATURATED), 24 G PROTEIN, 49 G CARB, 24 G SUGAR, 10 G FIBER, 78 MG SODIUM

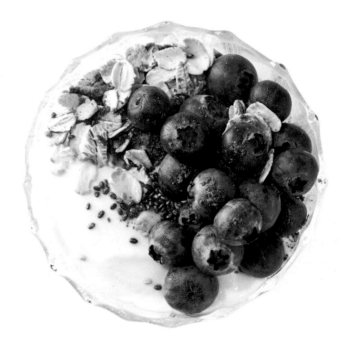

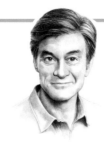

It's a Superfood

Blueberries are famous for packing an antioxidant punch. They're also linked to a lowered risk of heart disease.

Peach Smoothie

In a blender, combine the peaches, yogurt, banana, almond butter, flaxseed (if using), vanilla, ¼ cup ice, and ¼ cup water and puree until smooth.

---

411 CAL, 22 G FAT (5 G SATURATED), 24 G PROTEIN, 35 G CARB, 23 G SUGAR, 6 G FIBER, 139 MG SODIUM

EXTRA VEGGIE POWER! Toss in a handful of raw spinach or kale—you won't even taste it.

SERVES 1

8 wedges frozen peaches

¼ cup plain 2% Greek yogurt

½ medium banana

2 tablespoons almond butter

1 tablespoon ground flaxseed (optional)

½ teaspoon pure vanilla extract

Peanut Butter–Banana Overnight Oats

In a container, combine the milk, oats, peanut butter, banana, and chia seeds (if using). Cover and refrigerate overnight. Stir to combine in the morning.

---

340 CAL, 11 G FAT (4 G SATURATED), 15 G PROTEIN, 51 G CARB, 19 G SUGAR, 6 G FIBER, 133 MG SODIUM

SERVES 1

1 cup 2% milk

½ cup rolled oats

1 teaspoon peanut butter (or other nut butter)

½ small banana, sliced

1 tablespoon chia seeds or 1 tablespoon ground flaxseed (optional)

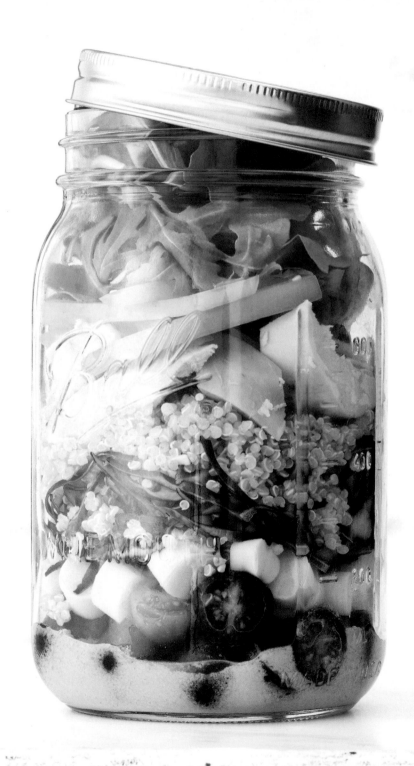

Salad in a Jar
(page 198)

LUNCH

Say good-bye to the midday slump
(and that wish to sneakily undo the
top button on your jeans). These meals
fuel you up without dragging you down.

All lunches serve one.

Salmon Power Bowl

½ cup cooked brown rice

3 ounces cooked salmon
(fillet or canned)

¼ (15-ounce) can black
beans, rinsed and drained

2 tablespoons salsa,
homemade (page 187)
or store-bought, with no
added sugar

Lime

Unlimited vegetables
of your choosing

In a bowl, top the rice with the salmon, beans, salsa, and a squeeze of lime juice. Add any vegetables from the unlimited veggie list (page 172).

Don't shy away from frozen salmon: It's less pricey and just as healthy as the fresh stuff. In a hurry: Thaw in a plastic bag submerged in cold water. In ten minutes it's ready to cook and will keep a good texture, especially if roasted.

---

302 CAL, 4 G FAT (1 G SATURATED), 25 G PROTEIN, 42 G CARB,
2 G SUGAR, 8 G FIBER, 609 MG SODIUM

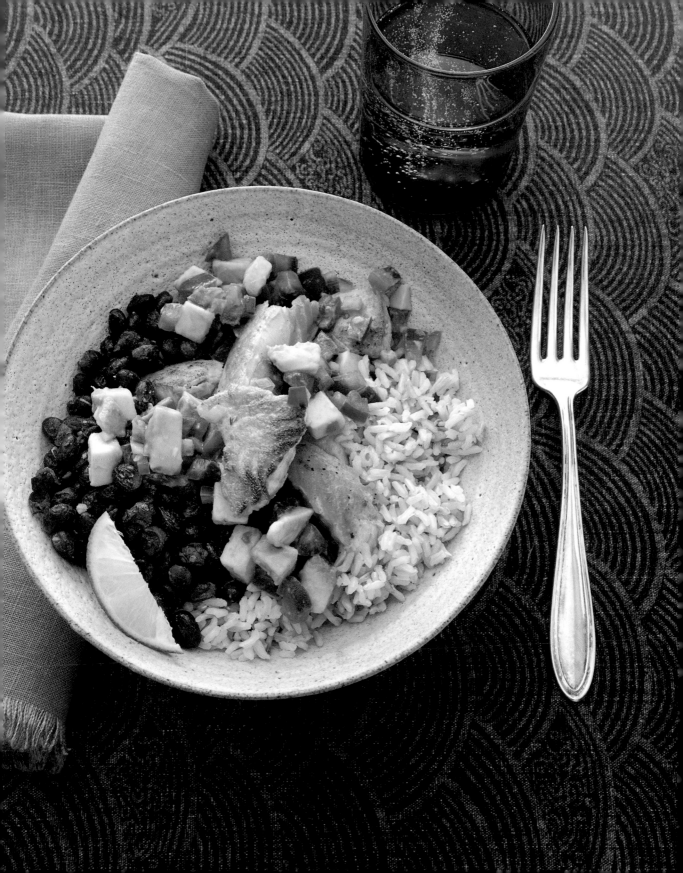

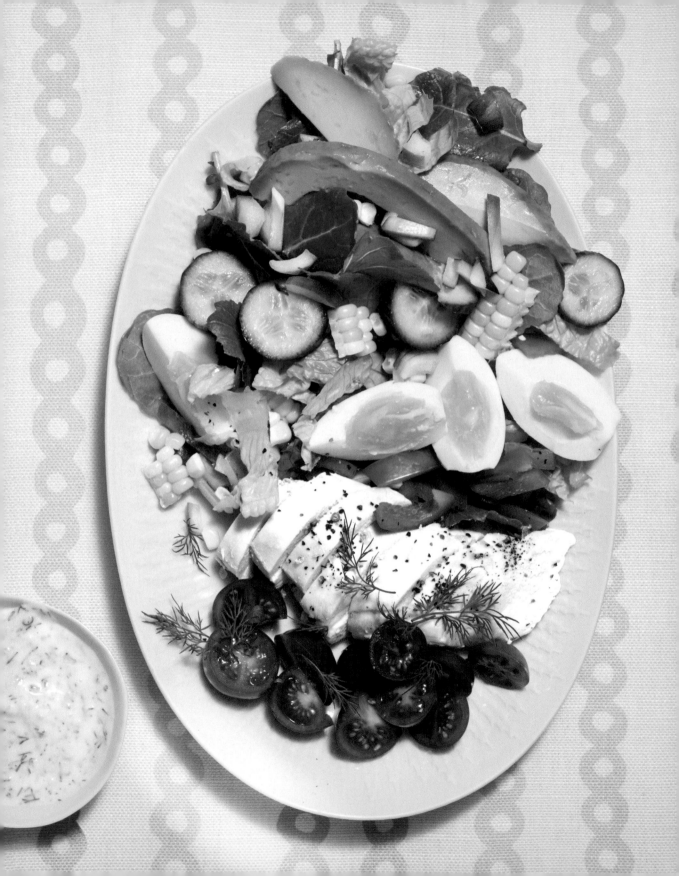

Rainbow Salad with Mixed Greens, Chicken, and Buttermilk Dressing

In a bowl or container, arrange the baby kale and romaine. Top with the chicken, egg, cherry tomatoes, bell pepper, corn, avocado, cucumber, and onion. Drizzle with the buttermilk dressing.

(WITHOUT DRESSING) 364 CAL, 16 G FAT (4 G SATURATED), 33 G PROTEIN, 25 G CARB, 10 G SUGAR, 8 G FIBER, 136 MG SODIUM

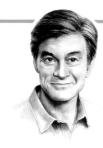

It's a Superfood

Eggs are the perfect pop of protein— they contain all nine of the essential amino acids your body needs.

SERVES 1

½ cup baby kale

½ cup chopped romaine hearts

½ cup sliced cooked chicken breast

1 hard-boiled large egg, quartered

½ cup halved cherry tomatoes

½ cup chopped bell pepper

¼ cup frozen corn, thawed

¼ avocado, sliced

½ cup sliced cucumber

¼ cup chopped red onion

Buttermilk Dressing (page 237)

Supergreen Salad with Chicken and Parmesan

SERVES 1

¼ cup packed fresh mint leaves

½ teaspoon olive oil

1 tablespoon fresh lemon juice

2 ounces boneless, skinless chicken breast

3 cups any leafy greens

¼ cup shaved Parmesan cheese (about 1 ounce)

2 tablespoons Sherry Vinegar Dressing (page 237)

Heat a ridged grill pan over medium-high heat or prepare an outdoor grill for direct grilling on medium-high.

Finely chop half the mint. Put the mint in a bowl and add the olive oil and lemon juice. Add the chicken to the bowl and rub with the mint mixture. Place the chicken on the grill pan and cook for 2 to 3 minutes on each side, or until the chicken just loses its pink color. Put the greens on a plate and top with the chicken. Add the cheese. Then, top it all off with sherry vinegar dressing and sprinkle with mint leaves for garnish.

(BEFORE DRESSING) 230 CAL, 12 G FAT (5 G SATURATED), 24 G PROTEIN, 7 G CARB, 24 G SUGAR, 10 G FIBER, 78 MG SODIUM

EXTRA VEGGIE POWER! Toss asparagus onto the grill with the chicken, then heap high.

Open-Faced Italian Turkey Sandwich

In a small bowl, whisk together the olive oil, mustard, lemon juice, chives, and parsley. Spread half the mustard mixture over the toast. Top with the turkey, roasted red peppers, and artichoke hearts. Drizzle with the remaining mustard mixture. Finish with red pepper flakes, to taste, if you like. Top with the lettuce leaves, using them as the "bread" on top.

---

385 CAL, 14 G FAT (3 G SATURATED), 32 G PROTEIN, 29 G CARB, 0 G SUGAR, 6 G FIBER, 862 MG SODIUM

EXTRA VEGGIE POWER! Throw on some sliced cucumbers, red onion, or radishes.

SERVES 1

2 teaspoons extra-virgin olive oil

2 teaspoons Dijon mustard

1 teaspoon fresh lemon juice

1 teaspoon chopped fresh chives

1 teaspoon chopped fresh flat-leaf parsley

1 slice whole-grain bread, toasted

3 ounces sliced turkey breast

¼ cup jarred roasted red peppers, drained

3 water-packed artichoke hearts, drained

Red pepper flakes (optional)

2 large lettuce leaves (such as radicchio or romaine)

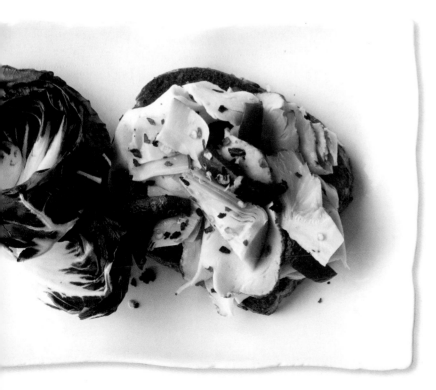

Salad in a Jar

SERVES 1

2 tablespoons Dijon Vinaigrette (page 236)

½ cup halved grape tomatoes

½ cup sliced hearts of palm

½ cup shredded red cabbage

½ cup cooked quinoa

3 ounces cooked boneless, skinless, chicken breast, diced

½ cup sliced bell pepper

1 cup baby arugula

In a quart-size jar or container, layer the ingredients in this order: dressing, grape tomatoes, hearts of palm, cabbage, quinoa, chicken, and bell pepper. Fill the rest of the jar with the baby arugula. Seal the jar and refrigerate until ready to serve. Shake to combine before serving.

See the photo on page 190.

421 CAL, 19 G FAT (3 G SATURATED), 29 G PROTEIN, 38 G CARB, 6 G SUGAR, 7 G FIBER, 867 MG SODIUM

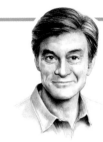

It's a Superfood

Lots of people think quinoa is a grain, but actually, it's a *seed*. It's loaded with protein, magnesium, phosphorous, and manganese.

Open-Faced Veggie Sandwich

In a small bowl using a fork, mash together the black beans, lime juice, cumin, salt, and olive oil. Spread on the toast. Top with the zucchini, cucumber, and sprouts (if using). Season with pepper. Top with lettuce and tomato.

---

258 CAL, 7 G FAT (1 G SATURATED), 12 G PROTEIN, 39 G CARB, 6 G SUGAR, 9 G FIBER, 416 MG SODIUM

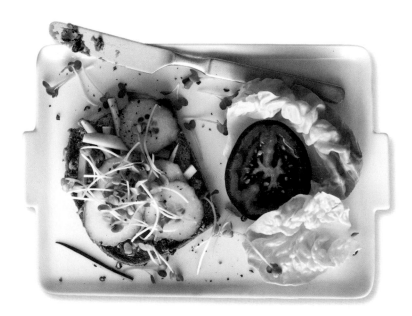

SERVES 1

⅓ cup canned black beans, rinsed and drained

Juice of 1 lime

¼ teaspoon ground cumin

Pinch of coarse salt

1 teaspoon extra-virgin olive oil

1 slice whole-grain bread, toasted

¼ cup shredded zucchini

6 slices cucumber

2 tablespoons sprouts of any kind (optional)

Freshly ground black pepper

Lettuce

Sliced tomato

Wild Rice Bowl with Egg

SERVES 1

½ cup wild rice

2 cups packed baby spinach

Coarse salt

Freshly ground black pepper

1 large egg, cooked sunny-side up

Cook the wild rice according to the package directions. When the rice is ready, take it off the heat, then add the spinach and stir until it has wilted. Season with salt and pepper. Top with the egg.

Note: You can cook a big batch of wild rice and sprinkle it over most anything for an extra hit of heartiness: soups, salads, even oatmeal.

---

305 CAL, 10 G FAT (2 G SATURATED), 14 G PROTEIN, 47 G CARB, 2 G SUGAR, 9 G FIBER, 530 MG SODIUM

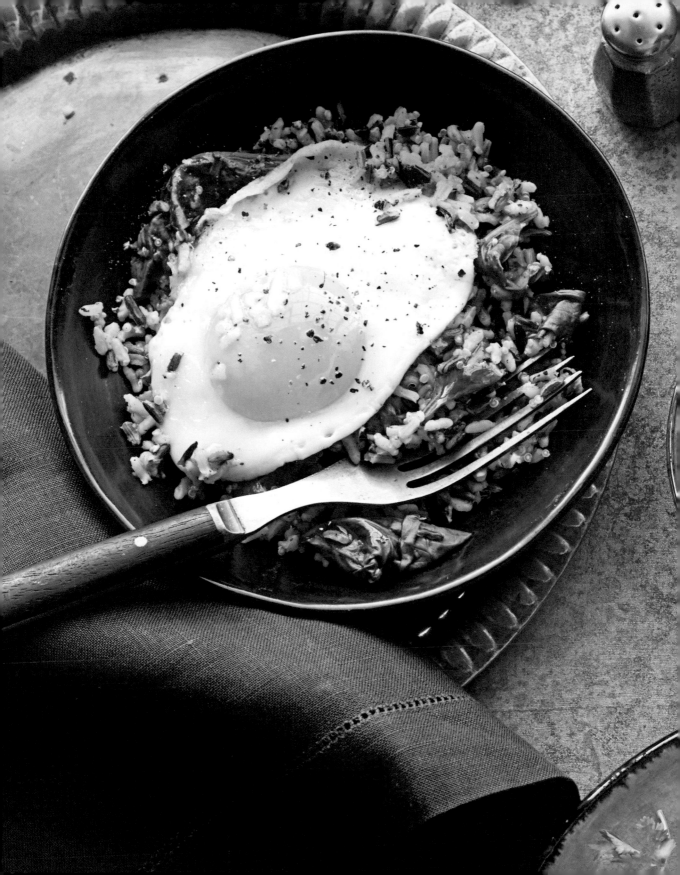

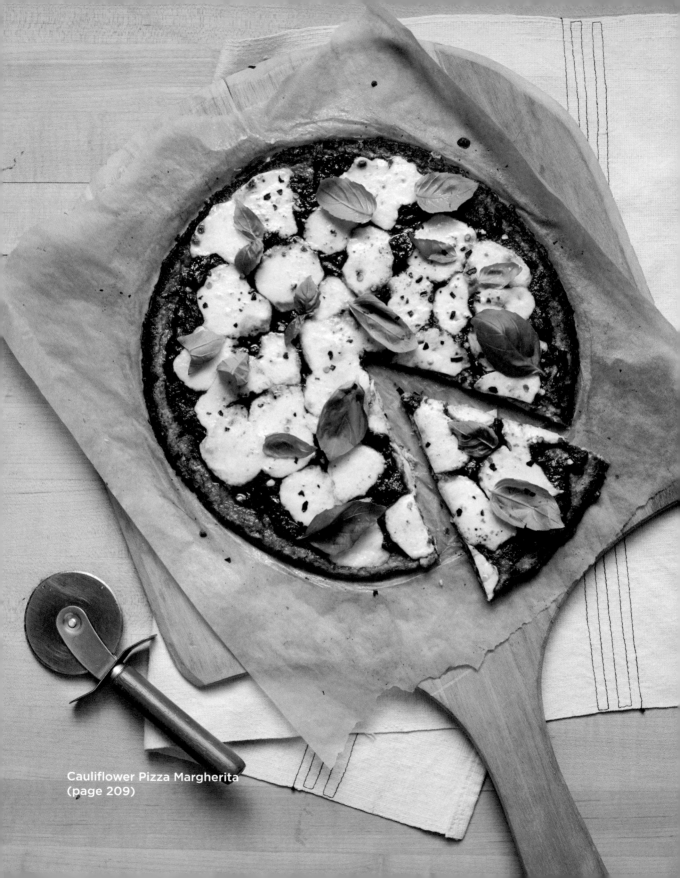

Cauliflower Pizza Margherita
(page 209)

DINNER

You're not the only one who'll love these twenty-one dinners. They're family- and friend-pleasers, too. Expect each plate to deliver the right balance of macronutrients, plus loads of flavor.

Dinners serve two or four—feel free to scale up or down, depending on who's coming to dinner or your affinity for leftovers.

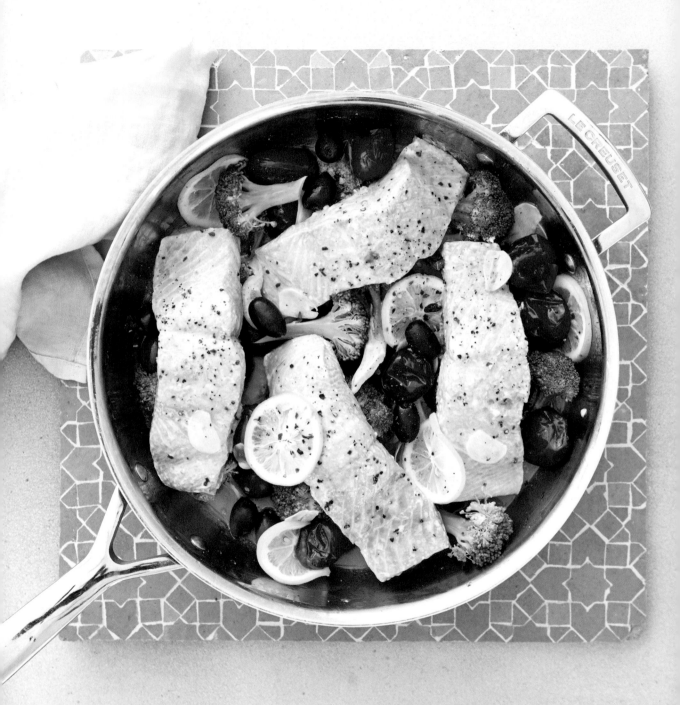

Lemony Salmon with Broccoli and Tomatoes

Juice 1 lemon into a small bowl to yield 2 tablespoons of juice, then whisk in the olive oil. Thinly slice the remaining lemon.

Place the broccoli, tomatoes, and garlic in one layer in a large, straight-sided skillet. Sprinkle with the red pepper flakes. Space the salmon fillets evenly on top. Season with the salt and black pepper to taste. Top with the sliced lemon. Pour half the lemon-oil mixture and 1 cup water into the skillet. Cover tightly. Bring to a boil, then reduce the heat to medium. Simmer gently, adjusting the heat as needed, until the fish is cooked through and the broccoli is tender, about 10 minutes. Scatter the olives on top. Spoon some of the pan sauce and remaining lemon-oil mixture over each serving.

---

390 CAL, 20 G FAT (3 G SATURATED), 40 G PROTEIN, 13 G CARB, 4 G SUGAR, 4 G FIBER, 511 MG SODIUM PER SERVING

SERVES 4

2 lemons

2 tablespoons olive oil

1 head broccoli (about 1 pound), trimmed and cut into 2½-inch-long pieces

10 ounces grape or cherry tomatoes (about 2 cups)

4 garlic cloves, thinly sliced

¼ teaspoon red pepper flakes

4 (6-ounce) skinless salmon fillets

½ teaspoon coarse salt

Freshly ground black pepper

1 cup pitted Kalamata olives

Whole Wheat Penne with Chicken

SERVES 2

4 ounces whole wheat penne pasta (about ⅔ cup)

2 tablespoons olive oil

3 cups cubed eggplant

Coarse salt

2 cups cubed zucchini

1 cup halved grape tomatoes

2 garlic cloves, minced

6 ounces cooked chicken breast, sliced

Freshly ground black pepper

Fresh or dried basil

---

515 CAL, 19 G FAT (3 G SATURATED), 39 G PROTEIN, 56 G CARB, 10 G SUGAR, 10 G FIBER, 798 MG SODIUM PER SERVING

Bring a large pot of salted water to a boil. Add the pasta and cook according to the package directions until al dente; reserve ⅔ cup of the pasta cooking water, then drain.

While the pasta is cooking, heat the olive oil in a skillet over medium-high heat. Add the eggplant and 4 pinches of salt. Cook, stirring, until golden, 4 to 5 minutes. Add the zucchini and 4 pinches of salt. Cook, stirring, until golden, 6 minutes. Add the tomatoes and garlic. Cook, stirring, until the tomatoes soften, 2 minutes. Add the chicken, reserved pasta water, and pasta. Cook over high heat, stirring, for 3 minutes. Season with pepper and 4 pinches of salt. Garnish with basil.

EXTRA VEGGIE POWER! After adding the olive oil to your skillet, throw in some chopped leeks. Stir a handful of arugula into the pasta before serving.

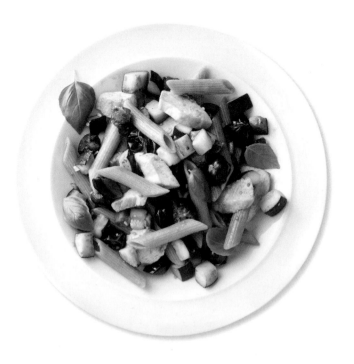

Spiced Lentils with Roasted Green Beans and Quinoa

Preheat the oven to 425°F.

In a small pot, combine the lentils and broth and bring to a boil. Cover and reduce the heat to medium-low. Simmer for 25 to 30 minutes, or until the lentils are tender; drain any excess liquid. Gently stir in the garlic powder, coriander, onion powder, chili powder, and a pinch each of salt and pepper.

While the lentils are cooking, in a large bowl, toss the green beans with the olive oil and a sprinkle each of salt and pepper. Spread the green beans over a rimmed baking sheet and roast, stirring occasionally, for about 20 minutes, or until tender.

Serve the lentils warm over the quinoa with a side of the roasted green beans.

SERVES 2

⅔ cup dried green lentils

2 cups low-sodium vegetable broth or water

1 teaspoon garlic powder

1 teaspoon ground coriander

½ teaspoon onion powder

½ teaspoon chili powder

Salt

Freshly ground black pepper

4 cups prewashed bagged green beans

2 teaspoons olive oil

1 cup cooked quinoa

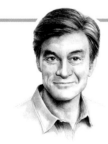

It's a Superfood

Just 1 cup of cooked lentils contains an amazing 16 grams of filling fiber.

380 CAL, 11 G FAT (0 G SATURATED), 19 G PROTEIN, 55 G CARB, 11 G SUGAR, 17 G FIBER, 290 MG SODIUM PER SERVING

Spicy Shrimp and Quinoa Bowl

SERVES 2

2 tablespoons olive oil

2½ cups sliced zucchini

2 garlic cloves, minced

6 ounces shrimp, peeled
and deveined

2 pinches of salt

2 pinches of red pepper
flakes

1 teaspoon dried oregano

1 cup halved grape
tomatoes

1 cup cooked quinoa

---

330 CAL, 17 G FAT
(2 G SATURATED),
18 G PROTEIN, 28 G CARB,
5 G SUGAR, 4 G FIBER,
616 MG SODIUM PER SERVING

Heat the olive oil in a medium skillet over medium heat. Add the zucchini and cook until it starts to turn golden, 2 to 4 minutes. Add the garlic and shrimp. Cook until the shrimp start to turn pink, about 2 minutes. Add the salt, red pepper flakes, oregano, and tomatoes. Cook until the tomatoes soften, 2 minutes. Serve over the quinoa.

EXTRA VEGGIE POWER! Before adding the zucchini, sauté sliced onions in the olive oil. Or when the shrimp is nearly done cooking, toss a handful or two of greens (kale, collards, or baby spinach) into the skillet.

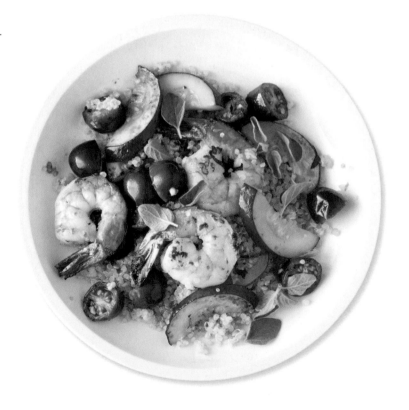

Cauliflower Pizza Margherita

Preheat the oven to 425°F. Line a baking sheet with parchment paper.

Cut the cauliflower florets from the stems. In batches, pulse the florets in a food processor until finely ground and fluffy. (Do not overprocess.) Transfer the cauliflower to a microwave-safe bowl and cover with plastic wrap; poke a few holes in the plastic. Microwave on high for 5 minutes. Uncover, stir, and let cool slightly. Gather the cauliflower in a clean dish towel and twist tightly to squeeze out as much moisture as possible. Transfer the cauliflower to a large bowl and add the egg, egg white, Parmesan, oregano, and salt. Stir well. Transfer to the baking sheet and pat out into a ¼-inch-thick circle (10 to 11 inches across). Bake until golden brown, about 25 minutes. Top with the sauce and mozzarella. Return to the oven and bake until the mozzarella has melted, 10 to 15 minutes more. Top with basil and sprinkle with red pepper flakes.

See the photo on page 202.

EXTRA VEGGIE POWER! Heat up a little olive oil in a pan (no more than 1 tablespoon), then sauté the mushrooms, bell peppers, or zucchini coins until tender. Add them to the pizza before baking.

SERVES 4

1 (2-pound) head cauliflower

1 large egg, lightly beaten

1 large egg white, lightly beaten

⅓ cup packed grated Parmesan cheese

¼ teaspoon dried oregano

½ teaspoon coarse salt

½ cup store-bought tomato sauce, no added sugar

6 ounces fresh whole-milk mozzarella cheese, sliced or torn into pieces

Fresh basil, for garnish

Red pepper flakes, for sprinkling

---

204 CAL, 13 G FAT
(7 G SATURATED),
14 G PROTEIN, 8 G CARB,
3 G SUGAR, 2 G FIBER,
524 MG SODIUM PER SERVING

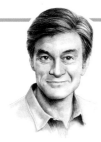

It's a Superfood

Low-cal cauliflower is the Transformer of veggies. Pizza crust, rice—it will shape-shift every which way. My favorite is zero-guilt mashed "potatoes"—just steam your cauliflower florets, drain, salt them, and mash 'em up.

Mustard and Quinoa–Crusted Salmon with Cauliflower Rice

SERVES 4

¼ cup white sesame seeds

¼ cup quinoa

4 teaspoons mustard seeds

4 teaspoons paprika

1 teaspoon coarse salt

1 teaspoon freshly ground black pepper

4 (6-ounce) skinless salmon fillets

¼ cup Dijon mustard

1 tablespoon plus 1 teaspoon olive oil

Preheat the oven to 400°F.

In a shallow bowl, mix together the sesame seeds, quinoa, mustard seeds, paprika, salt, and pepper. Coat the salmon with the mustard, then coat each fillet in the sesame seed mixture, patting it on carefully.

Heat the olive oil over medium-high heat in a large non-stick pan. Add the salmon and cook for 4 minutes per side, until the coating is browned. Transfer the salmon fillets to a rimmed baking sheet and bake for 8 minutes.

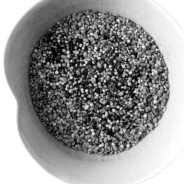

241 CAL, 7 G FAT
(0 G SATURATED),
5 G PROTEIN, 13 G CARB,
0 G SUGAR, 3 G FIBER,
854 MG SODIUM PER SERVING

Cauliflower Rice

SERVES 4

8 cups cauliflower florets

1 tablespoon olive oil

½ teaspoon coarse salt

Preheat the oven to 425°F.

Pulse the cauliflower florets in a food processor until rice-like (or grate on the large holes of a box grater). Toss with the olive oil and salt. Spread over a rimmed baking sheet and roast, stirring occasionally, for 20 to 30 minutes.

83 CAL, 4 G FAT (1 G SATURATED), 4 G PROTEIN, 11 G CARB,
4 G SUGAR, 4 G FIBER, 304 MG SODIUM PER SERVING

Salsa Turkey Burger with Baked Sweet Potato Fries

To make the salsa: Combine the tomatoes, cilantro, onion, jalapeño, lime juice, and salt. Set aside.

To make the burgers: Combine the ground turkey, chili powder, salt, and ½ cup of the tomato-salsa mixture. Form into 2 patties. Heat the olive oil in a nonstick skillet over medium-high heat. Cook the burgers, flipping once, until browned, 4 minutes, reduce the heat to low and cook through, covered, 5 minutes. Serve on lettuce with the remaining tomato-salsa mixture and more cilantro.

---

248 CAL, 13 G FAT (3 G SATURATED), 24 G PROTEIN, 10 G CARB, 5 G SUGAR, 3 G FIBER, 1,541 MG SODIUM PER SERVING

SERVES 2

For the salsa

2 medium tomatoes, finely chopped

1 cup loosely packed chopped fresh cilantro leaves, plus more for serving

¼ cup chopped red onion

2 tablespoons minced jalapeño (ribs and seeds removed)

Juice from 1 lime

1 teaspoon coarse salt

For the burgers

8 ounces ground turkey

½ teaspoon chili powder

½ teaspoon coarse salt

2 teaspoons olive oil

2 large lettuce leaves

Baked Sweet Potato Fries

Preheat the oven to 450°F.

Cut the sweet potato into ¼-inch-wide sticks; toss, on a large rimmed baking sheet, with the olive oil and salt. Roast for 20 to 25 minutes or until crisp, shaking once.

---

110 CAL, 7 G FAT (1 G SATURATED), 1 G PROTEIN, 12 G CARB, 4 G SUGAR, 2 G FIBER, 275 MG SODIUM PER SERVING

SERVES 2

1 medium sweet potato

1 tablespoon olive oil

¼ teaspoon salt

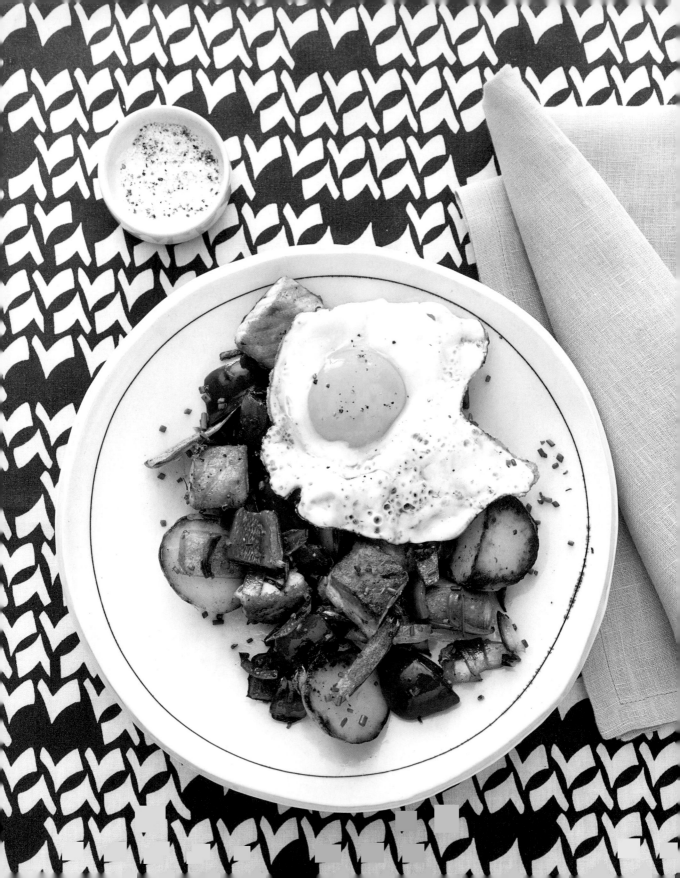

Salmon Hash with Sunny-Side-Up Eggs

Put the sweet potato in a small saucepan and add enough cold water to cover by 2 inches; simmer over medium heat until tender, about 12 minutes. Drain and cut into cubes.

Heat 1 tablespoon of the olive oil in a cast-iron or non-stick skillet over medium-high heat. Season the salmon with ¼ teaspoon each of the salt and black pepper. Cook in the skillet, turning, until golden, 3 to 4 minutes. Transfer to a plate. Add the sweet potato to the skillet. Cook over medium-high heat until golden, about 2 minutes. Stir in the onion, bell peppers, 2 tablespoons of the chives, and the remaining ¼ teaspoon each of salt and black pepper. Cook, stirring, until the vegetables are golden and tender, 4 to 8 minutes. Return the salmon to the skillet. Heat, stirring gently and letting the salmon flake, until cooked through, about 1 minute more. Transfer everything to a bowl; loosely cover with aluminum foil.

Wipe out the skillet and add the remaining 1 tablespoon olive oil. Cook the eggs over medium-low heat until the whites are set, about 3 minutes, or to your desired doneness. Divide the hash among four plates and top each with an egg. Sprinkle with the remaining 1 tablespoon chives before serving.

SERVES 4

1 large sweet potato, peeled

2 tablespoons olive oil

1 (1¼-pound) piece skinless salmon, cut into 2-inch chunks

½ teaspoon coarse salt

½ teaspoon freshly ground black pepper

1 small red onion, coarsely chopped

2 small bell peppers, coarsely chopped

3 tablespoons chopped fresh chives

4 large eggs

---

440 CAL, 26 G FAT (4 G SATURATED), 39 G PROTEIN, 12 G CARB, 5 G SUGAR, 2 G FIBER, 418 MG SODIUM PER SERVING

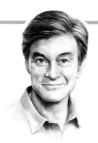

It's a Superfood

Sweet potatoes are a source of beta-carotene, a compound linked to eye health.

Black Bean Bowl

Canola oil cooking spray

½ cup frozen corn kernels

1 (5-ounce) boneless, skinless chicken breast (optional)

3 tablespoons diced tomato

2 tablespoons diced red onion

1 tablespoon fresh lime juice

1½ teaspoons plus 2 tablespoons chopped fresh cilantro

½ teaspoon minced jalapeño (ribs and seeds removed)

Pinch of ground cumin

Pinch of coarse salt

1 cup cooked brown rice

1 cup canned black beans, rinsed and drained

½ avocado, sliced, or ¼ cup prepared guacamole

¼ cup shredded cheddar cheese

Preheat the oven to 375°F.

Lightly spray a baking sheet with cooking spray. Spread the corn on the baking sheet and roast until golden brown, about 15 minutes.

In the meantime, heat a ridged grill pan over medium-high heat or preheat an outdoor grill to medium-high. Place the chicken (if using) on the grill and cook for 2 to 3 minutes on each side, or until the chicken just loses its pink color. Cut the chicken into cubes.

In a small bowl, combine the corn, tomato, onion, lime juice, the 1½ teaspoons cilantro, the jalapeño, cumin, and salt.

Spoon the rice, beans, chicken (if using), corn salsa, and avocado into two bowls. Top with the cheese and garnish with the remaining 2 tablespoons cilantro.

(WITHOUT CHICKEN) 391 CAL, 14 G FAT (4 G SATURATED), 15 G PROTEIN, 57 G CARB, 3 G SUGAR, 6 G FIBER, 433 MG SODIUM PER SERVING

(WITH CHICKEN) 467 CAL, 16 G FAT (4 G SATURATED), 29 G PROTEIN, 57 G CARB, 3 G SUGAR, 13 G FIBER, 468 MG SODIUM PER SERVING

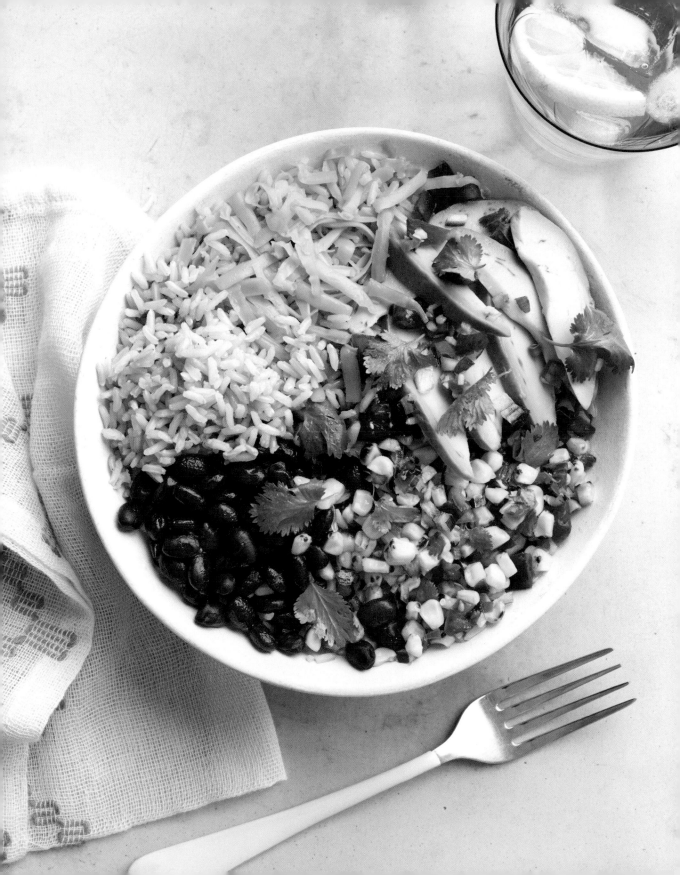

Pasta Salad with Shrimp and Herbs

SERVES 4

8 ounces whole wheat penne

¼ cup fresh lemon juice

3 tablespoons coarse-grain Dijon mustard

10 ounces large shrimp, peeled and deveined (about 16)

½ teaspoon coarse salt

Freshly ground black pepper

3 tablespoons extra-virgin olive oil

1 fennel bulb, thinly sliced crosswise, fronds reserved for garnish

⅓ cup chopped fresh chives

3 tablespoons chopped fresh tarragon (optional)

Bring a large pot of salted water to a boil. Add the penne and cook according to the package directions until al dente. Drain and let cool.

In a small bowl, mix together the lemon juice, mustard, and 2 tablespoons water. Set aside. Pat dry the shrimp. Season with ¼ teaspoon of the salt and pepper to taste. Heat 1 tablespoon of the olive oil in a large nonstick skillet over medium-high heat. Working in batches, cook the shrimp until golden brown, about 2 minutes per side. Add the shrimp to the pasta as they're cooked. Remove the skillet from the heat and stir in the mustard mixture, scraping up the browned bits from the bottom of the skillet. Toss the warmed sauce with the pasta. Refrigerate until cool. Add the fennel to the pasta, the remaining 2 tablespoons olive oil, the chives, tarragon (if using), and the remaining ¼ teaspoon salt. Toss well. Season with pepper. Garnish with fennel fronds, if desired.

---

378 CAL, 13 G FAT (2 G SATURATED), 16 G PROTEIN, 48 G CARB, 5 G SUGAR, 7 G FIBER, 900 MG SODIUM PER SERVING

EXTRA VEGGIE POWER! Plump it up with a handful of greens, such as arugula, baby spinach, or shredded kale.

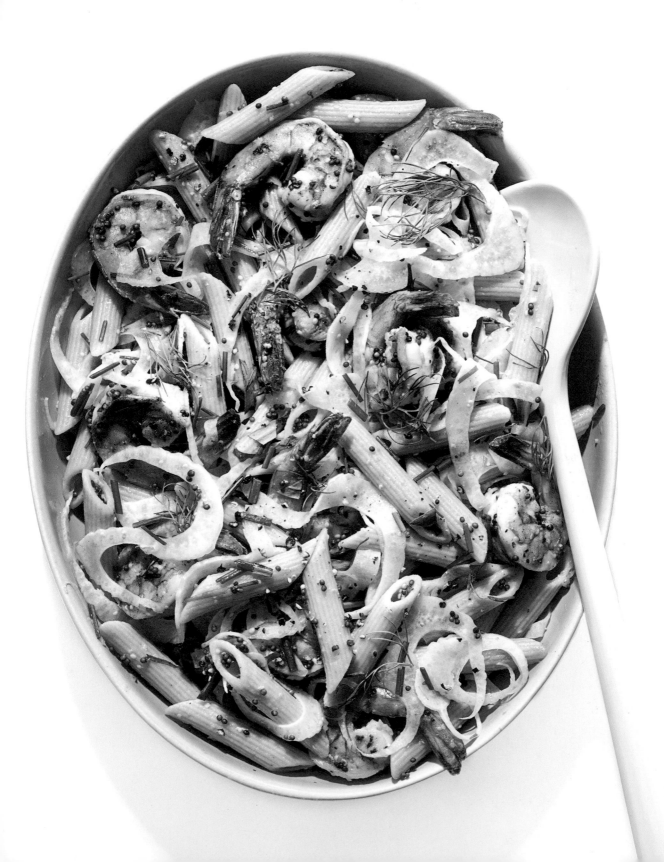

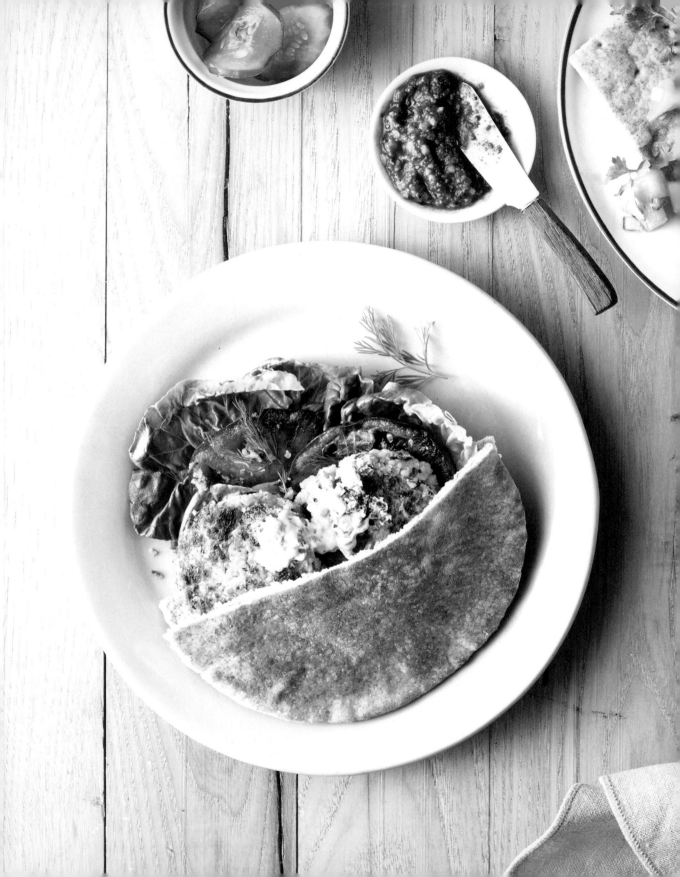

Mediterranean Chickpea Burger

Bring ⅔ cup water to a boil in a small saucepan. Add the bulgur. Cover; reduce the heat and simmer until the water has been absorbed, about 15 minutes.

Transfer the bulgur to a food processor, add the chickpeas, feta, egg, parsley, onion, lemon juice, cumin, salt, and pepper and pulse until well combined. Form the mixture into 8 patties (about 2 inches in diameter).

Heat the olive oil in a large nonstick skillet over medium heat. Cook the burgers, flipping once, until golden brown, 3 to 4 minutes per side. Serve 2 patties in each pita half.

333 CAL, 13 G FAT (3 G SATURATED), 13 G PROTEIN, 43 G CARB, 5 G SUGAR, 9 G FIBER, 663 MG SODIUM PER SERVING

EXTRA VEGGIE POWER! Top the burger with the usuals—lettuce, red onion, tomato, and cucumbers.

SERVES 4

¼ cup bulgur

1 (15-ounce) can chickpeas, rinsed and drained

½ cup crumbled feta cheese

1 large egg, lightly beaten

¼ cup chopped fresh flat-leaf parsley

3 tablespoons finely chopped red onion

2 tablespoons fresh lemon juice

1 teaspoon ground cumin

1 teaspoon coarse salt

½ teaspoon freshly ground black pepper

¼ cup olive oil

2 whole-grain pita pockets, halved

Whole Wheat Panko and Herb–Crusted Chicken

SERVES 2

6 tablespoons whole wheat panko bread crumbs

Zest of 1 lemon

2 tablespoons chopped fresh flat-leaf parsley

2 teaspoons freshly ground black pepper

½ teaspoon coarse salt

1 (12-ounce) boneless, skinless chicken breast, halved

2 large eggs, lightly beaten

2 teaspoons olive oil

Preheat the oven to 400°F.

In a shallow bowl, mix the panko, lemon zest, parsley, pepper, and salt. Dip the chicken into the egg, then coat with the panko mixture, patting it on carefully.

Heat the olive oil in a nonstick skillet over medium-high heat. Add the chicken and cook for 1 to 2 minutes per side. Transfer to a baking sheet and bake for 18 to 20 minutes. Serve with a big side salad.

Note: Whole wheat panko is good for more than just breading. Sprinkle it over slow-cooked dishes—such as chili or stews—to add a crisp, crunchy texture.

_____

(BEFORE SIDE SALAD) 354 CAL, 14 G FAT (3 G SATURATED), 43 G PROTEIN, 13 G CARB, <1 G SUGAR, 2 G FIBER, 652 MG SODIUM PER SERVING

EXTRA VEGGIE POWER! Serve with a nice helping of steamed green beans or asparagus.

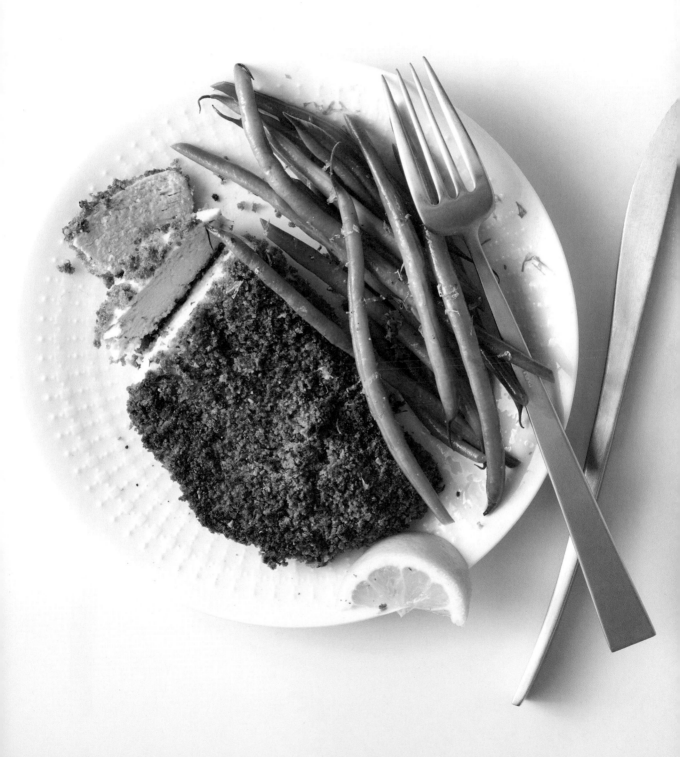

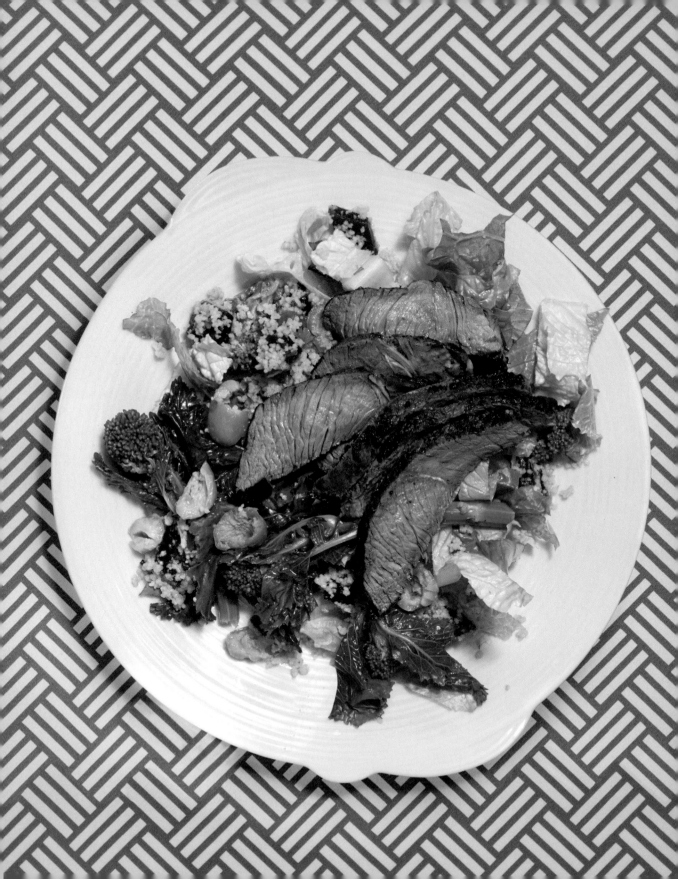

Steak Night Salad with Couscous

In a large bowl, toss together the couscous, romaine, bell pepper, olives, 4 tablespoons of the vinaigrette, the parsley, and ¼ teaspoon of the salt. Set aside.

Set a steamer basket over simmering water in a medium saucepan. Put the broccoli rabe in the steamer basket and cook, covered, until just tender, about 4 minutes. Let cool.

Season the steak with the remaining ¼ teaspoon salt and the black pepper. Heat the olive oil in a medium nonstick skillet over medium-high heat. Add the steak and cook, turning once, for 5 to 10 minutes for medium-rare (the timing will vary depending on the thickness). Let the steak rest 5 minutes, then slice.

Divide the couscous mixture, broccoli rabe, and steak among four plates. Drizzle with the remaining 2 tablespoons vinaigrette.

---

416 CAL, 20 G FAT (5 G SATURATED), 19 G PROTEIN, 39 G CARB, 4 G SUGAR, 9 G FIBER, 586 MG SODIUM PER SERVING

EXTRA VEGGIE POWER! Steam chopped cauliflower along with the broccoli rabe.

SERVES 4

3½ cups cooked whole wheat couscous

2 cups chopped romaine hearts

½ cup chopped roasted red bell pepper

¼ cup chopped pitted Kalamata olives

6 tablespoons Red Wine Vinaigrette (page 238)

2 tablespoons chopped fresh flat-leaf parsley

½ teaspoon coarse salt

8 ounces broccoli rabe, trimmed

8 ounces boneless sirloin steak

Freshly ground black pepper

1 tablespoon olive oil

Blackened Tilapia Tacos

SERVES 4

2 (6-ounce) tilapia fillets (if you don't like tilapia, you can substitute cod or another white fish)

2 teaspoons blackened spice rub

2 teaspoons olive oil

¾ cup frozen corn kernels, thawed (or fresh kernels cut from 1 ear)

1 medium red bell pepper, diced

8 (6-inch) corn or whole wheat tortillas, warmed

Lime, for serving

Heat a large nonstick skillet over medium-high heat for 1 minute. Coat the fillets with the spice rub. Add 1 teaspoon of the olive oil to the skillet, heat for another minute, then add the fish. Cook the fish until well browned and cooked through, 2 to 3 minutes per side for tilapia. Transfer to a plate.

Heat the remaining 1 teaspoon olive oil in the same skillet over high heat. Add the corn and bell pepper and cook, stirring once or twice, until the vegetables are browned, about 5 minutes. Slice each fillet into 4 pieces. Divide the tilapia and corn mixture among the tortillas. Serve with lime wedges.

See the photo on page 182.

---

246 CAL, 6 G FAT (1 G SATURATED), 20 G PROTEIN, 31 G CARB, 5 G SUGAR, 5 G FIBER, 120 MG SODIUM PER SERVING

EXTRA VEGGIE POWER! Top off your tacos with shredded cabbage or lettuce, sliced jalapeño, diced red onion, or sliced radishes.

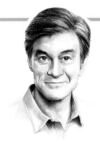

It's a Superfood

Corn gets a bad rap, nutritionally, but I'm a fan of the veggie. It's got fiber, and its natural sweetness can help crush your cravings for something sugary.

Quick Chicken Fried Rice

Heat 1 tablespoon of the canola oil in a large nonstick skillet over medium heat. Add the eggs and cook, stirring to scramble them, for 2 minutes; transfer to a plate.

In the same pan, heat the remaining 1 tablespoon canola oil. Add the rice, mixed vegetables, and snow peas and cook, stirring, for 3 minutes. Stir in the chicken, soy sauce, and scrambled eggs. Top with the scallion, if desired.

---

406 CAL, 20 G FAT (4 G SATURATED), 20 G PROTEIN, 43 G CARB, 4 G SUGAR, 5 G FIBER, 642 MG SODIUM PER SERVING

EXTRA VEGGIE POWER! Add sliced water chestnuts, sugar snap peas, and/or bamboo shoots.

SERVES 4

2 tablespoons canola oil

2 large eggs, beaten

3 cups cooked brown rice

1 (10-ounce) package frozen mixed vegetables

1 cup chopped snow peas

2 cups shredded cooked chicken (you can use rotisserie with the skin removed)

2 tablespoons low-sodium soy sauce

Chopped scallion, for garnish (optional)

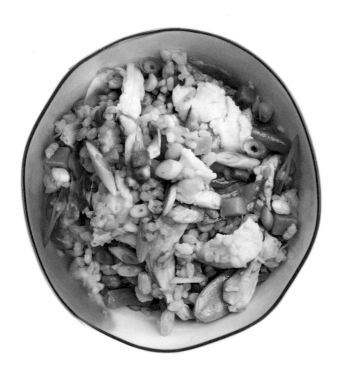

Asian Tofu Steak with Noodles

SERVES 2

2 heads baby bok choy

4 teaspoons canola oil

Red pepper flakes

6 ounces firm tofu, drained and patted dry

½ medium red bell pepper, thinly sliced

4 scallions, sliced, plus ¼ cup for garnish

2 teaspoons minced garlic

2 tablespoons low-sodium soy sauce

1 cup cooked whole wheat spaghetti

---

310 CAL, 15 G FAT
(1 G SATURATED),
16 G PROTEIN, 33 G CARB,
4 G SUGAR, 6 G FIBER,
653 MG SODIUM PER SERVING

Trim and chop the bok choy. Heat 2 teaspoons of the canola oil in a medium skillet over medium heat. Add the bok choy; cook, stirring, until the stalks are crisp-tender, 3 to 4 minutes. Transfer to a plate. Return the skillet to medium heat and add the remaining 2 teaspoons canola oil and a sprinkle of red pepper flakes. Add the tofu; sear, flipping once, for 1 minute per side. Add the bell pepper, scallions, and garlic. Cook, stirring, for 1 minute. Add the soy sauce, 2 tablespoons water, and the spaghetti. Stir the spaghetti to coat, about 1 minute. Serve with the bok choy. Top with the ¼ cup sliced scallion.

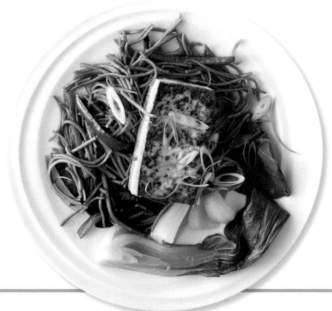

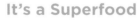

It's a Superfood

I'm a big fan of plant-based proteins like tofu. Plus, eating more of this soy-based staple may help you lose weight, according to one recent study.

Quick Whole Wheat Pasta with Broccoli Sauce

Bring a large pot of salted water to a boil. Add the rigatoni and cook according to the package directions until al dente; reserve ¼ cup of the pasta cooking water, then drain.

Heat the olive oil in a large skillet over medium heat. Add the garlic and cook for 1 minute. Add the broccoli florets and 1 cup water. Cook, covered, over medium-high heat for 7 minutes. Uncover. Cook, breaking up the broccoli, until the water has evaporated. Add the pasta, reserved pasta water, and the cheese. Season with the salt, black pepper, and a pinch of red pepper flakes.

EXTRA VEGGIE POWER! You can add cauliflower to the broccoli mix for more heft. Or serve with a simple side salad.

SERVES 4

12 ounces whole wheat rigatoni (other small shapes, such as shells or penne)

2 tablespoons olive oil

1 garlic clove, chopped

5 cups broccoli florets

¼ cup grated Parmesan cheese

¼ teaspoon coarse salt

¼ teaspoon freshly ground black pepper

Red pepper flakes

---

422 CAL, 11 G FAT
(2 G SATURATED),
15 G PROTEIN, 69 G CARB,
4 G SUGAR, 10 G FIBER,
309 MG SODIUM PER SERVING

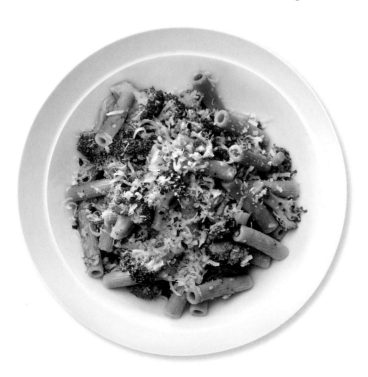

Arugula Salad with Fried Eggs and Asparagus

SERVES 4

8 ounces asparagus, trimmed

1 tablespoon olive oil

4 large eggs

8 cups baby arugula

¼ cup Chive Vinaigrette (page 238)

½ cup shaved Parmesan cheese

Chopped fresh chives, for garnish (optional)

Freshly ground black pepper

4 slices whole-grain bread, toasted

Set a steamer basket over simmering water in a medium saucepan. Put the asparagus in the steamer basket and cook, covered, until just tender, about 5 minutes. Let cool.

Heat the olive oil in a large nonstick skillet over medium heat. Add the eggs and fry until set, about 3 minutes. In a large bowl, toss the arugula with 3 tablespoons of the vinaigrette. Divide the arugula among 4 plates. Top each plate with the asparagus and an egg. Drizzle with the remaining vinaigrette. Sprinkle with the cheese, some chives (if using), and pepper to taste. Serve each salad with a slice of toast.

Yep, that's prosciutto on that salad—which isn't part of the 21-Day Plan. (It's not terrible for you in moderation—it even has a little iron—but it's a bit high in sodium.) I wanted you to see one example of how you can dress up these dishes when your three weeks are over. Just add one ingredient, and bam: It's a totally different meal. Culinary creativity!

(BEFORE VINAIGRETTE) 275 CAL, 15 G FAT (5 G SATURATED), 18 G PROTEIN, 17 G CARB, 5 G SUGAR, 4 G FIBER, 432 MG SODIUM PER SERVING

EXTRA VEGGIE POWER! Try making asparagus "noodles": Use a vegetable peeler on raw stalks to make long, thin strips. Add them to salads or your whole-grain pasta dishes.

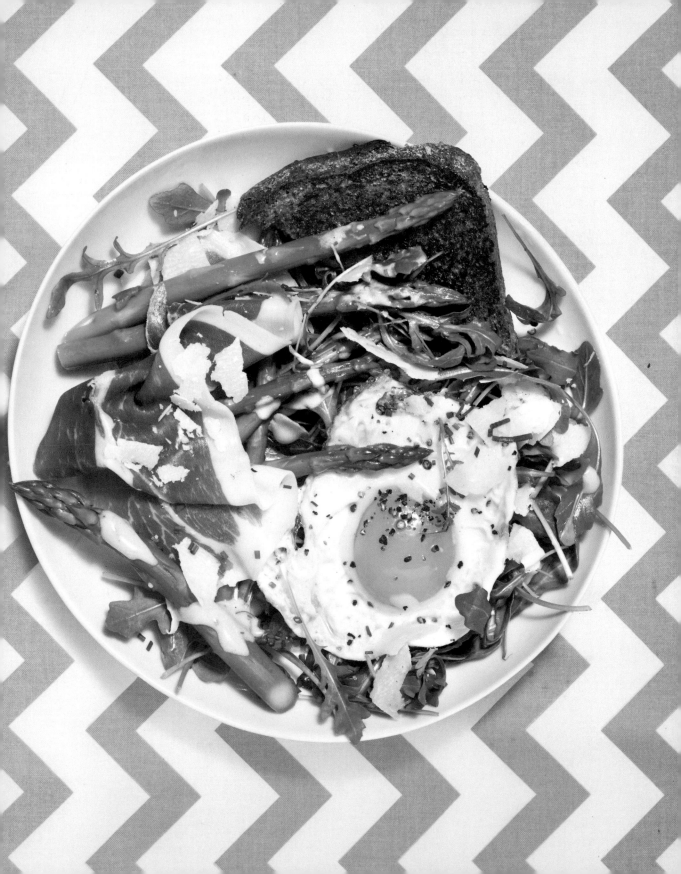

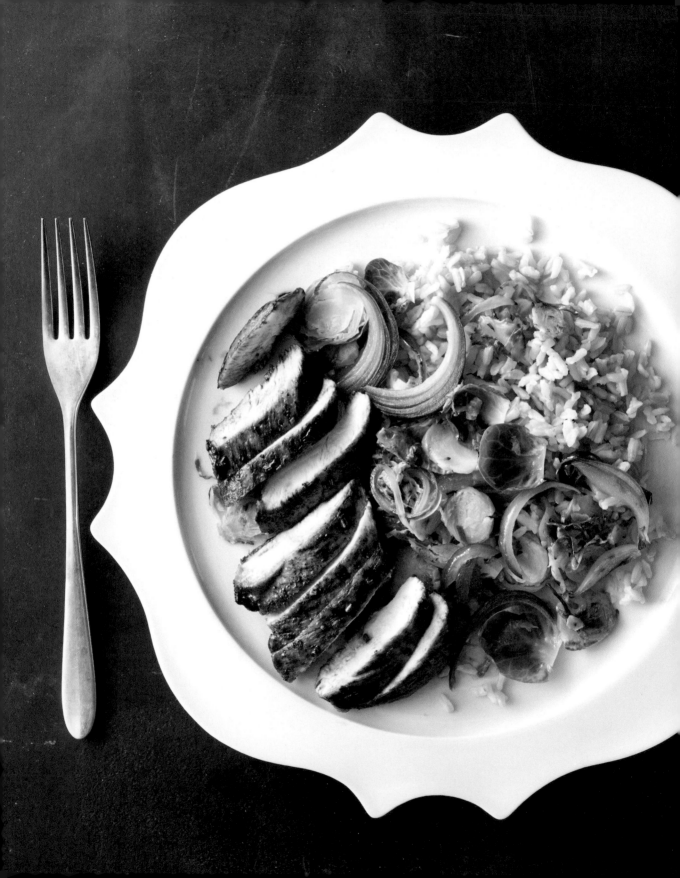

Balsamic-Glazed Chicken with Brussels Sprouts and Brown Rice

Heat a medium nonstick pan over medium-high heat. Season the chicken cutlets with the salt, rosemary, 1 teaspoon of the olive oil, and the pepper. Reduce the heat to medium and cook the chicken until cooked through, 2 to 3 minutes per side. Add the vinegar and cook for about 30 seconds more, turning the chicken to glaze it. Transfer to a plate; keep warm.

Rinse and dry the pan. Heat 2 teaspoons of the olive oil over medium heat and add the onion. Cook until the onion starts to soften, about 5 minutes. Add the remaining 2 teaspoons olive oil, the Brussels sprouts, and ¼ cup water. Toss to coat. Cover and cook for 1 minute. Uncover; raise the heat to high and cook until the sprouts are tender, 3 to 4 minutes more. Slice the chicken and serve with the sprouts and rice.

400 CAL, 15 G FAT (2 G SATURATED), 30 G PROTEIN, 34 G CARB, 5 G SUGAR, 5 G FIBER, 314 MG SODIUM PER SERVING

SERVES 2

2 (4-ounce) thin chicken breast cutlets

⅔ teaspoon coarse salt

2 teaspoons chopped fresh rosemary

5 teaspoons olive oil

Freshly ground black pepper

2 tablespoons balsamic vinegar

½ medium red onion, sliced

8 Brussels sprouts, thinly sliced

1 cup cooked brown rice

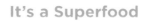

It's a Superfood

Brussels sprouts have a lot to boast about: They are rich in potassium, iron, and vitamins C and K.

Baked Eggs with Swiss Chard

2 tablespoons olive oil

1 cup sliced yellow onion

2 garlic cloves, minced

1 pound Swiss chard, washed, leaves stemmed and coarsely chopped (about 12 cups)

2 tablespoons plain 2% Greek yogurt

3 tablespoons grated Parmesan cheese

1 teaspoon fresh lemon juice

¼ teaspoon coarse salt, plus a pinch

Freshly ground black pepper

4 large eggs

4 whole-grain pita pockets or 4 slices whole-grain bread, toasted

Heat the olive oil in a medium ovenproof skillet over medium heat. Add the onion and garlic and cook, stirring, until tender, 4 minutes. Add the Swiss chard in batches and cook, tossing, until just tender, 5 minutes. Remove from the heat.

Stir in the yogurt, 1 tablespoon of the cheese, the lemon juice, the ¼ teaspoon salt, and the pepper to taste. Crack the eggs on top. Sprinkle with the remaining 2 tablespoons cheese and a pinch of salt. Bake until set, about 10 minutes. Serve with 1 slice each of the pita.

---

250 CAL, 14 G FAT (3 G SATURATED), 13 G PROTEIN, 19 G CARB, 4 G SUGAR, 4 G FIBER, 543 MG SODIUM PER SERVING

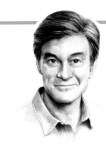

It's a Superfood

One serving of Swiss chard covers more than 100 percent of your daily vitamin K needs (a key nutrient for blood clotting).

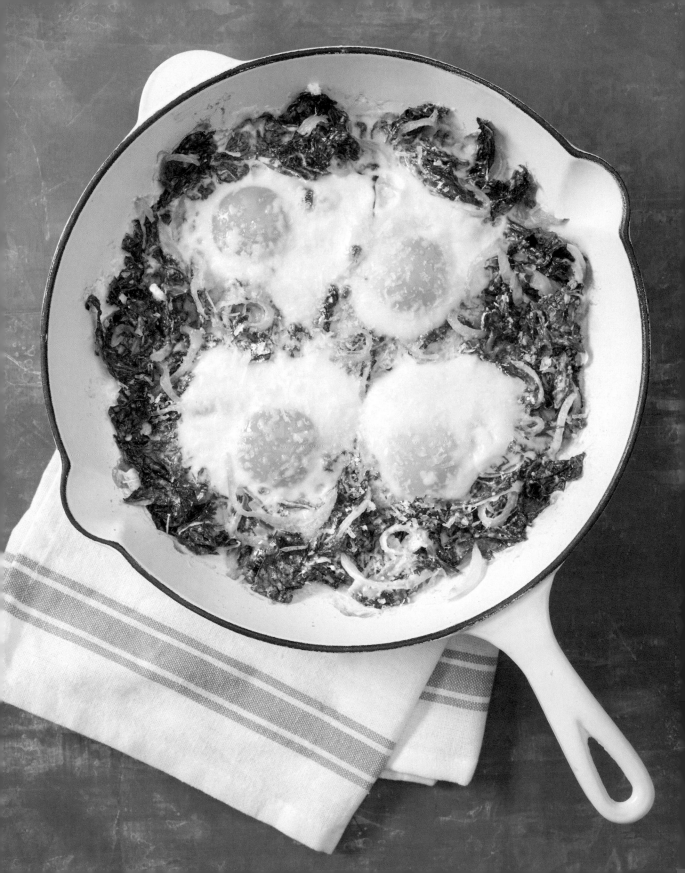

Quick Tuna Puttanesca

SERVES 4

12 ounces whole wheat penne

1 tablespoon olive oil

2 garlic cloves, chopped

¼ cup pitted and chopped Kalamata olives

1 tablespoon chopped capers

1 (28-ounce) can diced tomatoes

Red pepper flakes

1 (5-ounce) can oil-packed tuna, drained (water-packed tuna is also fine, though the oil-packed kind lends a little extra texture and richness to the dish. Note that the nutritional information was calculated with the oil-packed tuna.)

Bring a large pot of salted water to a boil. Add the penne and cook according to the package directions until al dente; drain.

Heat the olive oil in a large skillet over medium heat. Add the garlic, olives, and capers and cook for 3 minutes. Add the tomatoes with their juice and a pinch of red pepper flakes. Cook for 5 minutes. Toss the tomato sauce with the pasta and tuna.

461 CAL, 10 G FAT (1 G SATURATED), 19 G PROTEIN, 73 G CARB, 9 G SUGAR, 9 G FIBER, 797 MG SODIUM PER SERVING

EXTRA VEGGIE POWER! Add mushrooms to the skillet along with the garlic, olives, and capers. Or, after adding the tomatoes, stir in chopped artichoke hearts (packed in water).

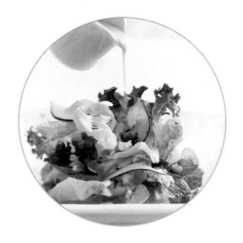

DRESSINGS

So easy to make, these dressings store well
in the refrigerator and will become your
go-to flavor enhancers when you want to add
a little punch to salads, pastas, and veggies.
Toss, dunk, and drizzle!

*The serving size for all the following
dressings is 2 tablespoons.*

Classic Vinaigrette

1 medium shallot, minced

3 tablespoons red wine vinegar

1 tablespoon Dijon mustard

½ teaspoon coarse salt

¼ teaspoon freshly ground black pepper

½ cup extra-virgin olive oil

In a small bowl, whisk together the shallot, vinegar, mustard, salt, and pepper. Add the olive oil. Whisk until emulsified. Refrigerate in a bottle or container. (The vinaigrette will keep in the fridge for up to 2 weeks.)

149 CAL, 18.01 G FAT (2.49 G SATURATED), .14 G PROTEIN, .92 G CARB, .39 G SUGAR, .18 G FIBER, 221.58 MG SODIUM PER SERVING

Dijon Vinaigrette

¼ cup fresh lemon juice

1 tablespoon plus 1 teaspoon coarse-grain Dijon mustard

½ cup extra-virgin olive oil

Pinch of coarse salt

Freshly ground black pepper to taste

In a small bowl, whisk together the lemon juice, mustard, olive oil, salt, and pepper to taste. Refrigerate in a bottle or container. (The vinaigrette will keep in the fridge for up to 2 weeks.)

126 CAL, 16.39 G FAT (2.26 G SATURATED), .04 G PROTEIN, .67 G CARB, .23 G SUGAR, .04 G FIBER, 90.61 MG SODIUM PER SERVING

Sherry Vinegar Dressing

In a small bowl, whisk together the vinegar, olive oil, mustard, shallot, parsley, salt, and pepper. Refrigerate in a bottle or container. (The vinaigrette will keep in the fridge for up to 2 weeks.)

---

156 CAL, 15.44 G FAT (2.13 G SATURATED), .06 G PROTEIN, .34 G CARB, .12 G SUGAR, .08 G FIBER, 172.74 MG SODIUM PER SERVING

MAKES ABOUT
7 SERVINGS

3 tablespoons sherry vinegar

½ cup extra-virgin olive oil

2 tablespoons coarse-grain Dijon mustard

1 tablespoon chopped shallot

1 tablespoon chopped fresh flat-leaf parsley

¼ teaspoon coarse salt

¼ teaspoon freshly ground black pepper

Buttermilk Dressing

In a small bowl, whisk together the buttermilk, yogurt, onion, garlic, dill, salt, and pepper. Refrigerate in a bottle or container. (The vinaigrette will keep in the fridge for up to 5 days.)

---

19 CAL, .36 G FAT (.23 G SATURATED), 1.48 G PROTEIN, 1.57 G CARB, 1.14 G SUGAR, .08 G FIBER, 113.59 MG SODIUM PER SERVING

MAKES ABOUT 7 SERVINGS

¼ cup low-fat buttermilk

¼ cup plain 2% Greek yogurt

1 tablespoon minced yellow onion

1 garlic clove, minced

2 tablespoons finely chopped fresh dill

¼ teaspoon coarse salt

¼ teaspoon freshly ground pepper

Red Wine Vinaigrette

MAKES ABOUT 8 SERVINGS

¼ cup plus 2 tablespoons red wine vinegar

2 teaspoons Dijon mustard

2 garlic cloves, minced

½ teaspoon coarse salt

½ teaspoon freshly ground black pepper

¼ cup plus 2 tablespoons extra-virgin olive oil

¼ cup chopped fresh flat-leaf parsley

In a small bowl, whisk together the vinegar, mustard, garlic, salt, and pepper. Whisk in the olive oil to combine well. Stir in the parsley. Refrigerate in a bottle or container. (The vinaigrette will keep in the fridge for up to 2 weeks.)

---

100 CAL, 10.15 G FAT (1.4 G SATURATED), .12 G PROTEIN, .49 G CARB, .02 G SUGAR, .11 G FIBER, 152.32 MG SODIUM PER SERVING

Chive Vinaigrette

MAKES ABOUT 8 SERVINGS

¼ cup white balsamic or white wine vinegar

2 tablespoons Dijon mustard

½ teaspoon freshly ground black pepper

¼ cup plus 2 tablespoons extra-virgin olive oil

2 tablespoons chopped fresh chives

In a small bowl, whisk together the vinegar, mustard, and pepper. Whisk in the olive oil to combine well. Stir in the chives. Refrigerate in a bottle or container. (The vinaigrette will keep in the fridge for up to 2 weeks.)

---

152 CAL, 12.47 G FAT (1.72 G SATURATED), .05 G PROTEIN, 1.25 G CARB, .02 G SUGAR, .07 G FIBER, 113.81 MG SODIUM PER SERVING

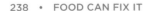

SNACKS

From super-fast to crowd-pleasing nibbles, these 21 recipes will keep you satisfied.

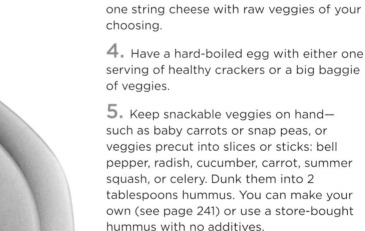

Grab-and-Go

Step 1: Stick hand in fridge. Step 2: Snack. It doesn't get easier than this.

1. Slice up an apple or pear, and enjoy with 2 tablespoons nut butter. Sprinkle with cinnamon, if you like.

2. Top ½ cup plain 2% Greek yogurt with nuts or berries.

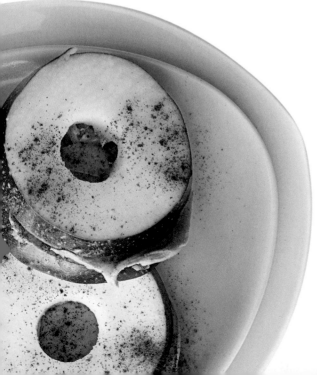

3. Keep string cheese handy. Have one piece with one serving of healthy crackers—either whole-grain, seed-based (such as Mary's Gone Crackers), or nut-based (such as Blue Diamond almond crackers). Or pair one string cheese with raw veggies of your choosing.

4. Have a hard-boiled egg with either one serving of healthy crackers or a big baggie of veggies.

5. Keep snackable veggies on hand—such as baby carrots or snap peas, or veggies precut into slices or sticks: bell pepper, radish, cucumber, carrot, summer squash, or celery. Dunk them into 2 tablespoons hummus. You can make your own (see page 241) or use a store-bought hummus with no additives.

6. Or dunk those same snackable veggies in 2 tablespoons nut butter.

7. Have a piece of fruit, such as an orange, apple, banana, or kiwi, with 1 ounce nuts.

Low Effort

These scrumptious snacks are worth a few minutes of chopping and seasoning.

1. Old Bay popcorn with super seeds: Toss 2 cups air-popped popcorn with ½ teaspoon extra-virgin olive oil. Sprinkle with ½ teaspoon Old Bay seasoning and 1 tablespoon toasted hulled sunflower seeds, and toss again.

2. Veggies with creamy avocado dip: Mash ¼ avocado with lime juice and a pinch of salt. If desired, add some chopped red onion. Then, dunk your snacking veggies.

3. Smoked paprika and almond popcorn: Toss 2 cups air-popped popcorn with 1 teaspoon extra-virgin olive oil. Sprinkle with 2 tablespoons toasted sliced almonds, ¼ teaspoon smoked paprika, and a couple of pinches of coarse salt, and toss again.

4. Tomato "pizzas": Halve 3 Campari or other midsize tomatoes and sprinkle with 1 tablespoon grated Parmesan cheese (or do a mix of Parmesan and shredded mozzarella). Broil until golden, 1 to 2 minutes. Drizzle with ½ teaspoon balsamic vinegar. Scatter 1 teaspoon sliced fresh basil leaves on top.

5. Curried-up carrot sticks: Toss about 1 cup carrot sticks with 1 tablespoon chopped fresh cilantro, 2 teaspoons fresh lime juice, ¼ teaspoon curry powder, ¼ teaspoon ground cumin, and a pinch of coarse salt.

6. Veggie rolls with nut butter: Spread 2 tablespoons nut butter over 6 stemmed Swiss chard leaves. Top with strips of bell pepper, cucumber, and celery. Sprinkle with chopped fresh cilantro and mint leaves. Drizzle with fresh lime juice. Roll to enclose and cut into vegetable rolls.

7. Frozen grapes with Greek yogurt: Top ¼ cup plain 2% Greek yogurt with ½ cup frozen red or green grapes. (Try them sprinkled with cinnamon.)

8. Brussels sprout chips: Trim the ends of 12 large Brussels sprouts and separate into single leaves. Toss with 2 teaspoons olive oil. Roast at 375°F on an oiled baking sheet, stirring occasionally, until crisp and browned, about 16 minutes. Toss with 1½ teaspoons low-sodium soy sauce.

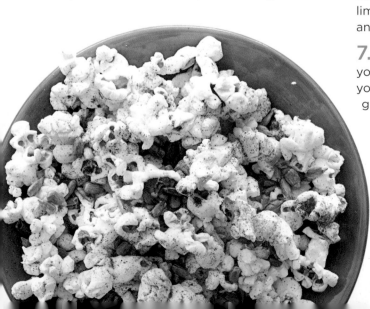

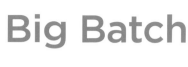

Big Batch

These each make four servings—enough to share with a crowd, or to keep just you snack-ready for a few days.

1. Chili-spiced pumpkin seeds: Toss 1 cup hulled pumpkin seeds with 2 teaspoons olive oil, ½ teaspoon chili powder, and ¼ teaspoon coarse salt. Spread on a rimmed baking sheet and toast in the oven at 375°F, stirring occasionally, until crisp, 8 to 10 minutes.

2. Creamy artichoke dip with cuke slices: Pulse in a food processor 1 (14-ounce) can artichoke hearts (rinsed and drained), 6 tablespoons grated Parmesan cheese, ¼ cup plain 2% Greek or regular yogurt, 2 teaspoons chopped fresh thyme, and ¼ teaspoon each coarse salt and freshly ground black pepper. Serve with cucumber rounds.

3. Edamame pesto dip with veggies: Puree in a food processor 1 cup thawed frozen shelled edamame; 2 tablespoons each extra-virgin olive oil, chopped fresh basil, sliced almonds, and grated Parmesan cheese; 1 tablespoon water; and ¼ teaspoon each coarse salt and freshly ground black pepper. Garnish with more basil. Serve with any veggies of your choosing.

4. Smoky hummus with veggies: Puree in a food processor 1 (15-ounce) can chickpeas (rinsed and drained), 2 tablespoons extra-virgin olive oil, 1 tablespoon fresh lemon juice, ½ teaspoon sriracha sauce (or similar hot sauce), and ½ teaspoon smoked paprika. Top with more smoked paprika. Serve with any veggies of your choosing.

5. Sweet potato strips: Use a vegetable peeler to slice 2 sweet potatoes lengthwise into thin strips. Toss with 4 teaspoons olive oil. Roast on an oiled nonstick baking sheet at 375°F until crisp and golden brown, 15 to 20 minutes. Season with a couple pinches of coarse salt. (Store leftovers in an airtight container for up to 3 days.)

6. Roasted chickpeas: Toss 1 (15-ounce) can chickpeas (rinsed and drained) with 1 tablespoon olive oil, 1 teaspoon ground turmeric, ½ teaspoon ground cumin, 1 minced garlic clove, and ¼ teaspoon coarse salt, plus freshly ground black pepper to taste. Spread the chickpeas on a rimmed baking sheet and roast at 425°F, shaking the baking sheet occasionally, for 18 minutes.

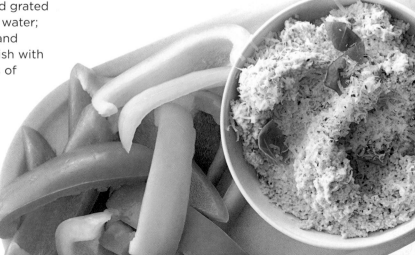

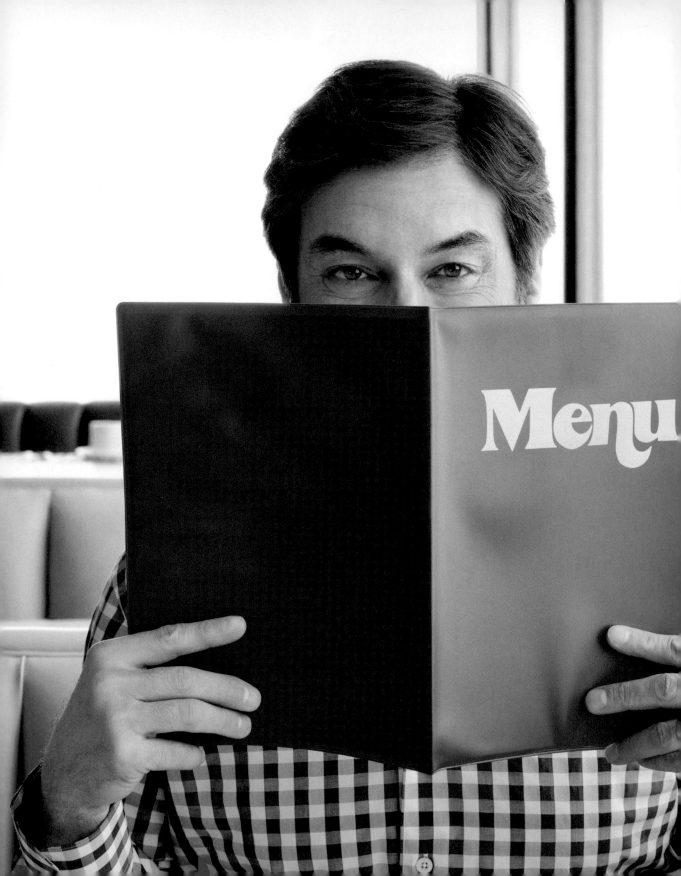

16.

Fix It!
Day 22 and Beyond

By now, you know a lot to get you going. You know how and why food can serve as preventive medicine. You know that nourishing food can be delicious food. You know why food means so much to me and my family. And you've kicked off your journey with the 21-Day Plan.

But what happens after that? How do you take what you've learned and apply it to the rest of your crazy life?

I'm willing to bet that the twenty-one days have engrained some new habits and inspired some new ideas for you. But ultimately, this plan is only marginally about the first twenty-one days. It's really about the thousands that come after that. What you do after this will be your recipe, your prescription, your family's tradition. Dreamed up by you. Made by you. Shared by you. And the key is being able to manage the three major eating environments you will encounter in your everyday life—eating in, eating out, and eating on the go.

Your emphasis will always be on eating in, because the greatest thing you can do to keep your healthy momentum going is to cook your own food. It's the only way to control what you're eating. That doesn't mean you'll never go to restaurants, but see if you can cut your frequency down to no more than three times a week. With the right recipe, cooking at home can feel just as celebratory as a night out. (You don't *always* have to make super-healthy food, either. I'd rather have you make chicken parm at home than have it at a restaurant. It's probably way healthier than the high-salt, high-calorie stuff you'd get served.)

You can still make the dishes you relied on during the 21-Day Plan, but now you can add the healthy and delicious recipes in this chapter. When you do eat out (or order takeout), use my restaurant guide to the healthiest options (starting on page 258). Also, the recipes in *Dr. Oz The Good Life* magazine are all healthful and based on the FIXES way of eating, so you'll find lots of great new ideas there, too.

Environment 1: Eating In

First, pat yourself on the back for completing the 21-Day Plan. Three weeks of home-cooked meals: That's no small feat. You've done a good thing for your body. Keep the benefits rolling with the following easy strategies. At first, they might feel like work, but give them a week or two and you'll be in the groove, noticing major benefits to your overall well-being.

1. Plan your weekly menu before grocery shopping. Decide what you're going to cook before you hit the supermarket, write up a shopping list, and bring it with you to stay on track. (A list can help you lighten up your weekly cart's calorie load without even trying—by 6,500 fewer calories, according to one study.) That'll help to prevent junky impulse buys—or that sad, sad moment two weeks later when you have to throw out armfuls of spoiled produce. (We've *all* gotten overambitious with salad greens.) Also, treat shopping as an opportunity to make healthy cooking easy on yourself because your supermarket is full of good-for-you convenience foods. Why suffer through cutting up a winter squash when the cubed kind is right there in the produce aisle? Load up your fridge, pantry, and freezer with other time-savers like precooked beets, cleaned and sliced mushrooms, fast-cooking whole grains, prepeeled

A SENSATIONAL START TO THE DAY

Ready to branch out at breakfast time? One of my favorite options is avocado toast. Mash half an avocado and spread it over one slice of whole wheat toast. Drizzle with lemon juice and olive oil and sprinkle with red pepper flakes. Add a slice of tomato, if you like. Delicious and satisfying, and it takes only a few minutes to make.

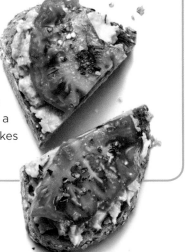

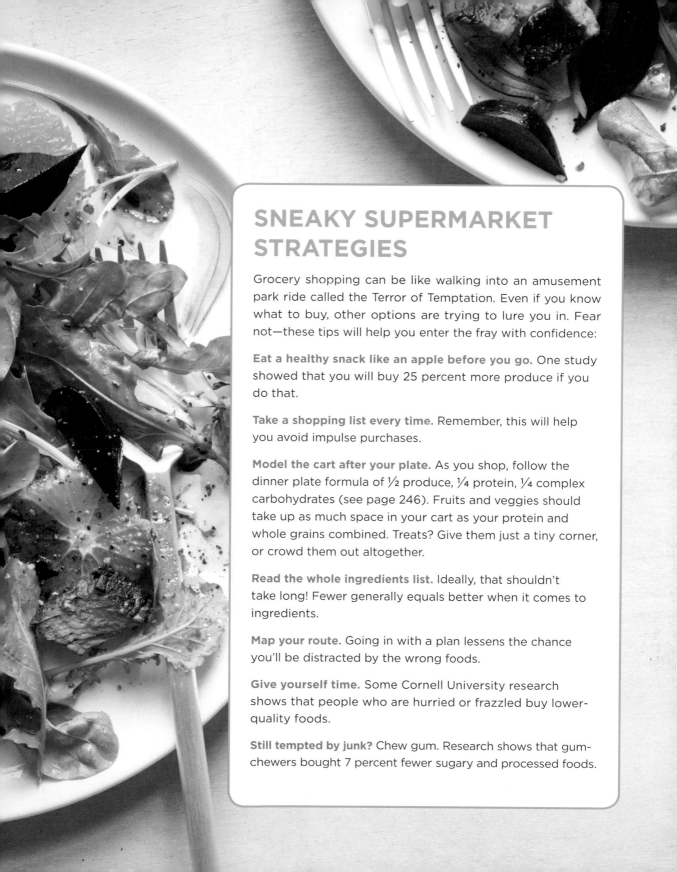

SNEAKY SUPERMARKET STRATEGIES

Grocery shopping can be like walking into an amusement park ride called the Terror of Temptation. Even if you know what to buy, other options are trying to lure you in. Fear not—these tips will help you enter the fray with confidence:

Eat a healthy snack like an apple before you go. One study showed that you will buy 25 percent more produce if you do that.

Take a shopping list every time. Remember, this will help you avoid impulse purchases.

Model the cart after your plate. As you shop, follow the dinner plate formula of ½ produce, ¼ protein, ¼ complex carbohydrates (see page 246). Fruits and veggies should take up as much space in your cart as your protein and whole grains combined. Treats? Give them just a tiny corner, or crowd them out altogether.

Read the whole ingredients list. Ideally, that shouldn't take long! Fewer generally equals better when it comes to ingredients.

Map your route. Going in with a plan lessens the chance you'll be distracted by the wrong foods.

Give yourself time. Some Cornell University research shows that people who are hurried or frazzled buy lower-quality foods.

Still tempted by junk? Chew gum. Research shows that gum-chewers bought 7 percent fewer sugary and processed foods.

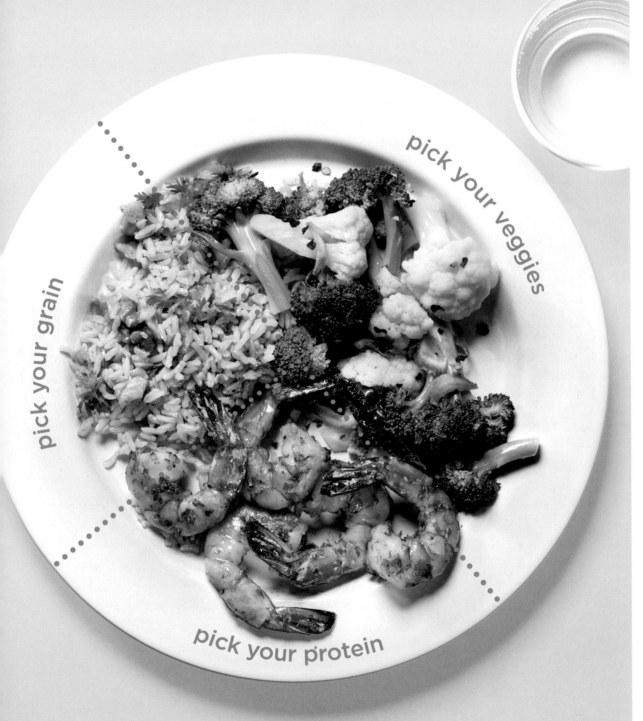

pick your veggies

pick your grain

pick your protein

Build a plate that's filled as follows: ½ produce,
¼ protein, and ¼ complex carbohydrates.

hard-boiled eggs, and refrigerated whole wheat pizza dough.

2. Automate your breakfasts. Find a breakfast or two you love, and eat them every day. The fewer options you give yourself to choose from, the easier it is to make a good decision.

3. Eat a salad. Every. Single. Day. This is a rule I live by. Truly, it's hard *not* to hit your daily veggie requirement—that's 2½ cups minimum—if there's a daily salad on the menu. And that doesn't always have to mean a big ol' leafy lunch. You can have a side salad with dinner, or a warm salad with grains and shredded greens. Have it any way you like, as long as you have it.

4. Do the No-Fail Dinner Formula. There's a lot riding on your dinner decision. So often, I see this meal become the diet definer: We've trained ourselves to view it as the major meal of the day, so it's easy to overeat; *plus*, it comes in the evening, when we're feeling tired and lazy and just want to sit down to an easy-to-fix bowl of something comforting. All these instincts can derail you, but there's a basic formula that helps. You always want your plate to look like this: ½ **produce,** ¼ **protein,** ¼ **complex carbohydrates**. It's that simple. Do this every night, and you'll be well on your way to getting the nutrients you need in the right proportions. One night you might combine a cupful of cooked whole wheat pasta mixed with the same amount of broccoli, topped with cubed chicken and served with a side salad. Another night, it might be a veggie-loaded stir-fry with tofu, served over brown rice. Or you could do a spinach salad topped with quinoa and salmon. There are a million ways to get there. You can start with my dinner spinner on page 250.

Environment 2: Eating on the Go

The joys of traveling are many: seeing new sights, setting out on adventures, quality time with family. Without question, eating is another one. Less wonderful? Bringing home a five-pound souvenir of bloat and pudge. I want you to enjoy your travels guilt-free and maybe have a few surprising nutritional *aha* moments. What I don't want is to see you revert to eating junk because it's your only option. Here's how Lisa and I find the happy medium:

BYOE: Bring Your Own Eats. Whether you're headed to the airport or buckling up for a long car ride, packing your own snacks is the way to go. My family's favorite healthy bites include single-serving packets of noshes, like pistachios, almond butter, and olives; zip-top bags of raw baby carrots, broccoli, and bell pepper strips; containers of hard-boiled eggs; and fruits with thick peels that don't need washing, like oranges, bananas, and kiwis.

Start the day right. When you're away from home, a smart breakfast routine is your best friend. My regular breakfast is plain 2% Greek yogurt with berries, and I take that basic yogurt-produce formula with me wherever I go. When I'm visiting my parents in Turkey, it's Turkish yogurt with cucumber and tomato wedges. At a hotel buffet, it's plain yogurt and a scoop of fruit salad. You get the picture. This helps me get off to a nutritious start—and if I want to go rogue at dinner and order (gasp!) a burger, I know the whole day wasn't a wash.

Don't forget to hydrate. Tote around a water bottle, and snack on produce with high water density. Watermelon, strawberries, and cukes are all good H2O sources.

Build healthy into your holiday. Kick off a day of sightseeing at the town farmers' market, gather a bushel of apples at a pick-your-own orchard, make a reservation at a farm-to-table restaurant, or take a picnic on a hike.

Use your hotel room "kitchen." I wouldn't go so far as to press panini with a hot iron (though I've seen it done), but I do tend to crowd the minifridge with my own picks, like bottles of coconut water, tubs of yogurt, and dinner leftovers. Another hack that comes in handy is using hot water from the electric kettle or coffeemaker to make instant oatmeal, whole-grain couscous, or tea. (I bring my favorite tea bags from home.)

Find foodies' favorite spots. Look near the sights you want to see by clicking through blogs, local websites, Yelp, and Instagram. Then you won't waste time and calories at a subpar tourist trap.

When in doubt, order the fish. My go-to— and generally a smart choice, so long as it's not deep-fried.

Get brave with produce. If you're given the chance to eat fruits or veggies in a new way, go for it. In California, I love seeing oranges

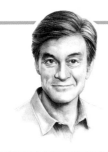

It's a Superfood

Eating 1½ cups or more of strawberries per week may help to lower your heart attack risk.

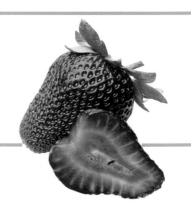

go savory in a salad with avocado and red onion. And southern succotash wows me; it has tomatoes and okra in addition to the lima beans and corn I'm used to. When you find a new favorite dish, take the recipe home.

Sip smart. A beer has around 150 calories, and science says that drinking it in moderation can reduce your heart attack risk. Wine has about 125 calories, plus artery-friendly antioxidants. A piña colada? You could be looking at more than 650 calories and 80 grams of sugar.

Slow down to really savor. One of the best parts of being on vacation is the luxury of time, so you can actually stop to enjoy meals instead of shoveling them down during a five-minute break. Even if you have a heavy day of sightseeing ahead, block off an hour for a real lunch break.

Go halfsies. You'll get to sample more if you split dishes. At restaurants, Lisa and I like to share two appetizers and a big main course, then have cappuccinos for dessert.

Go ahead, have that dessert. Just stick to one treat a day, and make it really phenomenal. Continental buffets will try to break you with the standard blueberry muffins and pastries, but just remember, you're holding out for something special. Which would you rather have: a stale muffin, or an exceptional slice of cherry pie à la mode later in the day?

Work produce into every meal. It doesn't have to be a side salad—though you know me, I won't say no to a salad. Get creative: If you're having barbecue, choosing a side of collard greens over mac and cheese could save you 150 calories. Topping pizza with peppers instead of sausage can lop off 50 calories a slice. Add chopped apple to your morning oatmeal. And opting for dark chocolate–dipped strawberries instead of a sundae can shave off hundreds of calories, and net you a dose of fiber and antioxidants.

Environment 3: Eating Out

I'm a big fan of home cooking, but everyone likes a restaurant night, and deserves one. In fact, Lisa and I have a weekly night out—she gets a break from cooking and we get to try some dishes we might not make for ourselves at home. Everyone wins.

It's true that restaurants are famous for sneaking extra butter and other fats, salt, and sugars into their foods, but if you order wisely, you can avoid those traps. I've rounded up a list of healthy restaurant choices you can enjoy without inadvertently undoing all the healthy, home-cooked progress you've made.

You can almost always eat well by ordering fish or chicken with steamed or roasted vegetables. Start with a salad (olive oil and vinegar), and ask them not to bring any bread. What about specialty places? Turn to page 258.

USE THE DINNER SPINNER

Drawing a blank on what to make for dinner? Follow this no-fail formula: a protein (¼ of your plate), a veggie (½ of your plate), and a grain (¼ of your plate). Then mix and match to build a healthy, quick, delicious meal.

You can use your favorite proteins from the 21-Day Plan, plus an easy-to-cook carb and a veggie. For example:

- Cook up quinoa-crusted salmon with some whole wheat couscous and a side of stewed cherry tomatoes.
- Serve balsamic chicken over a half cauliflower "rice," half quinoa mixture.
- Ladle spiced lentils over sautéed spinach; serve with a side of roasted sweet potatoes.
- Have the Asian tofu steak with a simple veggie stir-fry and a scoop of millet.

Or you can configure a restaurant order into its healthiest self:

- Order Chinese chicken and broccoli plus extra steamed veggies and brown rice.
- Pair whole wheat spaghetti and meatballs with a big side salad.
- Have salmon-and-avocado sushi rolls made with brown rice, then add a side of edamame.

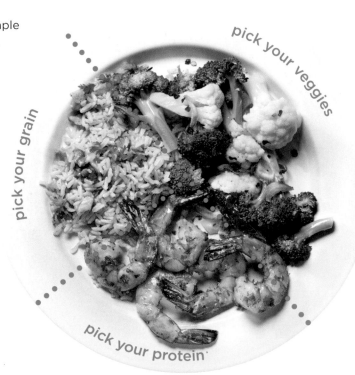

pick your grain

pick your veggies

pick your protein

Itching to try out a new (and weeknight-doable) dinner? Try this rotating roster of healthy recipes that lets you mix and match proteins, grains, and veggies to delicious effects. Once you have the formula down, it's easy to riff.

Proteins

Herbed Sautéed Shrimp

Chickpeas in Tomato Sauce

Chicken with Orange and Olives

Veggies

Sautéed Greens with Onions

Simple Roasted Veggies

Broccoli and Cauliflower Medley

Grains

Lemony Quinoa

Herby Millet with Walnuts

Farro Pilaf

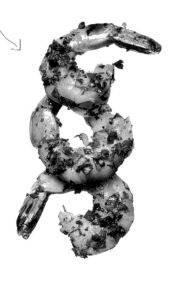

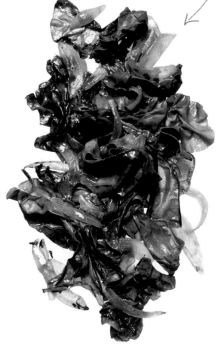

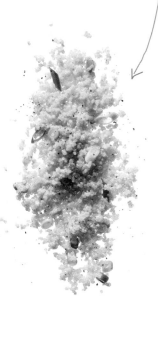

First, pick your protein.

Herbed Sautéed Shrimp

SERVES 4

1 tablespoon olive oil

1 teaspoon chopped garlic

1 pound large shrimp, peeled and deveined (about 20)

¼ cup chopped fresh flat-leaf parsley or cilantro

Salt

Freshly ground black pepper

Heat the olive oil in a large skillet over medium heat. Add the garlic and cook until golden, about 1 minute. Add the shrimp and cook, stirring, for 3 to 4 minutes, or until opaque. Add the parsley and season with salt and pepper.

---

113 CAL, 5 G FAT (1 G SATURATED), 16 G PROTEIN, 2 G CARB, 0 G SUGAR, 0 G FIBER, 644 MG SODIUM PER SERVING

Chickpeas in Tomato Sauce

SERVES 4

1 (15-ounce) can chickpeas, rinsed and drained

⅓ cup marinara sauce (homemade or store-bought, with no added sugar)

Red pepper flakes

¼ cup crumbled feta cheese (optional)

Put the chickpeas in a small saucepan or microwave-safe bowl and add the marinara sauce and red pepper flakes to taste. Heat through, either on the stovetop or in the micro-wave. Sprinkle with the feta (adds 1 g protein, 25 cal, and 2 g fat per serving), if using.

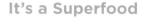

126 CAL, 4 G FAT (1 G SATURATED), 7 G PROTEIN, 17 G CARB, 4 G SUGAR, 5 G FIBER, 310 MG SODIUM PER SERVING

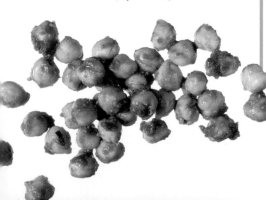

It's a Superfood

Beyond adding a nice amount of fiber and protein onto your plate, chickpeas also contain 10 to 25 percent of your daily iron needs, depending on your age.

Chicken with Orange and Olives

Preheat the oven to 350°F.

Heat the olive oil in a medium skillet with ovenproof handle over medium-high heat. Season the chicken breasts with salt and pepper and add them to the skillet. Cook for 2 to 3 minutes on each side until nicely browned. Transfer the skillet to the oven and bake for 15 minutes, or until the chicken is no longer pink in the center. Remove the chicken from the skillet and set aside; return the skillet to the stovetop. Add the orange zest and juice and bring to a boil over medium-high heat, scraping up any browned bits from the bottom of the skillet. Add the olives and cook until the mixture has thickened slightly, then return the chicken to the skillet to coat with the sauce.

---

171 CAL, 6 G FAT (1 G SATURATED), 24 G PROTEIN, 3 G CARB, 2 G SUGAR, 0 G FIBER, 254 MG SODIUM PER SERVING

SERVES 4

1 teaspoon olive oil

2 (8-ounce) boneless, skinless chicken breasts

Salt

Freshly ground black pepper

Zest and juice of 1 navel orange

¼ cup pitted Kalamata olives, chopped or sliced

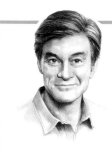

It's a Superfood

Olives are a great source of monounsaturated fatty acids, which help your heart by lowering the bad kind of cholesterol.

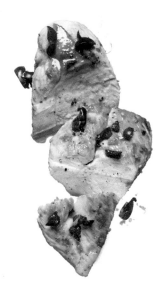

Next, pick your veggie.

Broccoli and Cauliflower Medley

SERVES 4

½ medium head broccoli, cut into florets

½ medium head cauliflower, cut into florets

1 tablespoon olive oil

2 garlic cloves, thinly sliced

½ lemon

Salt

Red pepper flakes

Place the broccoli and cauliflower florets in a steamer basket set over boiling water in a medium saucepan. Cover and steam until crisp-tender, about 4 minutes. (If you don't have fresh broccoli or cauliflower, you can microwave about 3½ cups frozen florets.)

Meanwhile, heat the olive oil in a small skillet over medium-low heat. Add the garlic to the skillet and cook, stirring occasionally, until golden, about 3 minutes. Remove the vegetables from the steamer, toss with the garlic and oil, and squeeze the lemon over the top. Season with salt and red pepper flakes.

63 CAL, 4 G FAT (1 G SATURATED), 3 G PROTEIN, 7 G CARB, 1 G SUGAR, 3 G FIBER, 32 MG SODIUM PER SERVING

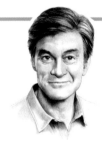

It's a Superfood

You get a surprisingly large vitamin C bonus in a cupful of cauliflower—more than half of your daily needs. The veg also contains good doses of fiber, vitamin K, and folate.

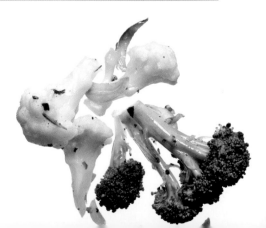

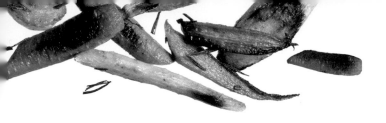

Simple Roasted Veggies

SERVES 4

Preheat the oven to 425°F.

In a large bowl, toss all the ingredients and spread out on a baking sheet. Roast for 25 minutes, then turn and roast until golden brown, about 10 minutes more.

1 bunch carrots, peeled and halved crosswise

3 parsnips, peeled, halved lengthwise, then halved crosswise

2 small turnips, cut into wedges

2 tablespoons olive oil

Salt

Freshly ground black pepper

½ teaspoon paprika

1 tablespoon chopped fresh rosemary (optional)

138 CAL, 7 G FAT (1 G SATURATED), 2 G PROTEIN, 18 G CARB,
7 G SUGAR, 5 G FIBER, 78 MG SODIUM PER SERVING

Sautéed Greens with Onions

SERVES 4

Heat the 2 teaspoons olive oil in a large skillet over medium-high heat. Add the onion and season with salt and pepper. Cook, stirring occasionally, until the onion is browned, 8 to 10 minutes. Add the stock, reduce the heat to medium-low, and simmer for 6 minutes. Transfer the onion to a bowl and return the skillet to a medium-high heat. Add the 1 tablespoon olive oil; then add the Swiss chard. Season lightly with salt and pepper and cook, tossing, for 2 to 3 minutes. Return the onion to the skillet, toss to combine, and serve.

1 tablespoon plus 2 teaspoons olive oil

1 small yellow onion, thinly sliced

Salt

Freshly ground black pepper

¼ cup low-sodium chicken stock

1½ pounds Swiss chard (1 large or 2 medium bunches), stemmed, leaves torn into large pieces (substitute other greens, if you like)

71 CAL, 6 G FAT (1 G SATURATED), 2 G PROTEIN, 4 G CARB,
2 G SUGAR, 1 G FIBER, 182 MG SODIUM PER SERVING

Finally, choose a grain.

Lemony Quinoa

SERVES 6

1¾ cups low-sodium chicken stock

1 cup quinoa

Juice of ½ lemon
(1 to 2 tablespoons)

1 tablespoon olive oil

4 scallions, thinly sliced

Salt

Freshly ground black pepper

In a small saucepan, bring the stock to a boil. Add the quinoa, reduce the heat to low, cover, and cook until the water has been absorbed, about 15 minutes. Fluff with a fork, transfer to a bowl, and stir in the lemon juice, olive oil, and scallions. Season with salt and pepper.

---

130 CAL, 4 G FAT (0 G SATURATED), 4 G PROTEIN, 19 G CARB, 0 G SUGAR, 2 G FIBER, 134 MG SODIUM PER SERVING

Herby Millet with Walnuts

SERVES 6

1 cup millet

⅓ cup coarsely chopped walnuts, toasted

¼ cup coarsely chopped fresh cilantro or flat-leaf parsley

¼ teaspoon salt

Freshly ground black pepper

In a medium saucepan, combine the millet and 2 cups water. Bring to a boil, then reduce the heat to low and cover the pot. Cook until the water has been absorbed, about 15 minutes. Remove from the heat and let sit, covered, for 10 minutes. Fluff with a fork, transfer to a bowl, and add the walnuts and cilantro. Season with salt and pepper.

---

148 CAL, 5 G FAT (1 G SATURATED), 3 G PROTEIN, 24 G CARB, 1 G SUGAR, 2 G FIBER, 100 MG SODIUM PER SERVING

Farro Pilaf

Heat the olive oil in a medium saucepan over medium-low heat. Add the onion and cook for 8 to 10 minutes, until soft and golden. Add the mushrooms and a sprinkle of salt and cook, stirring, until the mushrooms soften, 3 to 4 minutes more. Add the farro and cook, stirring, for 2 minutes. Add the stock and bring to a boil. Reduce the heat to maintain a simmer, and cook for 25 to 30 minutes, until all the liquid has been absorbed and the farro is tender.

---

144 CAL, 3 G FAT (0 G SATURATED), 5 G PROTEIN, 25 G CARB, 1 G SUGAR, 4 G FIBER, 201 MG SODIUM PER SERVING

SERVES 6

1 tablespoon olive oil

1 small yellow onion, chopped

1½ cups sliced cremini or button mushrooms

Salt

1 cup farro

2 cups low-sodium chicken stock

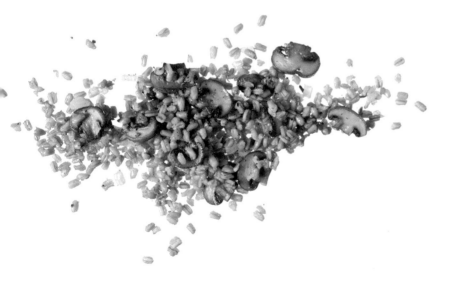

CHINESE

BEAN CURD WITH BROCCOLI

Bean curd, aka tofu, offers satisfying protein. Throw in a powerhouse vegetable like broccoli, and you get my seal of approval.

BUDDHA'S DELIGHT

This tofu-veggie dish won't leave you with a Buddha belly. It can come in around 300 calories.

DUMPLINGS

Steamed are less caloric than fried, but only by 10 to 30 calories an order. What's inside counts most: Choose veggie or shrimp, not pork, to cut nearly 100 calories per order.

FRIED RICE

Not as scary as it sounds, but only if you stick to a proper serving: a cupcake wrapper's worth of rice. Even better? Brown rice: Gram for gram, it contains four times more fiber than white rice.

MOO GOO GAI PAN

I love this chicken stir-fry loaded with mushrooms. The fungi are a source of B vitamins, which help our bodies turn food into fuel.

MOO SHU CHICKEN

An Oz-family favorite packed with cabbage, which has cancer-fighting potential. Skip the pancakes and ask for lettuce cups.

SAUTÉED BABY BOK CHOY

This green vegetable is bursting with nutrients and potential disease-fighting compounds.

SPARERIBS

Can't lie: These are a personal guilty pleasure. My trick? I eat only one or two. A whole portion of ribs has almost a day's worth of saturated fat.

STEAMED VEGETABLES

I load up on broccoli and string beans (or whatever other steamed veggies are on the menu).

WHOLE FISH

This is a good source of lean protein and a great dish to split. Go for grilled or steamed fish (not "crispy," aka fried).

WONTON SOUP

The wontons satisfy a craving for dumplings, and if you get a cup instead of a bowl, it's only about 70 calories.

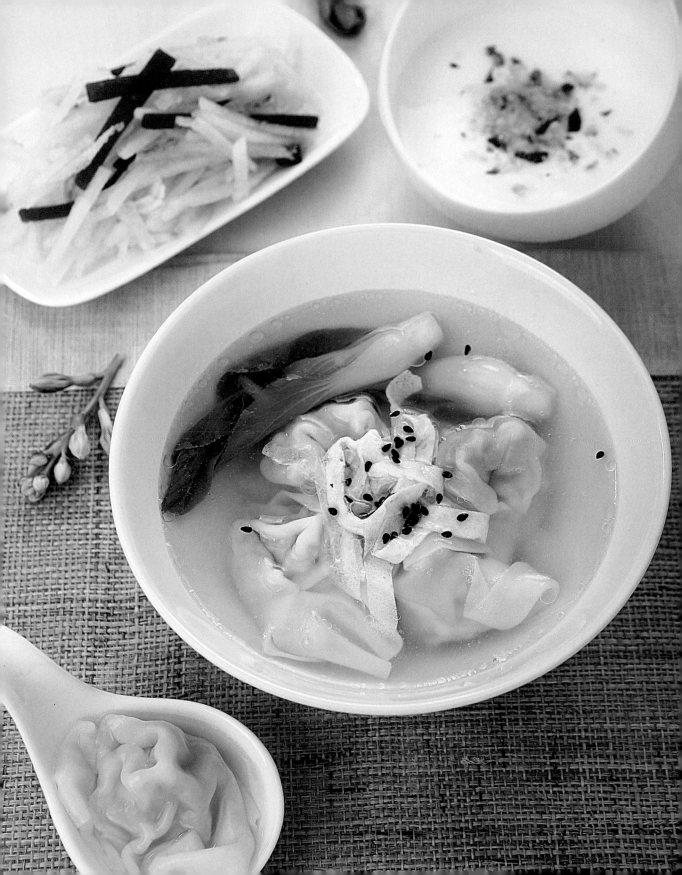

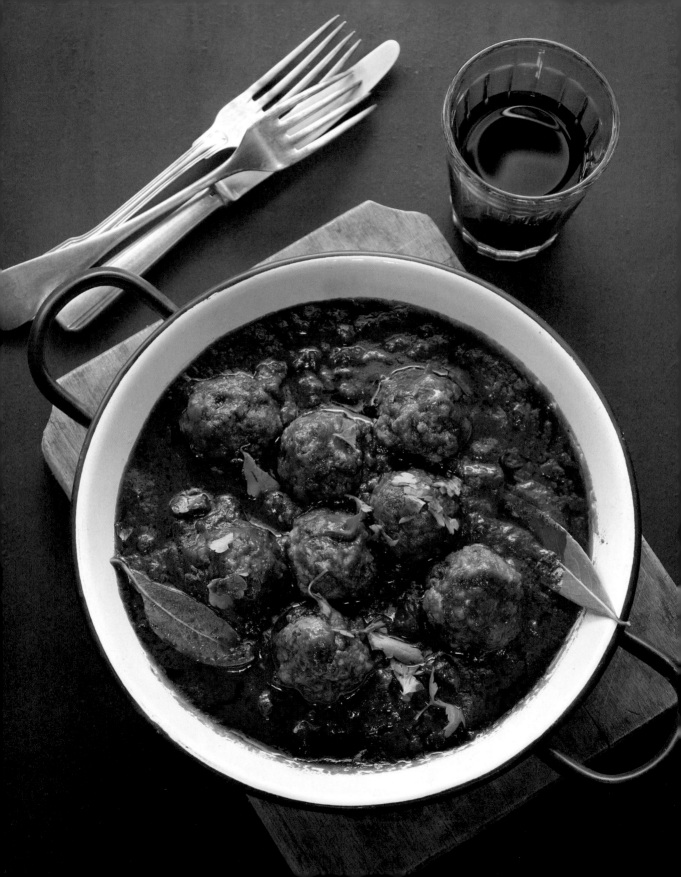

ITALIAN

ANTIPASTI

If you can get the kind with marinated vegetables and olives—not just meat and cheese—go for it. You don't have to worry about eating too much oil; you'll only wind up downing a few teaspoons of it (about 80 calories), and it's probably the heart-healthy kind, anyway.

CHICKEN CACCIATORE WITH MUSHROOMS

Lean protein and veggies—a smart pick.

GRILLED SALMON WITH AN HERBED CRUST

Salmon's pretty much my go-to entrée wherever I eat.

MEATBALLS IN MARINARA SAUCE

Split a side of these with the table. A small meatball has about 40 calories, and lots of hunger-squashing protein.

MINESTRONE

Starting your meal with broth-based soup can reduce your overall calorie intake. Plus, this usually has beans, which are rich in fiber and protein.

MUSSELS MARINARA

Mussels are high in protein and vitamin B. I like the kind in marinara sauce the best; the white wine sauce can sneak in too much butter.

SAUTÉED SPINACH IN GARLIC AND OLIVE OIL

This is one of my favorite appetizers. It's filling and usually has less than 100 calories.

SHRIMP SCAMPI

Not a bad option—ask for whole wheat pasta (it's often available), and eat more of the shrimp than the pasta.

MEXICAN

BLACK OR PINTO BEANS

Both kinds are fiber and protein powerhouses. I skip the refried kind, which can add extra fat.

BURRITO BOWLS

Another good one. I swap out the usual white rice base for lettuce or brown rice.

BURRITOS

If you go for one of these, nix the rice. It doesn't add flavor, and the tortilla has enough carbs on its own.

CHICKEN MOLE

Mole sauce is made with chiles, spices, seeds, and chocolate, so it's delicious and full of antioxidants. Pile on the veggie sides!

CHIPS AND GUACAMOLE

I love this appetizer! Avocados have healthy fats. Stick to two handfuls of chips.

FAJITAS

I like that these come with lots of peppers and onions. But don't feel as if you have to clean your plate: Too-big portions can drive up calories. (Besides, they make great leftovers.)

TACOS

Grilled chicken, grilled fish, or bean tacos are all great choices. I ask for any sauce on the side and use just a little.

SANGRIA

Mmm, antioxidants. Have a glass, and snack on the fruit for a fiber bonus.

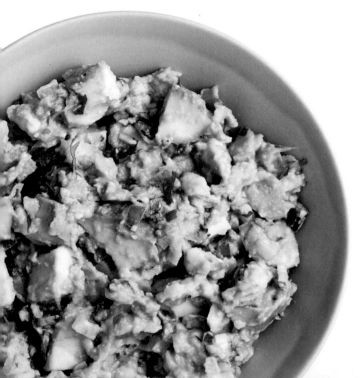

SALAD BAR

BASES

Mixed greens: Always a good bet, with next to no calories.

Red cabbage: "Leafy purples" may not have quite the same ring to it as "leafy greens," but don't hold that against red cabbage. The veggie's purple tint comes from heart-healthy compounds. These are extra good in make-ahead salads; they don't get as soggy as other bases.

Spinach or kale: My top choices when I can get them—they have so many nutrients, for nearly zero calories. I always go for the darkest greens available because they tend to have the most antioxidants.

PROTEINS

Chickpeas: Delicious plant-based protein.

Eggs: New science says that pairing raw vegetables with cooked eggs may help us absorb more of the veggies' nutrients.

Grilled chicken: Grilling adds flavor without loading on calories.

TOPPERS

Olives: They're loaded with healthy fats, and it only takes a few to pack your bowl with flavor.

Walnuts: I add crunch to every salad with nuts and seeds. Walnuts are one of my favorites—they're full of heart-healthy omega-3s. A serving size is 1 ounce—about ¼ cup.

VEGGIES

Carrots: There's a group of disease fighters called carotenoids, and if the name hasn't already tipped you off, carrots are full of 'em. (So are orange bell peppers.)

Red onions: Always a smart add, with plenty of flavor and almost no calories.

Tomatoes: I love that red tomatoes have lots of lycopene, which might lower the risk of heart disease and some forms of cancer.

Yellow bell peppers: These are antioxidant powerhouses. That's true of some other yellow and yellow-orange produce, too.

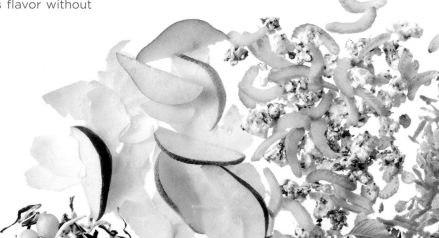

SANDWICH SHOP

EXTRAS

Avocados: Creamy and so heart-healthy.

Mayo: A spoonful is just fine. (Basically, it's eggs, oil, and lemon juice.) Also on my yes list: oil, vinegar, and all kinds of mustard.

MEAT AND CHEESE

Get grilled or roasted: Meat prepped that way beats a processed cold cut—those tend to have not-so-healthy additives and lots of sodium. (I'd choose roast beef over salami any day.) Chicken and turkey are my go-tos.

Use this calorie-cutting trick: Opt for meat or cheese—not both. Most cheeses are on par, nutritionally, so get your favorite and stick to no more than two slices.

THREE COMBOS I LOVE

A.C.L.T.: avocado, grilled chicken, lettuce, tomato, mustard, salt, and pepper.

Veggie sub: bell, banana, and/or jalapeño peppers; cucumbers; tomato; red onion; provolone; oil and vinegar.

The healthy meatball: meatballs, tomato sauce, sweet peppers, olives, spinach, and Italian seasoning.

VEGGIES

Raw veggies: The more, the merrier—heck, just throw a whole salad on there. (So what if you need a fork to eat it?) Cucumbers, red onion, bell pepper, tomato . . .

Green means go: Lettuce is great; spinach is even better. Whichever greens you choose to fill your sandwich with, get a double order.

Hot peppers: These add tons of flavor for not a lot of calories. But pickling can sneak in sodium, so keep it to just one kind of pepper.

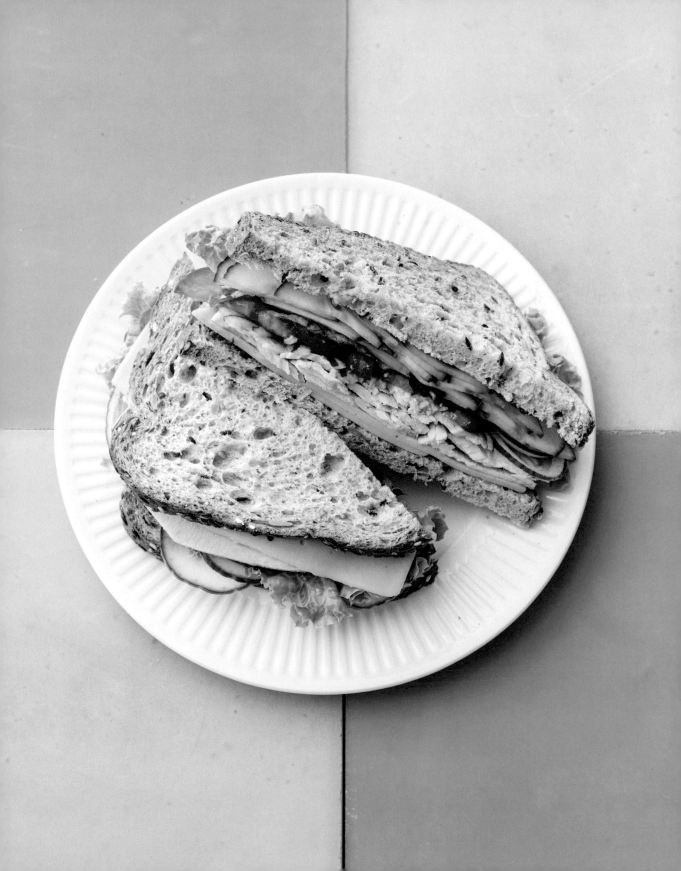

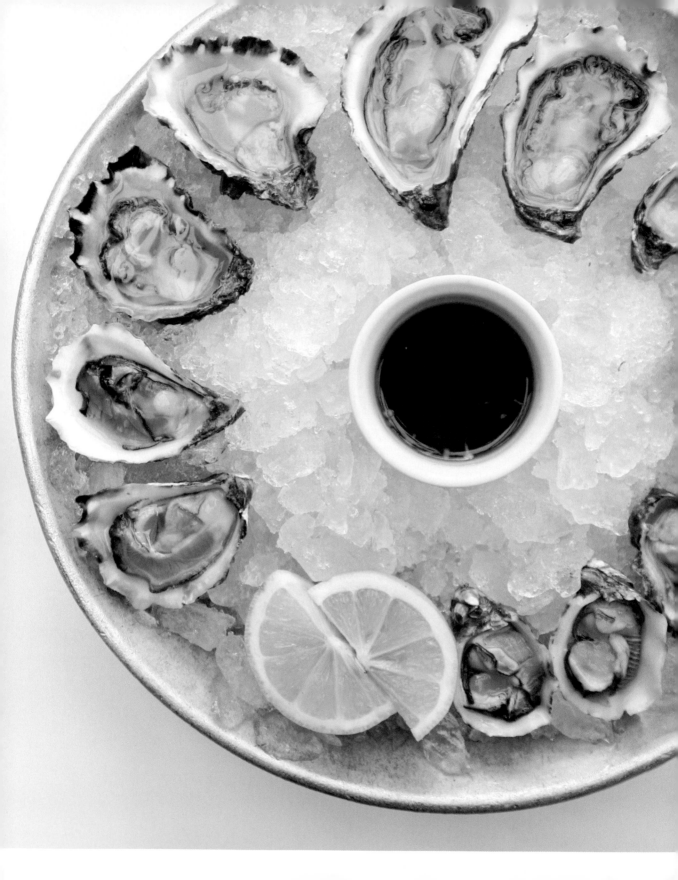

SEAFOOD

BLACKENED CATFISH

A smart and tasty order, with healthy fats, vitamins, and plenty of filling protein.

CATCH OF THE DAY

The type of fish matters less than how it's prepped. If you can get it grilled, it's one of the healthiest dishes on the menu.

CRAB LEGS

Just one leg packs in about 25 grams of protein, plus important nutrients like zinc and selenium.

LOBSTER ROLL

Sure, there's mayo or butter in the lobster salad, but this isn't likely to break the calorie bank. One chain's clocks in at 320 calories.

MANHATTAN CLAM CHOWDER

A cup of chowder will help fill you up— Manhattan-style is my pick. It's got about two-thirds the calories of the creamy New England kind.

OYSTERS

A nutrient-rich pick with iron and zinc. Get 'em raw or grilled. Broiled oysters tend to go heavy on butter and oil, and deep-fried can load on the calories scary-fast. (Avoid anything deep-fried as a rule. A plate of fish-and-chips at one major restaurant chain contains a truly staggering 1,990 calories.)

SHRIMP COCKTAIL

A zero-guilt treat (six big shrimp = about 60 calories). Douse them with lemon juice for extra flavor.

STEAMED CLAMS

One serving of these healthy little guys (about 10 small clams) covers 130 percent of your daily iron needs, plus plenty of vitamin B12.

STEAMED LOBSTER

Get crackin'. Even with buttery dip, a 1¼-pound lobster still weighs in at less than 550 calories.

SOUP SPOT

BLACK BEAN

A warming winner—it's low in calories and has tons of fiber and protein. (I'm also a fan of its tasty cousin, lentil soup.)

MINESTRONE

This low-cal soup has a high-fiber medley of vegetables, pasta, and beans. Plus, it packs in a healthy dose of vitamin A.

TOMATO

It has lots of antioxidants, like cancer-fighting lycopene. I treat this as the veggie portion of the meal and pair it with protein and starch.

VEGETABLE BISQUE

It's worth asking some what's-in-there questions. Bisque with cream can be a meal in its own right, caloriewise; straight-up veggie puree is more of a starter.

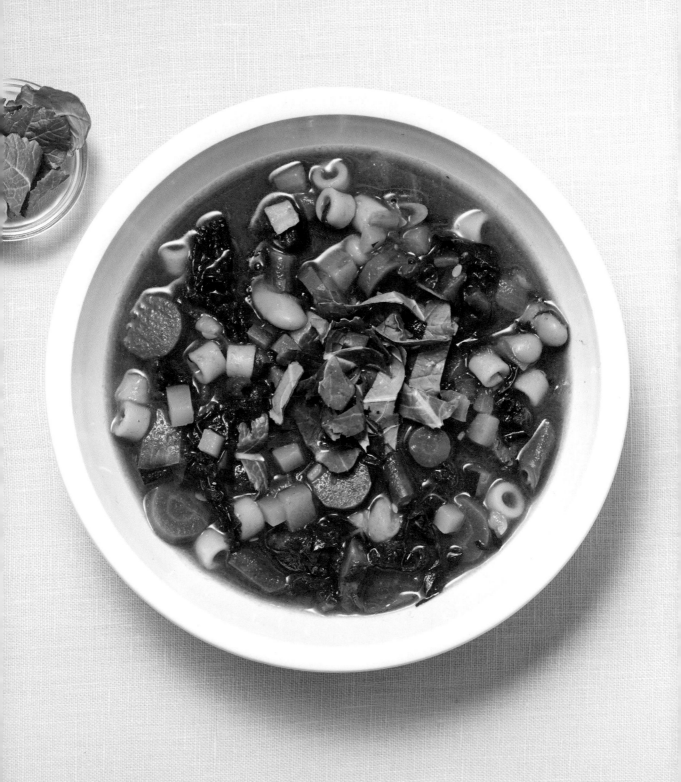

JUICE AND SMOOTHIE BAR

Beet juice: This root veggie is full of folate, and raw beets have more of it than cooked or canned beets.

Berry-yogurt smoothie: A great call if it's made with plain yogurt—bonus points for Greek—and real berries. (Some places use frozen yogurt or sherbet—not as healthy.)

Carrot juice: A small glass meets your daily vitamin A needs for nearly a week.

Green juice: Greens are always nutritional powerhouses, but juices with them are often sweetened up with sugary pineapple, orange, or apple juice. If fruit juice isn't the main ingredient, go for it.

Peanut butter–banana smoothie: Look for a simple ingredients list. If it's really just banana, nut butter, and maybe some milk or yogurt, you're good to go. When chocolate and fro-yo start to sneak in, that's a tip-off that this may be more of a dessert than a healthy snack or breakfast.

ADD-INS

Chia seeds: A 2 tablespoon serving of this super seed has about 8 grams of fiber, so I like to add it to juice, which tends to be low in fiber. This way, you'll stay full longer.

Ginger: Beyond adding a spicy kick to your drink, ginger may also lower your cholesterol.

Greens: Lots of smoothie spots will throw a handful or two of greens into anything you order. It's well worth it—they blend right in, flavorwise, and bring nutritional heft to your order.

Wheatgrass: This rock star plant packs a healthy punch with amino acids, vitamins, and minerals.

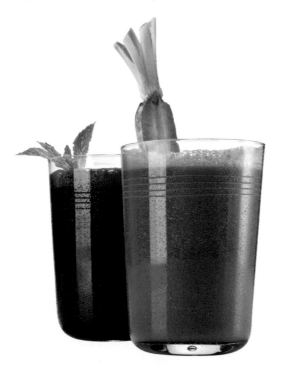

COFFEE SHOP

The trick to ordering healthily at a coffee shop? Actually ordering *coffee*. Regular coffee. You can't go wrong with plain ol' java and a big splash of milk. Try adding cinnamon instead of sugar, and you've got a pick-me-up for around 25 calories. (And if you need sugar, it's hardly the end of the world. Even if you add two packets, your drink still rings in at about 50 calories.)

Skip the lattes. Even the "skinny" ones. Sure, they're made with nonfat milk—but *a lot* of it. (A 16-ounce one at a major chain has 120 calories.) Instead, try a café au lait—half coffee, half milk, and about half the calories.

Cappuccinos are made with foamed milk instead of steamed, so it's literally airier—and lower-cal. An 8-ounce one made with 2% milk only sets you back 80 calories.

As a rule, **avoid flavored syrup.** At one chain, each pump injects about 20 calories—and those add up quickly.

Go no whip. A dollop of whipped cream can tack on at least 70 calories and 8 grams of fat. That's more than an Oreo.

Looking to grab breakfast on the fly? **Pick up a breakfast sandwich.** Most major chains have options that ring in around 300 calories or fewer. Protein from eggs hits the spot.

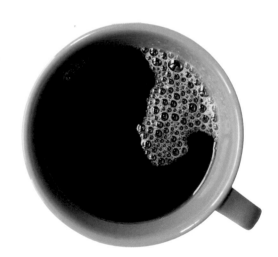

WHAT TO EAT AT A
COCKTAIL PARTY

Those stuffed mushroom caps and salmon puffs look so small when you're snagging them off a tray or buffet table, but they add up. Follow my tips to work a party the smart way.

SAY YES TO ALL THESE:

Bruschetta: Olive oil and tomatoes are a power duo. Just watch portions: If the toasts are open-faced-sandwich-size, I have only one piece.

Cheese plate: A little bit is just fine; stick to a cube or two. And if you see grapes on the platter, grab 'em. Garnish or not, they're fair game.

Chicken skewers: Tasty and filling. A full serving of chicken is about the amount that would cover your palm.

Chocolate-covered strawberries: Only about 50 calories a pop!

Crudités: No one's shocked when I put a big dent in the veg tray. (Also good: veggie skewers and olives.) If they come with dip, I keep it to two spoonfuls.

Deviled eggs: True, they're higher in calories than regular eggs, but they've still got protein and a vital nutrient called choline, which has been linked to brain health. Not really so devilish.

Mini quiches: These offer nutritional benefits from eggs and a few veggies, but the buttery crust makes them more of a treat.

Mixed nuts: Have a handful to fill up.

Shrimp cocktail: High in nutrients, low in calories. Stick to six (or three, if you're having another protein).

Smoked salmon and cream cheese rolls: Heart-healthy salmon is always welcome on my plate, and I love this flavor combo.

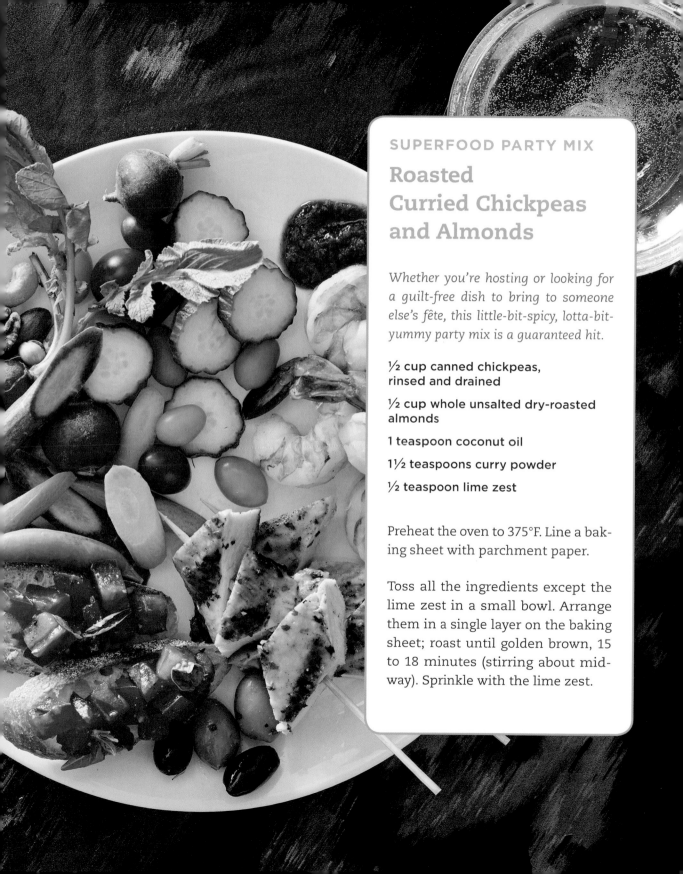

Roasted Curried Chickpeas and Almonds

Whether you're hosting or looking for a guilt-free dish to bring to someone else's fête, this little-bit-spicy, lotta-bit-yummy party mix is a guaranteed hit.

½ cup canned chickpeas, rinsed and drained

½ cup whole unsalted dry-roasted almonds

1 teaspoon coconut oil

1½ teaspoons curry powder

½ teaspoon lime zest

Preheat the oven to 375°F. Line a baking sheet with parchment paper.

Toss all the ingredients except the lime zest in a small bowl. Arrange them in a single layer on the baking sheet; roast until golden brown, 15 to 18 minutes (stirring about midway). Sprinkle with the lime zest.

FAST ACTION EATS

Surprise: You *can* score a healthy meal at a fast-food spot or chain restaurant. I've scoured the menus at twenty of America's favorites to find the healthiest picks at each.

Applebee's

Classic Turkey Breast Sandwich, 560 calories: Thanks to a healthy, keep-you-satisfied hit of protein, two-thirds of what you need in a day, the turkey breast sandwich gets my vote. Even with a little mayo, it's still good on calories, and I like that lettuce and tomato on top.

Grilled Chicken Caesar Salad with dressing (half size), 400 calories: A half portion of chicken Caesar salad will fill you up with greens, chicken, and cheese.

Burger King

MorningStar Veggie Burger with lettuce, tomatoes, onion, and ketchup on a sesame seed bun, hold the mayo—310 calories: It's got plenty of protein, plus satisfying fiber.

The Cheesecake Factory

Tuscan Chicken, served with tomatoes, artichokes, capers, fresh basil, and balsamic vinaigrette, over fresh vegetables and farro, 590 calories: I love to see farro, a nutrient-dense whole grain, hitting the big time here, served up next to grilled chicken and so many great veggies.

SkinnyLicious Grilled Turkey Burger with grilled onions, lettuce, tomato, mayo, and a green salad, 580 calories: You'll satisfy your burger craving and work in some veggie goodness with the side salad.

Chili's

Cup of Terlingua Chili, 230 calories, plus house salad (hold the dressing and drizzle with olive oil and vinegar), 243 calories: Their beef chili is surprisingly low in calories and sodium— and you get extra credit if you round things out with a salad or other veggie.

Chipotle

Burrito Bowl with black beans and fajita veggies, brown rice, and fresh tomato salsa, 375 calories: Their terrific vegetarian rice-and-bean combo provides half or more of your daily fiber quota.

Burrito Bowl with steak and fajita veggies, brown rice, and tomatillo green chili salsa, 395 calories: The steak bowl is also an unexpectedly good choice—and the veggies and salsa help with your quota of vitamin C.

Domino's

Medium (12-inch) Thin-Crust Veggie Pizza with fresh baby spinach, fresh mushrooms, black olives, and diced tomatoes (3 slices), 435 calories: The secret is to go for the thin-crust pizzas, which are made with a smaller portion of cheese. More good news: Less crust also means less sodium. (Plus, pizza's a great vehicle for all those veggies.)

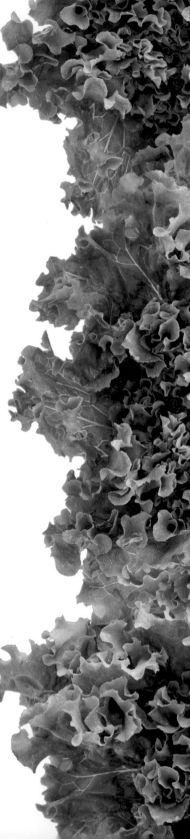

Bacon, Egg, and Cheese on English Muffin, 350 calories, plus medium coffee with milk (iced or hot), 40 calories: A breakfast sandwich can be a smart splurge, as long as you stick to this trick: Order it on an English muffin instead of other breads, and you'll save close to 200 calories.

2 Eggs, Any Style (I like sunny-side up), 220 calories, plus seasonal mixed fruit, 60 calories, plus English muffin with pat of butter, 180 calories: I go for the eggs and leave the yolks in. (The latest science shows they're highly nutritious, so no need to stick to just the whites.) Add a couple of sides, and you've got a substantial meal with a balance of protein, fruit, and carbs.

Chili Bowl (hold the cheese—it adds 110 calories), 380 calories: It's got 14 grams of protein—a good helper for appetite control.

Artisan Grilled Chicken Sandwich, 380 calories: This satisfying pick hits the spot better than one of their salads, and it's got a very respectable 37 grams of protein to keep you fuller longer.

Herb Grilled Salmon, served with steamed garlic broccoli, 480 calories: A protein-rich pick with lots of omega-3s.

Outback Special Sirloin (6 ounce) and asparagus (premium side) and sweet potato, 603 calories: As long as it's an occasional feast, steak is fine by me. Pair the meat with a big serving of veggies for a protein-and-fiber combo that will stave off hunger.

Grilled Teriyaki Chicken with a half serving of brown rice and a half serving of steamed mixed veggies, 526 calories: Your tasty plan of attack here is to lean on the lean proteins—like chicken—for the main dish, then ramp up the meal's fiber with brown rice and steamed veggies as your sides.

Half Napa Almond Chicken Salad Sandwich on sesame semolina, 350 calories, plus half classic salad with standard dressing, 90 calories: Divide and conquer—that's the secret to sandwich success. Order this sandwich by the half, and you'll still get a good-size portion while slashing calories and sodium.

Oven-Broiled Wild-Caught Flounder, 420 calories, plus broccoli and baked potato, 250 calories: When it comes to seafood, broiled or grilled is the way to go, not battered and fried. This meal keeps things simple while providing more than a day's worth of protein and a good measure of veggies, thanks to the sides.

Hearty Veggie and Brown Rice Salad Bowl, 430 calories, plus tall 2%-milk cappuccino, 90 calories: The vegetarian salad—packed with a rainbow of colorful produce—supplies your full daily requirement (and then some) of vitamins A and C.

Protein Bistro Box with hard-cooked egg, cheese, multigrain bread, fruit, and peanut butter–honey spread, 370 calories, plus tall 2%-milk cappuccino, 90 calories: With more than 25 percent of your daily dose of protein, this box lives up to its name.

6-inch Black Forest Ham on nine-grain wheat with cucumbers, green peppers, lettuce, red onions, and tomatoes with olive-oil-blend dressing, 290 calories: Who knew a ham sub could be so heart-healthy? Pile the veggies high.

Cheesy Bean and Rice Burrito, 420 calories: While you'd never guess it from the name, the burrito is a smart choice with 6 grams of fiber.

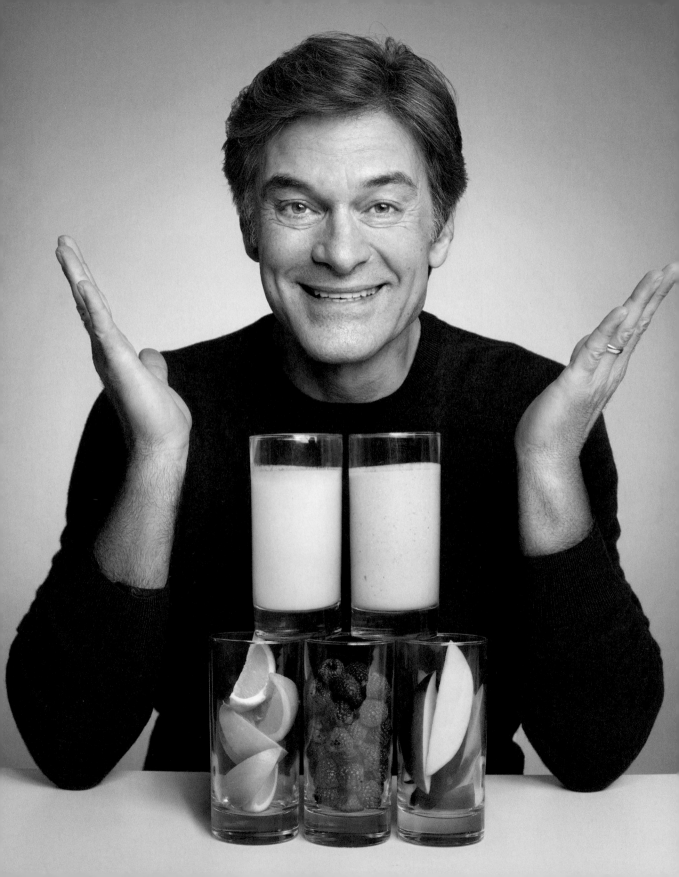

17

The 3-Day
Fix-It Cleanse

Think of how good you feel in a clean and freshly scrubbed environment, whether it's your kitchen, when all the cooking splatter gets wiped away with shine and lemon scents, or your car, when the wrappers, pebbles, and trash are vacuumed up and outta there. Or even your newly organized closet—when you've winnowed down, made your donations, and turned that cramped storage space into a tidy cove of serenity.

That's what dietary cleanses do: They help to remove the grit and grime from your innards, reboot all of your systems, and set you up to speed through the green lights of life.

Once you've completed the 21-Day Plan and you've graduated to eating the FIXES way, every day, you may still feel the need for a cleanse every so often. Think of it as a kind of dietary temp worker. It comes in occasionally for three days, gets some necessary work done, then may return sometime down the road. I do a cleanse four times a year—once every time the seasons change—as a way to reenergize and keep myself nutritionally inspired. You may choose to cleanse as often as once every two months (I wouldn't do it more frequently than that), or immediately following a few days of straying, like after a vacation, the holidays, or a particularly indulgent weekend.

The purpose is to give your systems a quick jolt by feeding your organs a strong dose of healthy foods and zero doses of unhealthy ones, by restricting your calories a bit to help your stomach realize it doesn't need as much food as you think, and by making you *feel* cleaner because you're eating cleaner. In other words, a cleanse helps you out of a junk funk and puts you back on track to healthier eating.

You are not going to lose dramatic amounts of weight on my three-day cleanse (though you may certainly see some movement on the scale for a variety of reasons). But this nutritional nudge will set you off in the right direction. I've outlined specifically what to eat during these three days, but first, some general guidelines:

Restrict your calories, but do not starve. This regimen contains around 1,250 calories per day, which is nearly 20 percent less than you eat in my 21-Day Plan. But you are not denying your body nutrients like you would in a deprivation-based cleanse; instead, you are delivering only good nutrients to your body. This is about cleansing, not enduring three days of hunger that makes you want to gnaw on a coffee table. So while you may be a little bit uncomfortable because you're hungry, you won't be *starving*.

Be rigid. While I don't think your general eating life should follow strict rules (after all, the "S" in FIXES stands for Special-occasion sugar), a seventy-two-hour cleanse is an exception: no added sugar, no heavily processed foods, no alcohol, no caffeine. (If you are prone to experiencing caffeine withdrawal, you might want to prepare your body by cutting back a little bit a few weeks before starting a cleanse: Cut your original intake by 25 percent the first week, 50 percent the second week, and 75 percent the third week. By the time you're ready to begin the cleanse, you should be able to go cold turkey.) That's a key part of the intestinal spruce-up. With the clean ingredients that you will be eating, your organs will feel like they're swimming in Caribbean waters.

Speaking of waters, stick to drinking water and decaffeinated herbal tea. During these three days, I want you to make hydrating a priority. (Sparkling water is fine; if you need a little flavor, add a squeeze of lemon.)

Say a simple mantra: repair and rejuvenate. This is what the cleansing foods will do as they begin to get your organs, systems, tissues, and blood flow working the way they should.

Here, my three-day kick in the pants.

Cleanse Menu

No weird ingredients, no fancy equipment— just good, simple, healthy food. You have two options: You can eat a mix of solid foods and sippable options, or you can opt for an all-liquid cleanse. The benefit to all-liquid is that it reduces the load on your intestines, giving them a short respite. If that sounds appealing, go the liquids-only route. Otherwise, a mix of smoothies and chewable meals should be just fine.

The 3-Day Fix-It Cleanse

Here's your plan. Plus, sip on a nourishing broth anytime you're hungry—
have as much as you like on each day (page 284).

DAY 1	DAY 2	DAY 3
Breakfast		
Scrambled eggs with sliced fruit	Steel-cut oats with apples and almonds	Rev-up blueberry smoothie
OR	OR	
Citrus fuel smoothie	Apple-almond super juice	
Lunch		
Arugula-quinoa salad	Broccoli soup with white beans	Mega-greens smoothie
OR	OR	
Spinach-avocado smoothie	Kale salad with avocado, citrus, and nuts	
Dinner		
Curried carrot soup	Vegetarian chili with brown rice	Veggie-loaded lentil soup
	OR	
	Kale and cuke super juice	
Snack		
Any grab-and-go snack (page 239)	Any grab-and-go snack (page 239)	Any grab-and-go snack (page 239)
OR	OR	OR
Blueberry-peach snack smoothie	Blackberry-honeydew snack smoothie	Nectarine-carrot snack smoothie

Breakfast

Scrambled Eggs with Sliced Fruit

SERVES 1

Canola oil cooking spray

1 large tomato, diced

1 large egg

2 large egg whites

Salt

Freshly ground black pepper

1 small banana, sliced

1 small orange, peeled and sliced into rounds

1 tablespoon ground flaxseed

¼ teaspoon ground cinnamon

Mist a small skillet with cooking spray and place it over medium heat. Add the tomato and sauté until soft, about 2 minutes. In a small bowl, whisk together the egg and egg whites; add to the skillet and scramble. Season with salt and pepper. Serve alongside the banana and orange, topped with the flaxseed and cinnamon.

---

330 CAL, 8 G FAT (2 G SATURATED), 14 G PROTEIN, 57 G CARB, 35 G SUGAR, 10 G FIBER, 125 MG SODIUM

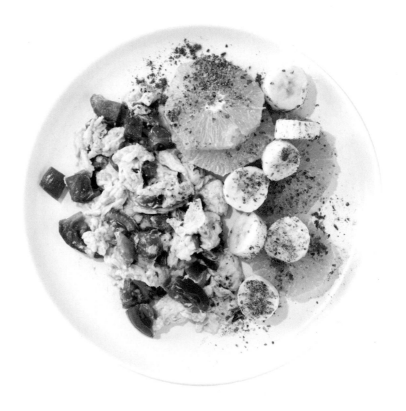

Citrus Fuel Smoothie

Combine all the ingredients in a blender with ½ cup ice and puree until smooth.

295 CAL, 8 G FAT, 14 G PROTEIN, 47 G CARB, 29 G SUGAR, 9 G FIBER, 220 MG SODIUM

SERVES 1

1 small banana, quartered

1 orange, peeled, quartered, and seeded

½ teaspoon ground cinnamon

½ cup plain 2% Greek yogurt

1 cup unsweetened almond milk

2 teaspoons ground flaxseed

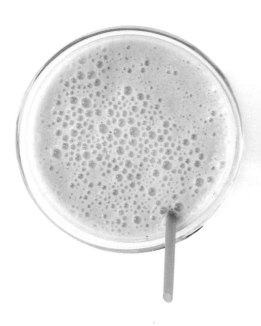

Steel Cut Oats with Apples and Almonds

SERVES 1

1 cup cooked steel cut oats

1 apple, cored and diced

1 tablespoon chia seeds

1 tablespoon slivered raw almonds

½ teaspoon ground cinnamon

Top the oats with the apple, chia seeds, almonds, and cinnamon.

---

350 CAL, 13 G FAT,
10 G PROTEIN, 57 G CARB,
17 G SUGAR, 16 G FIBER,
15 MG SODIUM

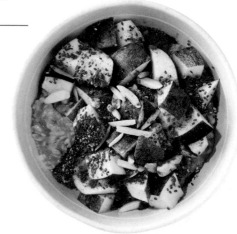

Apple-Almond Super Juice

SERVES 1

1 Granny Smith apple, peeled, cored, and chopped

½ small banana

5 almonds

1 tablespoon peanut butter

1 cup unsweetened almond milk

1 tablespoon chia seeds

½ teaspoon ground cinnamon

Combine all the ingredients in a blender with ½ cup ice and puree until smooth.

---

347 CAL, 18 G FAT, 9 G PROTEIN, 44 G CARB, 24 G SUGAR,
10 G FIBER, 251 MG SODIUM

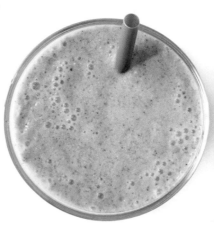

Rev-Up Blueberry Smoothie

Combine all the ingredients in a blender (with two or three ice cubes, if you like a slushier texture) and puree until smooth.

---

313 CAL, 11 G FAT (2 G SATURATED), 14 G PROTEIN, 45 G CARB, 25 G SUGAR, 11 G FIBER, 278 MG SODIUM

SERVES 1

1¼ cups unsweetened almond milk

1 cup frozen blueberries

½ cup plain 2% Greek yogurt

1 tablespoon chia seeds

¼ teaspoon ground cinnamon

½ medium frozen banana

½ cup spinach

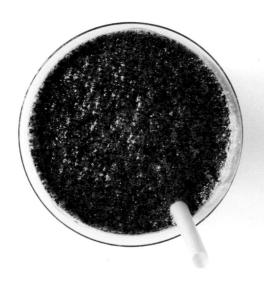

Between Meals

Lisa's Tides-You-Over Veggie Broth

MAKES ABOUT 12 CUPS

2 tablespoons olive oil

2 leeks, chopped and washed well

2 medium carrots, peeled and chopped

2 celery stalks, chopped

1 potato, peeled and cut into 1-inch cubes

1 ounce dried mushrooms, rinsed

1 head garlic, peeled and halved

1 (1-inch) piece fresh ginger, peeled and chopped

2 tablespoons chopped fresh cilantro

1 (3-inch) strip lemon zest

¾ cup light coconut milk

⅓ cup white miso paste

2 tablespoons low-sodium soy sauce

½ teaspoon cayenne pepper

½ teaspoon ground coriander

When we're doing the liquids-only thing, Lisa and I rely on her light but filling broth to hold us between mealtimes (or even to swap in for a meal or two). It's easy to make, and brings your mind away from that dark "I would kill for a sandwich" place. Fill up a thermos and sip whenever hunger pangs strike.

Heat the olive oil in a large pot over medium heat. Add the leeks, carrots, and celery and cook, stirring occasionally, for 5 minutes. Add 1½ gallons water, then add the remaining ingredients. Bring to a boil, then reduce the heat to maintain a simmer and cook for 2½ hours. Strain into a large bowl; discard the solids. Refrigerate or freeze for 2 to 3 months.

---

55 CAL, 3.5 G FAT (1 G SATURATED), 1 G PROTEIN, 5 G CARB, 2 G SUGAR, 0 G FIBER, 313 MG SODIUM

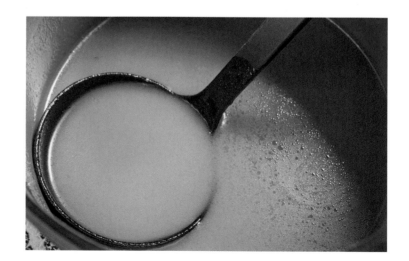

Lunch

Arugula-Quinoa Salad

In a serving bowl, toss together the vegetables, cheese, quinoa, and dressing.

(INCLUDING VINAIGRETTE) 428 CAL, 9 G FAT, 14 G PROTEIN, 40 G CARB, 13 G SUGAR, 9 G FIBER, 281 MG SODIUM

SERVES 1

3 cups baby arugula

1 celery stalk, sliced

1 medium carrot, peeled and coarsely grated

½ cup chopped precooked beets (from an 8-ounce package)

¼ cup crumbled goat cheese

½ cup cooked quinoa

1½ tablespoons Classic Vinaigrette (page 236)

Spinach-Avocado Smoothie

Combine all the ingredients in a blender with 1 cup water and 4 or 5 ice cubes and puree until smooth.

368 CAL, 26 G FAT (4 G SATURATED), 17 G PROTEIN, 22 G CARB, 8 G SUGAR, 11 G FIBER, 83 MG SODIUM

SERVES 1

1½ cups spinach

1 cup cucumber, peeled and seeded

15 almonds

½ avocado, pitted and peeled

½ cup plain 2% Greek yogurt

1 teaspoon fresh lemon juice

Pinch of cayenne pepper

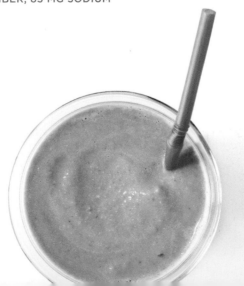

Broccoli Soup with White Beans

SERVES 1

½ teaspoon olive oil

¼ cup chopped yellow onion

½ garlic clove, minced

1½ cups low-sodium vegetable broth

¾ cup canned cannellini beans, rinsed and drained

2 cups broccoli florets

1½ teaspoons fresh lemon juice

Small pinch of cayenne pepper

Pinch of salt

Pinch of freshly ground black pepper

Side salad, for serving

Heat the olive oil in a medium pot. Add the onion, cover, and cook until softened, 5 to 7 minutes. Add the garlic, broth, beans, and broccoli. Bring to a boil, then reduce the heat to medium-low and simmer for 30 minutes. Season with the lemon juice, cayenne, salt, and black pepper. Carefully transfer the soup to a blender and puree until smooth. Serve with a simple side salad.

(EXCLUDING SIDE SALAD) 290 CAL, 3.5 G FAT, 21 G PROTEIN, 49 G CARB, 3 G SUGAR, 15 G FIBER, 188 MG SODIUM

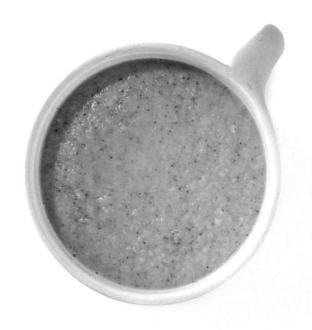

Kale Salad with Avocado, Citrus, and Nuts

In a large bowl, combine the kale, lemon juice, olive oil, salt, and pepper. Massage the kale with your hands to mix and tenderize the leaves. Top with the avocado, citrus fruit, and pecans.

358 CAL, 23 G FAT (3 G SATURATED), 9 G PROTEIN, 38 G CARB, 1 G SUGAR, 10 G FIBER, 206 MG SODIUM

SERVES 1

3 cups stemmed and shredded kale leaves

1½ teaspoons fresh lemon juice

1½ teaspoons olive oil

Pinch of coarse salt

Pinch of freshly ground black pepper

¼ avocado, pitted, peeled, and chopped

½ citrus fruit (such as pink grapefruit or orange), peeled, seeded, and sliced

⅛ cup pecans, chopped and toasted

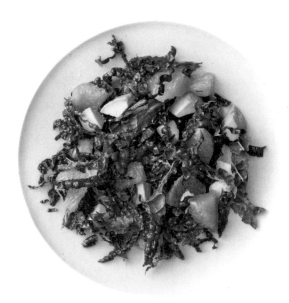

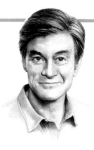

Massage Your Kale, People!

You don't have to go full-on shiatsu. But when it comes to this tough green, a little bit of pampering goes a long way. Massaging these fibrous leaves make them easier to chew and digest. Just knead the stemmed leaves—like you would bread dough—for a few minutes with oil and lemon juice until they feel less stiff and turn a brighter shade of green.

Mega-Greens Smoothie

SERVES 1

½ cup stemmed and chopped kale leaves

½ cup spinach

1 cup frozen pineapple chunks

1¼ cups unsweetened almond milk

½ teaspoon ground cinnamon

2 teaspoons chia seeds

½ teaspoon fresh lemon juice

½ cup plain 2% Greek yogurt

Combine all the ingredients in a blender and puree until smooth.

_____

264 CAL, 8 G FAT (2 G SATURATED), 14 G PROTEIN, 36 G CARB, 9 G SUGAR, 8 G FIBER, 279 MG SODIUM

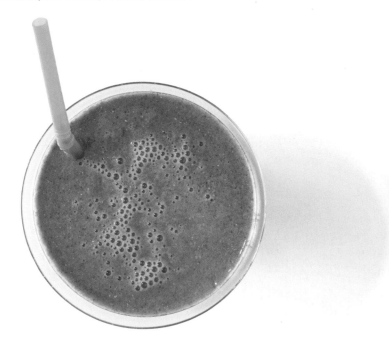

Dinner

Curried Carrot Soup

Heat the olive oil in a medium saucepan over medium-low heat. Add the garlic and onion; sauté for 2 to 5 minutes. Add the carrots, curry paste, stock, salt, and pepper. Bring to a boil, then cover, reduce the heat to medium-low, and simmer for 20 to 25 minutes. Remove from the heat and add the coconut milk. Carefully transfer the soup to a blender and puree until smooth. Swirl in the yogurt before serving.

300 CAL, 12 G FAT, 18 G PROTEIN, 32 G CARB, 17 G SUGAR, 7 G FIBER, 190 MG SODIUM

SERVES 1

2 teaspoons olive oil

2 garlic cloves, chopped

½ medium yellow onion, chopped

1½ cups peeled and chopped carrots

1 teaspoon red curry paste

1 cup low-sodium chicken stock or vegetable broth

Pinch of salt

Pinch of freshly ground black pepper

½ cup light coconut milk

⅓ cup plain 2% Greek yogurt

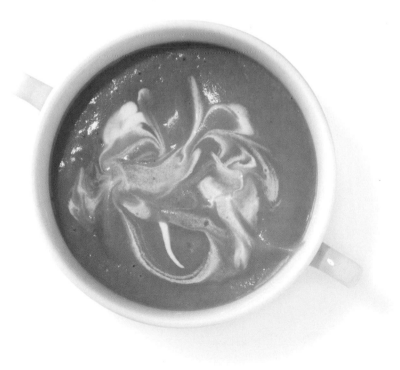

Vegetarian Chili with Brown Rice

SERVES 1

1 tablespoon olive oil

¾ cup chopped yellow onion

1 teaspoon minced garlic

1½ teaspoons chili powder

1 teaspoon ground cumin

1 medium red bell pepper, chopped

1 (15-ounce) can kidney beans, rinsed and drained

1 (15-ounce) can diced tomatoes

1 cup cooked brown rice

2 tablespoons plain 2% Greek yogurt

Heat the olive oil in a medium pot over medium heat. Add the onion, garlic, chili powder, and cumin and cook until the onion is softened, about 7 minutes. Add the bell pepper, beans, and tomatoes and cook until the bell pepper is soft. Serve over the rice, topped with the yogurt.

456 CAL, 10 G FAT (2 G SATURATED), 19 G PROTEIN, 74 G CARB, 12 G SUGAR, 15 G FIBER, 846 MG SODIUM

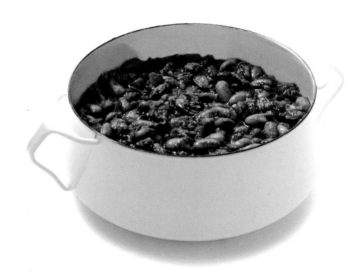

Kale and Cuke Super Juice

Combine all the ingredients in a blender with ½ cup cold water and ½ cup ice cubes and puree until smooth.

---

234 CAL, 5 G FAT (2 G SATURATED), 13 G PROTEIN, 37 G CARB, 25 G SUGAR, 8 G FIBER, 49 MG SODIUM

Spice up this staple veg with an Asian-style cucumber salad: Toss cucumber slices with a splash each of soy sauce and white vinegar and season with red pepper flakes.

½ cup chopped kale

¼ cup chopped red cabbage

½ green apple, cored and chopped

½ cup frozen blueberries

½ cup plain 2% Greek yogurt

⅓ cup chopped cucumber

2 teaspoons chia seeds

¼ cup fresh orange juice

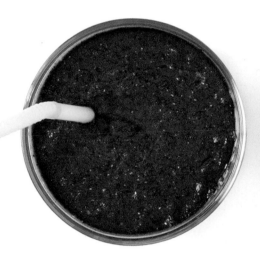

Veggie-Loaded Lentil Soup

SERVES 1

1 teaspoon olive oil

¼ chopped yellow onion

½ medium carrot, peeled and diced

½ celery stalk, diced

½ medium zucchini, diced

4 green beans, halved

2½ tablespoons dried green lentils

½ teaspoon dried basil

½ teaspoon dried thyme

½ teaspoon dried oregano

½ (15-ounce) can crushed tomatoes

1 cup low-sodium vegetable broth

2 Swiss chard leaves, torn (baby spinach also works)

Salt

Freshly ground black pepper

Heat the olive oil in a medium pot over medium heat. Add the onion, carrot, and celery and sauté for 3 to 4 minutes. Add the zucchini and green beans and sauté for 2 to 3 minutes. Stir in the lentils, herbs, tomatoes, and broth; bring to a boil. Cover, reduce the heat to medium-low, and simmer for 25 to 30 minutes, until the lentils are tender. Toss in the Swiss chard and season with salt and pepper. Carefully transfer the soup to a blender and puree.

340 CAL, 6 G FAT, 17 G PROTEIN, 56 G CARB, 13 G SUGAR, 14 G FIBER, 250 MG SODIUM

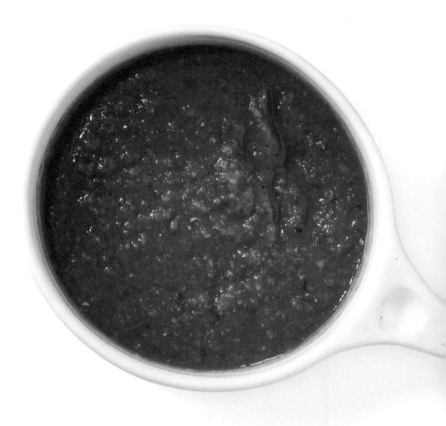

Snack Smoothies

Blueberry-Peach Snack Smoothie

Combine all the ingredients in a blender and puree until smooth.

___

140 CAL, 3 G FAT, 5 G PROTEIN, 26 G CARB, 20 G SUGAR, 3 G FIBER, 59 MG SODIUM

SERVES 1

¾ cup blueberries (fresh or frozen)

¼ cup fresh (or thawed frozen) sliced peaches

½ cup 2% milk

1 teaspoon fresh lemon juice

Blackberry-Honeydew Smoothie

Combine all the ingredients in a blender and puree until smooth.

___

139 CAL, 3 G FAT, 6 G PROTEIN, 25 G CARB, 20 G SUGAR, 5 G FIBER, 81 MG SODIUM

SERVES 1

¾ cup honeydew

½ cup blackberries

½ cup 2% milk

1 teaspoon fresh lime juice

Nectarine-Carrot Smoothie

Combine all the ingredients in a blender and puree until smooth.

___

196 CAL, 2 G FAT, 8 G PROTEIN, 41 G CARB, 30 G SUGAR, 5 G FIBER, 62 MG SODIUM

SERVES 1

1 cup sliced nectarine

½ cup sliced peeled carrot

½ cup diced pineapple

¼ cup fresh orange juice

¼ cup plain 2% Greek yogurt

¼ teaspoon turmeric

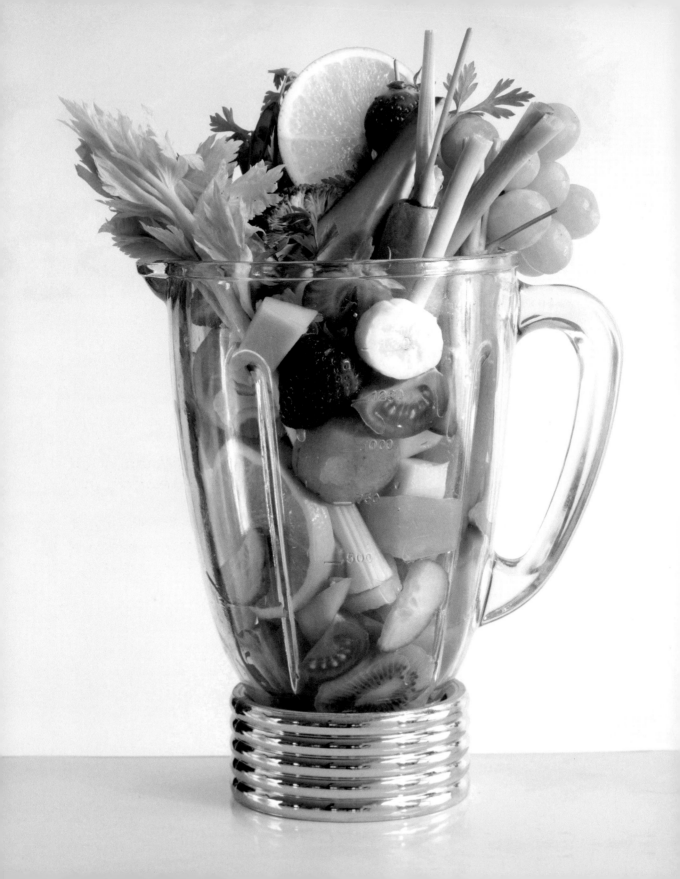

18.

The Fix-It Blender: Even More Tips, Tricks, and Tactics!

We love our blender. We can throw in a whole bunch of ingredients, press a button, and get rewarded with something healthy and delicious, whether it's smoothies, sauces, or spicy vegetable juices.

This chapter is my version of an *information* blender, where I'm throwing in an array of useful ingredients. Take from it whatever appeals and seems likely to improve your eating life. You'll find some recipes, a few tactics, and plenty of ideas to help make your kitchen fix-it central.

Spice It Up

It's not a pantry without shakeable seasoning magic. Whatever you do, don't let these spices get dusty at the back of your cabinet.

The right spices can elevate both the taste and health cred of whatever you're cooking for next to no calories. So flip open those little jars and tins, and try some of my healthy ideas. Start with the ones that have exact measurements; then, once you get the hang of that, channel your inner chef with the "little bit of this, little bit of that" inspirations. When you're really into the swing of things, you can even ditch the recipes altogether. Just *play*.

BLACK PEPPER

More than a seasoning basic, pepper can also be the star of the show.

Lemon-Pepper Shrimp: Cook 1¼ pounds peeled and deveined shrimp in 2 tablespoons olive oil with 2 teaspoons minced garlic, ¾ teaspoon freshly ground black pepper, and ½ teaspoon coarse salt over medium-high heat for 4 minutes. Stir in 1 teaspoon lemon zest and 1 tablespoon fresh lemon juice. Serve the shrimp with lemon wedges. *Serves 4, 165 calories*

Hot and Sweet Roasted Pineapple: Mix 3 tablespoons pure maple syrup with ½ teaspoon freshly ground black pepper and ½ teaspoon pure vanilla extract. Toss ½-inch-thick slices of fresh pineapple (4 cups) with half the syrup. Roast at 450°F for 10 minutes. Brush with the rest of the syrup and roast for 10 minutes more. Serve for dessert with plain 2% Greek yogurt. *Serves 4, 142 calories*

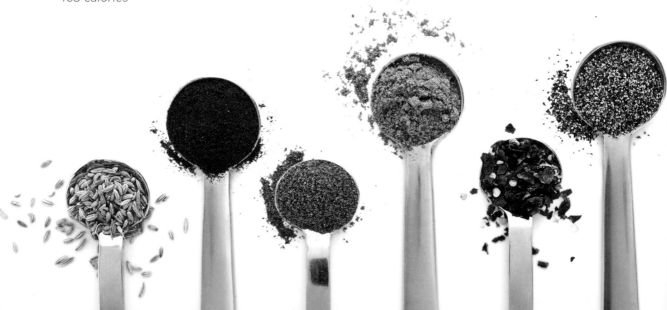

CINNAMON

The fragrant powder you swirl into your
A.M. oatmeal could come with a side of
health benefits. In some studies, daily
cinnamon supplements lowered blood
sugar levels.

Banana-Date Smoothies: Puree in a
blender 1 large banana, ½ cup plain 2%
Greek yogurt, 1 cup ice, 2 tablespoons
chopped dates, and 1 teaspoon
ground cinnamon until smooth.
Serves 2, 129 calories

Quinoa Breakfast Porridge:
Reheat leftover cooked quinoa
with 2% milk stirred in to desired
thickness. Sprinkle with ground
cinnamon and top with dried
fruit and a drizzle of pure
maple syrup.

CUMIN

The secret ingredient of many chili powders,
cumin is brilliant in bean dishes and also a
good spice for anything Indian- or Mexican-
inspired.

Chickpea and Pita Sandwich: Puree in a
food processor 1 (15-ounce) can chickpeas,
rinsed and drained, 3 tablespoons extra-virgin
olive oil, 2 tablespoons fresh lemon juice, 1
teaspoon ground cumin, ½ teaspoon coarse
salt, and freshly ground black pepper to
taste. Serve in whole wheat pita halves with
tomato and arugula. *Serves 4, 293 calories*

Soups: Add sprinkles of ground cumin to
bean soup (or any soup that could use a
flavor kick).

Spiced Salad Dressing: Make an olive
oil and lime juice dressing with a drizzle of
honey and up to ½ teaspoon ground cumin.
Toss with avocado or bean salad.

FENNEL SEEDS

These have a licorice-like flavor that makes all
sorts of foods sing. To crush the seeds, use
the flat side of a chef's knife.

Fennel-Carrot Soup: Cook 1 cup chopped
yellow onion in 2 tablespoons olive oil with 1
minced garlic clove, 1 ½ teaspoons crushed
fennel seeds, and ½ teaspoon coarse salt,
plus freshly ground black pepper to taste,
over medium heat for 3 minutes. Add 1 pound
carrots (cut into 1-inch pieces; 2½ cups)
and 2½ cups low-sodium vegetable broth.
Simmer, covered, for 20 minutes. Carefully
transfer to a blender and puree. Dollop with
plain 2% Greek yogurt. *Serves 4, 146 calories*

Tomato-Fennel Pasta: Add up to 1½
teaspoons crushed fennel seeds to marinara
sauce. Toss with whole wheat pasta and
grated Parmesan cheese.

Fennel-Coated Salmon: Crush 1 ½
teaspoons fennel seeds. Mix with olive oil,
lemon zest, coarse salt, and freshly ground
black pepper. Use as a rub for salmon fillets,
then bake.

GINGER

You might know the spice best as the magic
in gingerbread cookies, but it also makes
a delish addition to veggie side dishes and
hot drinks. Scientists have also been testing
different forms of ginger as an alternative to
drugs for arthritis pain, menstrual cramps,
and migraines.

Roasted Spiced Squash: Toss 1½ pounds cubed butternut squash (5 cups) with 1½ tablespoons olive oil, 1 minced garlic clove, 1 teaspoon ground ginger, ½ teaspoon ground cumin, ½ teaspoon coarse salt, ¼ teaspoon ground cinnamon, and freshly ground black pepper to taste. Roast at 425°F, stirring once, for 30 minutes. *Serves 4, 107 calories*

Ginger Tea: Bring 2 cups water, 1 tablespoon fresh lemon juice, 1 tablespoon honey, ¾ teaspoon ground ginger, ¼ teaspoon ground turmeric, and a pinch of cayenne pepper to a boil. *Serves 2, 37 calories*

Gingered Green Beans: Boil green beans until crisp-tender. Heat some chopped garlic and ground ginger in olive oil, then add the green beans and toss to coat. Sprinkle with a pinch of coarse salt and a squeeze of fresh lemon juice.

NUTMEG

Don't wait for the once-a-year eggnog; nutmeg can flavor up both sweet and savory dishes.

Caramelized Pears: Cut 2 pears into wedges and core. Melt 1 tablespoon unsalted butter with 1 tablespoon honey, 1½ teaspoons pure vanilla extract, ⅛ teaspoon grated nutmeg, and ⅛ teaspoon ground cinnamon over medium-high heat. Add the pears and cook until glazed, about 7 minutes, turning in the syrup. Serve over plain 2% Greek yogurt. *Serves 4, 97 calories*

Sautéed Baby Spinach: Sauté baby spinach with garlic in olive oil. Sprinkle with nutmeg to taste and toss with fresh lemon juice.

Spiced Mashed Potatoes: Sprinkle nutmeg to taste over mashed sweet or white potatoes.

RED PEPPER FLAKES

Not for pizza night only—use these any time you crave a bit of heat.

Hot-Pepper Carrots: Toss 2 pounds carrots, halved lengthwise, with 1½ tablespoons olive oil, 1 teaspoon coarse salt, and ½ teaspoon red pepper flakes. Roast at 425°F for 30 minutes. *Serves 4, 138 calories*

Spiced Mango: Sprinkle cubed mango with lime juice and red pepper flakes.

Feta Toasts: Top slices of whole-grain toast with crumbled feta cheese, red pepper flakes, thyme, and honey.

SAFFRON

A little flowery and bitter—in a good way. This spice may help ease depression, because each pinch delivers an antioxidant called crocin. Quickly soak saffron threads in water before adding to the pot. This brings out the flavor and helps give dishes like rice a great golden color.

Saffron Shrimp: Soak ¼ teaspoon crushed saffron in 1 tablespoon warm water for 3 minutes. Cook 1 cup chopped yellow onion in 2 tablespoons olive oil with 2 teaspoons minced garlic, the saffron water, and ½ teaspoon coarse salt, plus freshly ground black pepper to taste, over medium-high heat for 4 minutes. Add 1 pound peeled and deveined shrimp and cook for 4 minutes. Stir in 2 tablespoons fresh lime juice. *Serves 4, 160 calories*

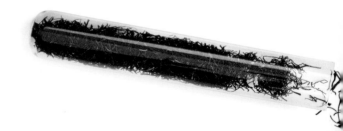

Flavor Up Rice: Soak a pinch or two of crushed saffron in 1 tablespoon warm water for 3 minutes. Stir into risotto or other rice dishes.

Soup Boost: Soak a pinch or two of crushed saffron in 1 tablespoon warm water for 3 minutes. Stir into tomato soup, fish chowder, or minestrone.

SMOKED PAPRIKA

With its addictive hints of char, this spice turns simple meals into standouts.

Spiced Sweet Potatoes: Cut 1 ¾ pounds sweet potatoes (about 3) into ½-inch-thick wedges and toss with 2 tablespoons olive oil, 2 teaspoons smoked paprika, 2 minced garlic cloves, 1 teaspoon coarse salt, and ½ teaspoon freshly ground black pepper. Roast at 450°F for 25 minutes. *Serves 4, 219 calories*

Red Pepper Sauce: Puree in a food processor 1 (12-ounce) jar roasted red peppers, drained; ½ cup sliced almonds; ½ cup grated Parmesan cheese; 1 tablespoon extra-virgin olive oil; 1 tablespoon red wine vinegar; 1 teaspoon smoked paprika; 1 minced garlic clove; and 2 teaspoons coarse salt, plus freshly ground black pepper to taste. Serve with broiled fish or roasted meat. *66 calories per 2 tablespoons*

Smoky Scrambled Eggs: For every 2 large eggs, beat in ⅛ teaspoon smoked paprika and a generous pinch each of coarse salt and freshly ground black pepper, and cook.

Smoked Paprika Roast Chicken: Using your favorite basic roast chicken recipe, rub chicken with 1 tablespoon olive oil mixed with 2 teaspoons smoked paprika, 1 teaspoon coarse salt, and ½ teaspoon freshly ground black pepper.

TURMERIC

The spice aisle's overachiever, turmeric is full of the antioxidant curcumin, which may be a weapon against cancer, suggests a 2015 review in the journal *Molecules*. (Curcumin could also ease arthritis symptoms.) Team turmeric with black pepper and your body may absorb even more of that curcumin goodness.

Cauliflower-Coconut Soup: Cook 1½ cups chopped yellow onion in 2 tablespoons olive oil with 3 minced garlic cloves, 1 teaspoon ground turmeric, and ¾ teaspoon coarse salt, plus freshly ground black pepper to taste, over medium-high heat for 4 minutes. Stir in 2 cups water, 1 ¾ pounds cauliflower florets (9 cups), and 1 cup light coconut milk. Simmer for 15 minutes. Carefully transfer to a blender and puree. *Serves 4, 173 calories*

Spiced Scrambled Eggs: For every 2 large eggs, beat in ¼ teaspoon ground cumin and ⅛ teaspoon ground turmeric. Add a generous pinch each of coarse salt and freshly ground black pepper, and cook.

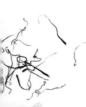

HOW TO CHOOSE BOOZE

If you remember my stories about Luigi and the folks who live in the Blue Zones (see page 25), you already know how I feel about alcohol. It's fine in moderation and it's a part of life that people enjoy. Some alcohol even contains ingredients that promote health and longevity. Moderation, of course, can be difficult, depending on the situation (weddings, happy hours, and TGIF nights have especially notorious reputations). Many, many people eat fairly well but can't seem to lose weight, and the culprit often lies with the amount of alcohol they consume. If you're a social drinker prone to having "one too many," then try some of these tricks:

- Don't order tonic water in your mixed drinks. It has 62 calories and 16 grams of sugar per serving. Better to go with club soda.

- Champagne and sparkling wines have less than 90 calories per 4-ounce glass. Not bad for celebratory bubbles.

- Order a glass of water with whatever you're drinking. Either alternate sips or alternate drinks—for every alcoholic beverage you have, down a glass of water before the next one.

- If you're going with a more exotic mixed drink like a margarita or whiskey sour, ask the bartender to go light on the simple syrup (which is loaded with sugar). The drink will still taste sweet, but it'll have fewer calories than the regular version.

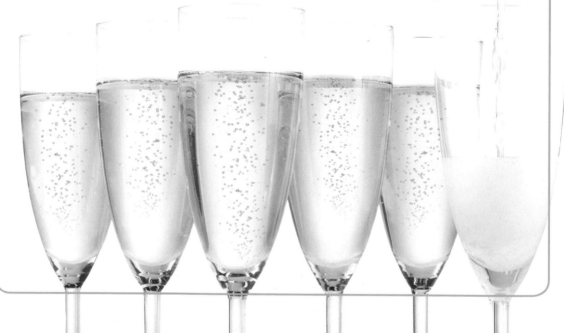

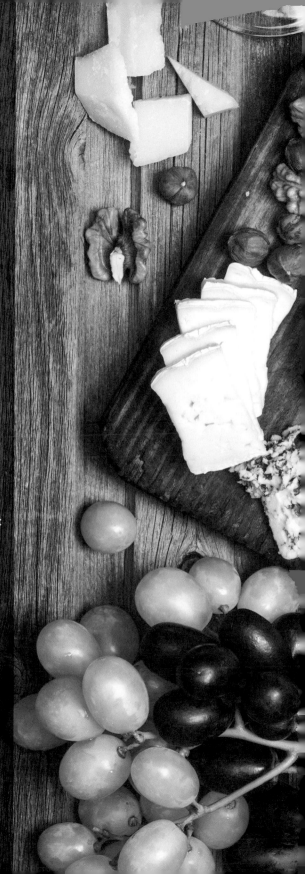

GIVE CHEESE A CHANCE

Vegetarians love and rely on cheese for protein and calcium, foodies relish it for its creamy taste, but cheese maintains near-devil status in most dieters' minds. That's because it's almost the ubiquitous punch line of so many bad-for-you foods—cheese fries, cheese pizza, cheese quesadillas, cheesecake, on and on. With high levels of sodium, calories, and saturated fat, you don't see many well-respected diets that include Brie.

Does that mean you need to eliminate cheese completely? No. And if you want to indulge from time to time, just integrate it into your rotation in moderation. Some ways to do that:

- Cheese lovers: Limit yourself to one serving a day, and get clear on what a serving is. (For most cheeses, that's 1.5 to 2 ounces—the packaging is a good guideline.) So if you want to sprinkle some shredded cheese on a salad, make sure it's just a sprinkle and not a truck load. For cheddar, a serving is about the size of a wine cork. For feta, it's the size of two golf balls.

- In general, choose softer cheeses like mozzarella and Brie because they contain more liquid and fewer calories.

- Grate it. A little bit goes a long way if you distribute it all over your dish. You'll find that you don't need a whole heck of a lot to get some of that cheesy flavor.

- Protein-packed cottage cheese is endlessly versatile. It always pairs well with fruit. For a savory twist, add chopped olives and fresh herbs (such as parsley), plus a drizzle of balsamic vinegar.

Stock Up

Sure, you can buy a carton of vegetable broth at the supermarket—but this homemade one comes together nearly as easily, and tastes way better (in my unbiased opinion).

Lisa's Famous Vegetable Broth

MAKES ABOUT
10 CUPS

2 tablespoons olive oil

2 leeks, chopped and washed well

2 medium carrots, peeled and chopped

2 celery stalks, chopped

1 potato, peeled and cut into 1-inch cubes

1 ounce dried mushrooms, rinsed

1 whole head garlic, peeled and halved

8 sprigs fresh flat-leaf parsley, coarsely chopped

½ teaspoon dried oregano

¼ teaspoon freshly ground black pepper

1 bay leaf

Lisa boils up a cauldron of this stuff every other week or so, and then uses it to add oomph to soups, sauces, whole grains, and more. You can freeze leftovers for two to three months so you always have it on hand when you're ready to cook—try pouring into ice cube trays for DIY "bouillon cubes." Feel free to use this in any of the recipes that call for vegetable broth. (You'll notice that it's not quite as rich as her cleanse broth on page 284.)

Heat the olive oil in a large pot over medium heat. Add the leeks, carrots, and celery and cook, stirring occasionally, for 5 minutes. Add 1 gallon water and the remaining ingredients. Bring to a boil, then reduce the heat to maintain a simmer and cook for 1½ hours. Strain into a large bowl; discard the solids. Refrigerate or freeze.

243 CAL, 3 G FAT, 0 G PROTEIN, 2 G CARB, 1 G SUGAR, 0 G FIBER, 10 MG SODIUM PER CUP

Feed a Cold

The only good thing about having a cold in our house is getting to enjoy this delicious and nourishing chicken soup.

The Oz Family Chicken Soup

Cook the farro according to the package instructions and set aside.

Preheat the oven to 400°F.

Cut the garlic heads crosswise to remove the tops and expose the cloves. Place them on a large piece of aluminum foil; drizzle with olive oil and sprinkle with salt. Gather the edges of the foil and press together to enclose the garlic. Roast for 30 minutes. Remove the garlic from the oven and carefully open the foil. Let cool, then squeeze out the softened cloves, discarding the papery skins.

In a blender, combine the roasted garlic and stock and puree. Set aside.

Heat 2 tablespoons of the olive oil in a large Dutch oven over medium heat. Add the onion and carrots and sauté until the onion is translucent. Add the jalapeño and cook for 2 minutes, or until soft. Stir in the ginger and cook just until fragrant. Stir in the stock and the parsley, if using. Add the farro, chicken, and lemon juice. Taste and adjust the seasoning. Serve warm.

---

451 CAL, 11 G FAT (2 G SATURATED), 34 G PROTEIN, 58 G CARB, 3 G SUGAR, 0.5 G FIBER, 198 MG SODIUM

SERVES 4

1 ½ cups farro

2 heads garlic

Olive oil

Salt

6 cups low-sodium chicken stock

1 medium yellow onion, diced

2 medium carrots, peeled and sliced into coins

1 jalapeño, thinly sliced (ribs and seeds removed)

1 (1-inch) piece fresh ginger, minced

½ cup chopped fresh flat-leaf parsley (optional)

2 cups shredded cooked chicken breast

Juice of 1 lemon

ANY WAY YOU SLICE IT

What's the one food I hear over and over as something that people "just can't give up"? Has to be pizza. After all, it's become our symbol for convenience, it's easy to order for a gathering, and—not gonna argue—tasty. (As a whole, America eats somewhere in the neighborhood of 350 slices per second.) There's just something about the sauce, crust, and cheese combo . . . While the tomato sauce certainly has health benefits, many kinds of crust and an over-load of cheese (not to mention the heaps of processed meats that might top things off) don't exactly make pizza a high-prior-ity health food.

That said, I do love the idea of families making pizza together—everyone hanging out in the kitchen and customizing personal pies. And it's sweet when couples have a traditional Friday-night wine-and-pizza meal. The connections that happen over those pies far outweigh the negative effects. I also think there's a happy medium—a way to enjoy a slice more often, without sacrificing taste:

Order or use a premade crust that's whole wheat. The flavors of sauce and toppings muscle out the bread for the most part anyway, so you might as well make the structural layer as healthy as possible. Also, the thinner the crust, the better, from a calorie perspective.

You already know what I'm going to say here: veggies, veggies, and more veggies. Treat pizza like a nice, flat plate to pile with peppers, mushrooms, artichoke hearts, spinach, and more. When you order the veggie works, you get vitamins, minerals, and fiber without lots of extra calories. Load them up. If you're really feeling the need for pepperoni, try going with a turkey substitute or maybe firing up a few slices of bacon and sprinkling bits of it over the pie.

Choose a tomato sauce that's low in sugar. Many brands are filled with added sugars, so take some time to find one that's not brimming with the sweet stuff.

On every pizza night, commit to ordering or making a big salad and have it before the pie arrives. You'll pack in your produce and go a long way in satisfying your stomach so you're good with one slice. How big should that slice be? About the size of your hand with the fingers spread as if you're giving a high-five.

YOUR STEALTH SNACK

It's the hard-boiled egg! Each one is filled with amino acids and 6 grams of protein to keep you full. Folks used to avoid them because eggs had a false rep for raising cholesterol, but no need to worry—eggs actually contain magnesium, which aids in keeping blood pressure and cholesterol in check. Plus, eggs are naturally portable, so you can easily bring one to work and stick it in the office fridge.

And don't skip the yolks. Though it's true that they're where most of the egg's calories come from, the yellow stuff is full of important nutrients—folate, which helps reduce heart disease and stroke risk, and vitamins B_6 and B_{12}, which fend off fatigue and memory loss. There's also vitamins A, E, K, and D (that last one promotes bone health, and can even help reduce hypertension); choline, which is key for brain and liver function; and eye-health helpers, such as lutein and zeaxanthin.

To vary the taste, try one with hummus and whole-grain crackers. Or spice one up with salt, pepper, and paprika. Or dice one into your vegetables as a way to add a little protein and different flavor to your usual side dish. And now you'll find them cooked, peeled, and ready-to-scarf at your supermarket.

Behold, your perfect soft-to-hard-boiled egg guide.

Drop into boiling water and choose the cooking time you like best.

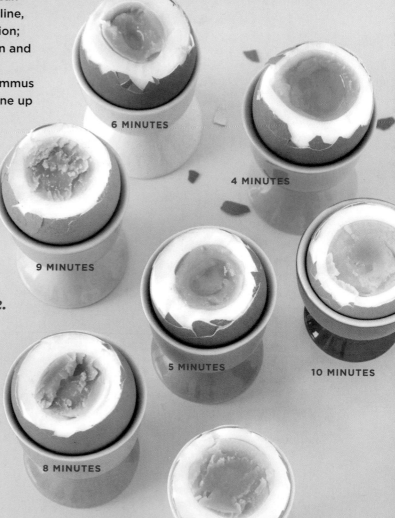

6 MINUTES

4 MINUTES

9 MINUTES

5 MINUTES

10 MINUTES

8 MINUTES

7 MINUTES

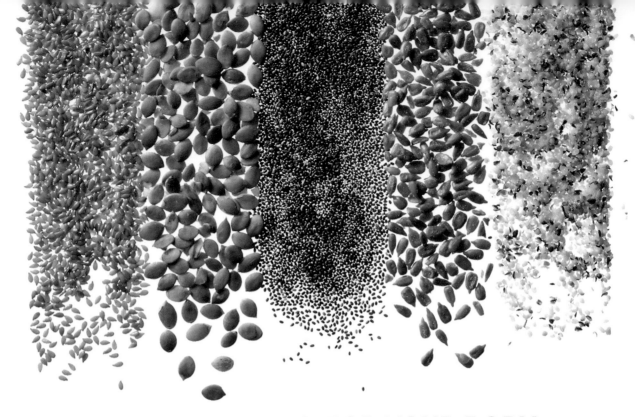

WHAT SEEDS CAN DO FOR YOUR BODY

Tiny seeds are big on protein and healthy fats—making them a great snack or a nice add-on to salads. You can even blend them into smoothies for extra nutritional punch. Some of my favorites:

FLAXSEED: BEST FOR FISH AVOIDERS

An original superfood, flax is brimming with fiber, cholesterol-lowering compounds called lignans, and healthy omega-3 fats (like you get from fish). Try in yogurt or a crumb coating for chicken. Buy them ground so you get all the nutrients inside the hard outer coating.

PUMPKIN SEEDS: BEST FOR FENDING OFF DIABETES

Pumpkin seeds, often called pepitas, are a good source of magnesium (a tablespoon has as much as a large banana), a mineral many people don't get enough of and one that can help lower your risk of heart disease, stroke, and diabetes.

CHIA SEEDS: BEST FOR BOOSTING FIBER

The soluble fiber in chia seeds swells in your gut to create a sense of fullness that helps keep your hand out of the junk food drawer. These seeds start out crunchy, then get jellylike in liquids like smoothies and yogurt.

SUNFLOWER SEEDS: BEST FOR YOUR GROCERY BILL

The inexpensive kernels are a stellar source of vitamin E (a tablespoon gives you a fifth of a day's needs). Look for shelled seeds labeled "raw"— they're not roasted in the oils that can hike up the calories.

HEMP SEEDS: BEST FOR BOOSTING PROTEIN

These nutty-tasting seeds, or "hearts," from the hemp plant get props for their high protein content and omega-3s. Don't confuse them with their cannabis cousin grown for marijuana—this stuff doesn't come with a high. Sprinkle into smoothies and cereals.

A MORE TENDER TENDER

You can have chicken tenders without succumbing to processed and fried meat. Make them yourself with healthy ingredients: Crushed, puffed brown rice cereal works nicely for a coating, as does cooked quinoa. Or you can try this part bread crumbs, part nuts formula: Mix together ½ cup finely chopped nuts (such as pecans, pistachios, almonds, or walnuts), ¼ cup healthy bread crumbs (such as whole wheat bread crumbs or whole wheat panko), and ¼ cup of any of the flavor-booster combos listed here (the ratio is up to you). Then use your fingers to press them on top of your chicken, and bake until the tenders are cooked through and the crust is golden.

FLAVOR BLENDS

- Chopped rosemary + lemon juice + lemon zest + garlic + salt
- Chopped scallions + prepared horseradish + salt
- Chopped cilantro + lime juice + cumin + garlic
- Lemon juice + lemon zest + chopped chives + capers

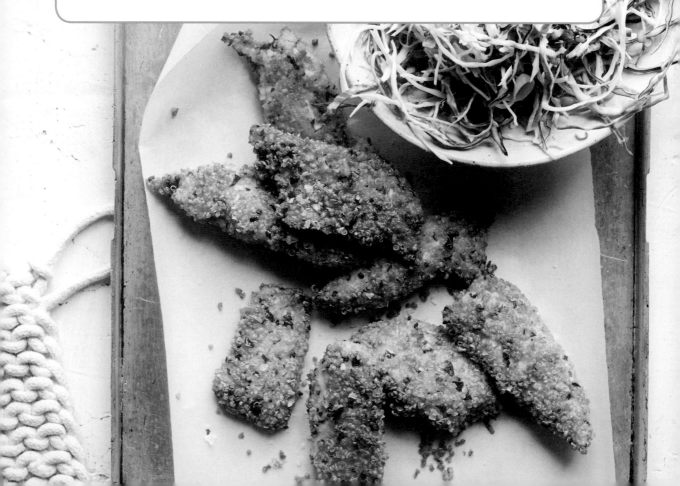

SUPERCHARGE YOUR PLATES

By all means, keep loading on the veggies—but know that they're not the only plate pumper-uppers. Here are a few low-calorie, high-volume options that help your meal feel like more.

- **Strawberries:** Make a diced-strawberry salsa with jalapeño, cilantro, lime juice, red onion, and salt, then sling all that deliciousness on grilled chicken.
- **Air-popped popcorn:** Add popped kernels to your next homemade trail mix. Or toss into salads or over soup, then skip croutons and crackers.
- **Popped quinoa:** Yep—you can "pop" quinoa like popcorn, in a dry pot, shaking it over a burner. Then stir the little puffed seeds into yogurt for cereal-like crackle, scatter popped quinoa over roasted sweet potatoes with a simple yogurt sauce and fresh herbs, or crunch up your hummus with a few sprinkles.
- **White beans:** If you're making soup, replace heavy cream with low-fat milk and make up the richness with pureed white beans.

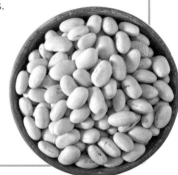

HEALTHIFY ANYTHING!

Yes, even bacon. Here are some ways to enjoy indulgent foods a little bit more healthfully.

- **Bacon:** It only takes a bit to jazz up anything. Crumble it up and add to roasted veggies, a leafy green salad, or a bowlful of whole grains.
- **Burgers:** Mix finely chopped vegetables, such as mushrooms, onions, or cauliflower, into your ground meat to help slash calories.
- **Butter:** A portion size is 1 teaspoon. The more flavor it has, the less you'll need to use so amp up the taste with these great add-ins. Let a stick of butter come to room temperature, work in extras, and chill. Three great combos: cilantro + lime juice + chipotle powder, chives + dill, lemon juice + Old Bay seasoning. (A spoonful or two of each should do it.)
- **Mayo:** This spread's high in calories, but just a little isn't so bad for you. You can mix up a spread that's half mayo, half plain 2% Greek yogurt, and get more gloop-factor for fewer calories. Or better yet, you can make your own (see page 34).

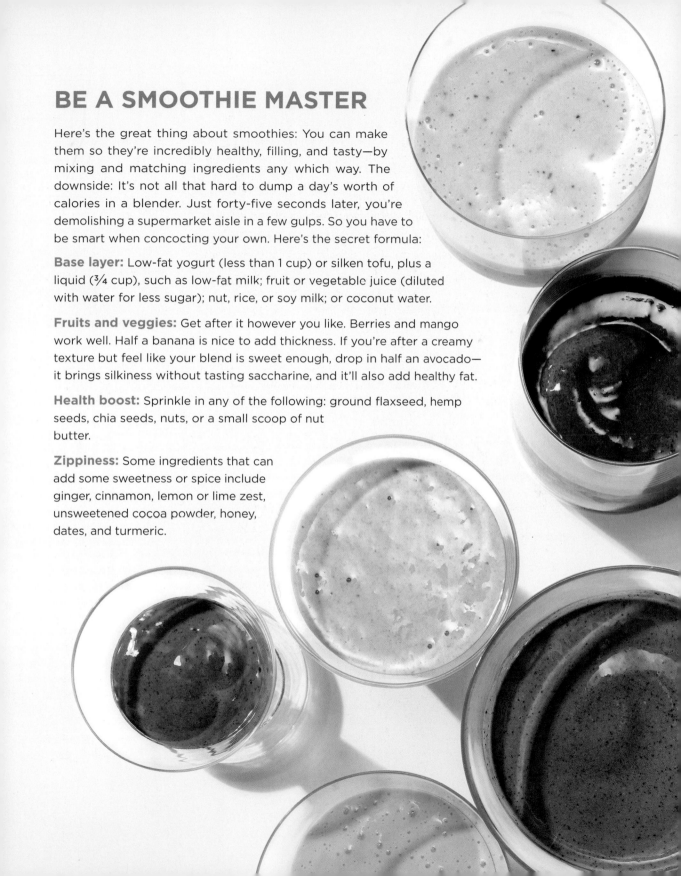

BE A SMOOTHIE MASTER

Here's the great thing about smoothies: You can make them so they're incredibly healthy, filling, and tasty—by mixing and matching ingredients any which way. The downside: It's not all that hard to dump a day's worth of calories in a blender. Just forty-five seconds later, you're demolishing a supermarket aisle in a few gulps. So you have to be smart when concocting your own. Here's the secret formula:

Base layer: Low-fat yogurt (less than 1 cup) or silken tofu, plus a liquid (¾ cup), such as low-fat milk; fruit or vegetable juice (diluted with water for less sugar); nut, rice, or soy milk; or coconut water.

Fruits and veggies: Get after it however you like. Berries and mango work well. Half a banana is nice to add thickness. If you're after a creamy texture but feel like your blend is sweet enough, drop in half an avocado—it brings silkiness without tasting saccharine, and it'll also add healthy fat.

Health boost: Sprinkle in any of the following: ground flaxseed, hemp seeds, chia seeds, nuts, or a small scoop of nut butter.

Zippiness: Some ingredients that can add some sweetness or spice include ginger, cinnamon, lemon or lime zest, unsweetened cocoa powder, honey, dates, and turmeric.

The Weekender Breakfast

Baking and slicing up a nice big frittata or omelet is a weekend staple for my family. Start with this basic recipe, but don't feel beholden to it—the nice thing about frittatas is that they're basically a happy home for any on-the-verge-of-wilting veggies in your fridge. Omelets do the job, too.

Spinach-Mushroom Omelet

SERVES 4

1 tablespoon olive oil

1 small yellow onion, chopped

8 ounces mushrooms, trimmed and thinly sliced

2 ounces baby spinach, washed

8 large eggs

½ teaspoon salt

4 teaspoons unsalted butter

¼ teaspoon coarse salt

⅛ teaspoon freshly ground black pepper

Heat the olive oil in a large nonstick skillet over medium heat. Add the onion and mushrooms and sauté until the mushrooms are browned, about 7 minutes. Add the spinach; cook until wilted, about 4 minutes. Set aside in a strainer (to help drain excess liquid off the spinach). Wipe the pan clean.

In a medium bowl, beat the eggs and the salt with ½ cup water. Add 1 teaspoon of the butter to the skillet and heat over medium-high heat. Pour in ½ cup of the egg mixture. Cook, gently lifting the edge of the eggs with a spatula and tilting the pan to allow the uncooked eggs to run underneath, until the eggs are set, about 1 minute. Spoon ¼ of the mushroom-spinach mix into the omelet, fold the unfilled half of the omelet over the filling, and slide onto a warm plate. Repeat with the remaining butter, egg mixture, and filling until you have four omelets. Top with the coarse salt and pepper.

---

229 CAL, 17 G FAT (6 G SATURATED), 15 G PROTEIN, 5 G CARB, 2 G SUGAR, 1 G FIBER, 523 MG SODIUM PER SERVING

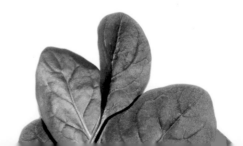

Frittata with Bell Peppers and Onions

Preheat the oven to 375°F.

In a medium bowl, whisk together the eggs, egg whites, milk, and lemon juice. Heat the olive oil in an 8-inch non-stick ovenproof skillet over medium-high heat. Add the onion, bell peppers, salt, and black pepper. Cook, stirring, until the onion is tender, about 3 minutes. Stir the vegetables and cheese into the egg mixture, then pour the mixture into the skillet. Bake the frittata until just set in the middle and the cheese has melted, 20 to 25 minutes. Let cool for 4 to 5 minutes, then cut into four wedges and serve.

179 CAL, 10 G FAT (5 G SATURATED), 17 G PROTEIN, 4 G CARB, 3 G SUGAR, 1 G FIBER, 293 MG SODIUM PER SERVING

SERVES 4

4 large eggs

1 cup egg whites (about 8 large egg whites)

2 tablespoons 2% milk

¼ teaspoon fresh lemon juice

⅛ teaspoon olive oil

½ cup chopped red or yellow onion

½ cup chopped mixed red and yellow bell peppers

Pinch of coarse salt

Pinch of freshly ground black pepper

½ cup shredded cheddar cheese

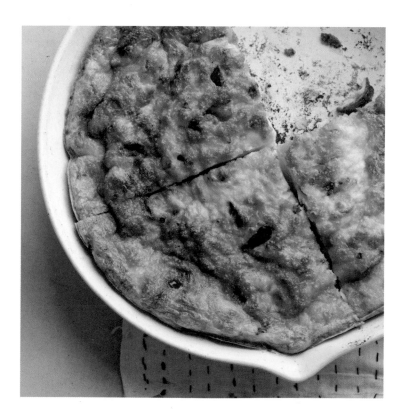

Special-Occasion Veggies

When you're having a crowd for a holiday feast, serve veggies in their fanciest party dresses. You'll love these sides so much, you'll want to make them your mains.

Roasted Brussels Sprouts with Grapes

SERVES 8

1½ pounds Brussels sprouts, trimmed and halved

3 tablespoons olive oil

½ teaspoon coarse salt

¼ teaspoon freshly ground black pepper

3 large shallots, sliced ¼ inch thick

2 cups red seedless grapes

1 tablespoon red wine vinegar

⅛ cup unsalted roasted almonds, coarsely chopped

Preheat the oven to 425°F.

On a rimmed baking sheet, toss the Brussels sprouts with 2 tablespoons of the olive oil, the salt, and pepper.

On a separate rimmed baking sheet, toss the shallots and grapes with the remaining 1 tablespoon olive oil. Roast the sprouts and grapes, turning when browned on one side (about 20 minutes for sprouts, 15 minutes for grapes), and roast until browned all over, 25 to 35 minutes total.

Combine the vinegar with 1 tablespoon water and add to the baking sheet with the grapes. As it steams, deglaze the pan, stirring up any browned bits from the pan with a wooden spoon. Toss the grape mixture and sprouts together, and top with the almonds.

149 CAL, 8 G FAT (1 G SATURATED), 4 G PROTEIN, 17 G CARB, 9 G SUGAR, 4 G FIBER, 142 MG SODIUM PER SERVING

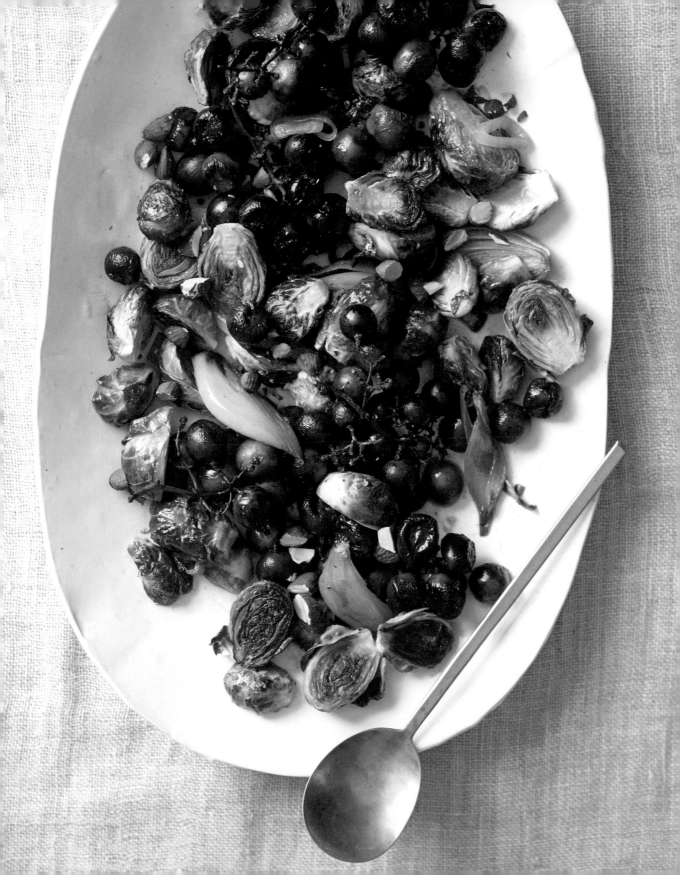

Stuffed Acorn Squash with Farro

SERVES 8

5 acorn squashes, halved and seeded

2 tablespoons extra-virgin olive oil, plus more for drizzling

1 teaspoon coarse salt

½ teaspoon freshly ground black pepper

4 cups white button mushrooms, trimmed and sliced

1 large yellow onion, diced

1 tablespoon chopped fresh rosemary

4 cups stemmed and chopped Tuscan kale leaves

3 cups cooked farro

1 ¼ cups crumbled goat cheese

1 tablespoon chopped fresh flat-leaf parsley for sprinkling

Red pepper flakes, for sprinkling

Preheat the oven to 375°F.

Drizzle the squashes with 1 tablespoon of the olive oil and season with ½ teaspoon of the salt and ¼ teaspoon of the black pepper. Arrange the squashes, cut sides down, on two rimmed baking sheets. Pour ¼ cup water into each sheet. Bake until just tender, 25 to 45 minutes. Remove from the oven but leave the oven on. Turn the squashes over and let cool. Scrape the flesh from 8 halves into a bowl with a fork, leaving a wall at least ¼ inch thick. Scrape the remaining 2 halves completely and discard the shells.

Heat the remaining 1 tablespoon olive oil in a large non-stick skillet over medium-high heat. Add the mushrooms, onion, and rosemary and cook, stirring, until the onion is soft, about 6 minutes. Add the kale and cook until wilted, 1 to 2 minutes. Stir in the farro and squash flesh. Season with the remaining ½ teaspoon salt and ¼ teaspoon black pepper. Remove from the heat. Fold the cheese into the filling. Divide among the 8 squash shells and bake on the rimmed baking sheets until golden, 35 to 45 minutes. Drizzle with the olive oil and sprinkle with the parsley and red pepper flakes.

309 CAL, 9 G FAT (4 G SATURATED), 11 G PROTEIN, 51 G CARB, 1 G SUGAR, 8 G FIBER, 363 MG SODIUM PER SERVING

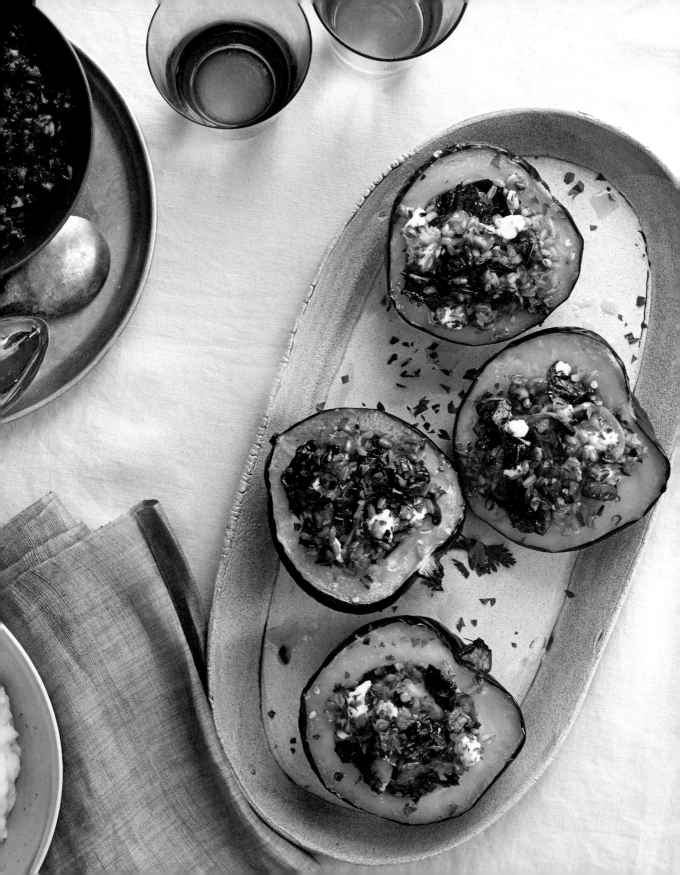

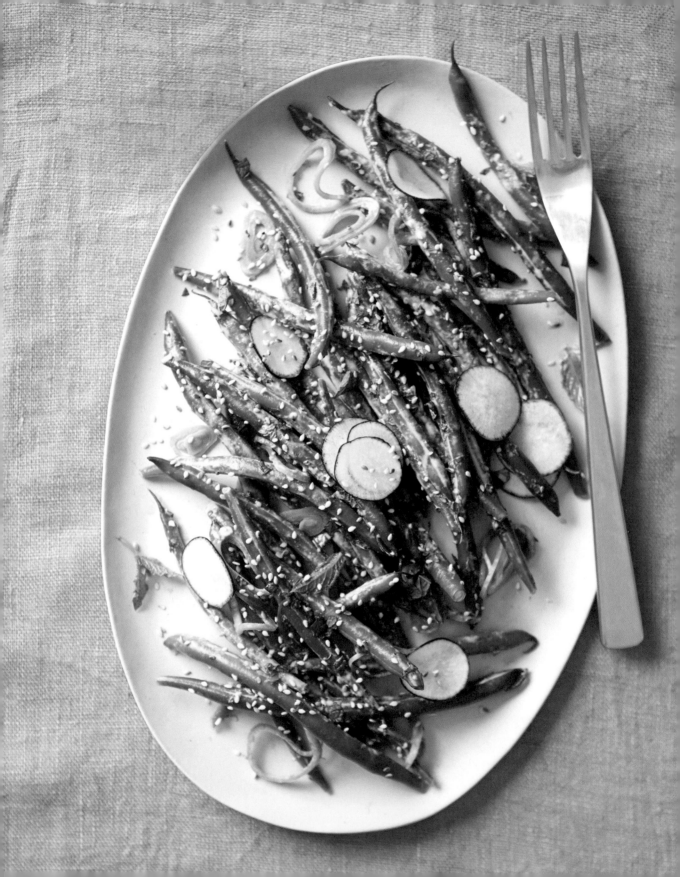

Green Beans with Tahini

Bring a large pot of water to a boil. Cook the green beans until bright green and crisp-tender, 2 to 3 minutes. Drain and plunge into a bowl of ice water. Once cooled, drain again and blot dry.

In a small bowl, whisk together the tahini, lemon juice, garlic, cayenne, olive oil, ¼ teaspoon of the salt, and 3 tablespoons water.

Heat the vinegar in the microwave until hot, about 20 seconds. Pour over the shallot. Let it pickle until cool, about 10 minutes. Drain. Toss the green beans with the dressing, the remaining ¼ teaspoon salt, the black pepper, mint, and sesame seeds. Top with the shallot and radish.

Tip: Instead of a butter-and-flour roux, use tahini to thicken soups (say, a creamy bisque) and add a delicious nutty note. Stir it in while the soup is cooking; aim for a spoonful or two of tahini per serving.

---

109 CAL, 8 G FAT (1 G SATURATED), 3 G PROTEIN, 7 G CARB, 3 G SUGAR, 2 G FIBER, 129 MG SODIUM PER SERVING

SERVES 8

1 ¼ pounds green beans, trimmed

¼ cup tahini

2 tablespoons fresh lemon juice

1 small garlic clove, minced

Pinch of cayenne pepper

2 tablespoons extra-virgin olive oil

½ teaspoon coarse salt

¼ cup red wine vinegar

1 large shallot, thinly sliced

¼ teaspoon freshly ground black pepper

2 tablespoons chopped fresh mint

1 tablespoon sesame seeds, toasted

Sliced radish, for garnish

Roasted Sweet Potatoes with Ginger and Curry

SERVES 8

6 medium sweet potatoes, cut into 1 ½-inch pieces

1 (3-inch) piece fresh ginger, peeled and cut into thin matchsticks

½ cup orange juice (preferably fresh)

2 tablespoons olive oil

½ teaspoon coarse salt

¼ teaspoon freshly ground black pepper

1 teaspoon curry powder

½ cup pecans

Preheat the oven to 425°F.

Toss together the sweet potatoes, ginger, orange juice, olive oil, salt, pepper, and curry powder. Spread out on a rimmed baking sheet. Roast for 20 minutes. Stir and add the pecans. Roast, stirring occasionally, until tender and slightly browned, 20 to 30 minutes more.

202 CAL, 8 G FAT (1 G SATURATED), 3 G PROTEIN, 30 G CARB, 10 G SUGAR, 5 G FIBER, 201 MG SODIUM PER SERVING

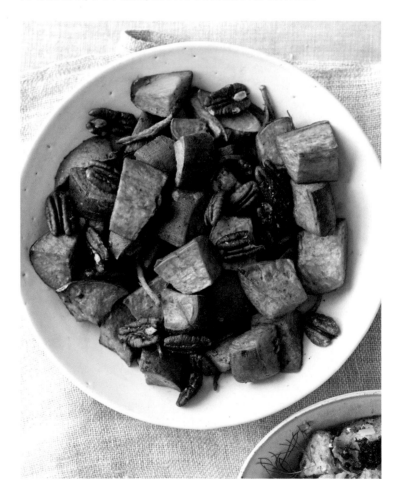

Kale, Cranberry, and Hazelnut Salad

In a blender, combine the buttermilk, yogurt, tarragon, parsley, lemon juice, garlic, and a generous pinch each of salt and pepper; blend until smooth. Wash the kale leaves and trim away any thick, tough stems; pat dry and tear into small pieces (you'll end up with about 10 cups of kale). Using tongs, toss the kale with the dressing until well combined. Place the kale on a platter and top with the cranberries and hazelnuts.

---

122 CAL, 6 G FAT (2 G SATURATED), 6 G PROTEIN, 14 G CARB, 7 G SUGAR, 3 G FIBER, 70 MG SODIUM PER SERVING

SERVES 10

½ cup low-fat buttermilk

1 (7-ounce) container plain whole-milk Greek yogurt

¼ cup loosely packed fresh tarragon leaves

¼ cup fresh flat-leaf parsley leaves

2 tablespoons fresh lemon juice

1 small garlic clove

Coarse salt

Freshly ground black pepper

2 bunches kale (preferably Tuscan; about 30 leaves, stems removed)

½ cup plump dried cranberries, coarsely chopped

½ cup toasted hazelnuts, coarsely chopped

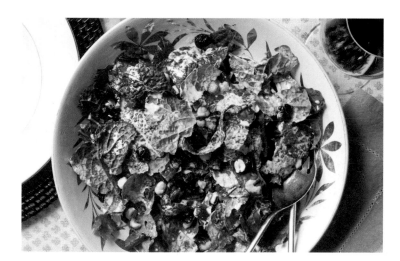

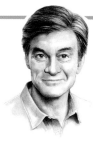

It's a Superfood

Hazelnuts contain plenty of folate, a nutrient essential for building strong bones and preventing birth defects. Eat the skin for an extra-powerful dose of antioxidants. About 90 percent of the world's supply is grown in my ancestral home of Turkey. Most of that is probably used in Nutella. But I recommend them in salads, sprinkled on cottage cheese, or toasted and spiced as snacks. Eat them my way, please!

Roasted Veggies with Olive Dressing

SERVES 10

2 pounds parsnips, peeled, thin ends trimmed away, halved or quartered lengthwise (depending on thickness)

5 tablespoons extra-virgin olive oil

2 teaspoons coarse salt

2 pounds sweet potatoes, peeled (it's okay if some peel is left on), ends trimmed, cut lengthwise into wedges

½ cup coarsely chopped pitted black, green, or Kalamata olives (or a combination)

3 tablespoons fresh lemon juice

1 tablespoon finely chopped shallot

1 small garlic clove, finely chopped

½ cup loosely packed fresh mint leaves, coarsely chopped

½ cup fresh cilantro leaves, coarsely chopped

Preheat the oven to 375°F.

Toss the parsnips with 1 tablespoon of the olive oil and 1 teaspoon of the salt on a rimmed baking sheet; arrange in a single layer. Toss the sweet potatoes with 1 tablespoon of the olive oil and the remaining 1 teaspoon salt; arrange in a single layer on a separate rimmed baking sheet. Roast the parsnips for 10 minutes; remove and gently stir. Then place the parsnips back in the oven and add the sheet of sweet potatoes. Roast the vegetables, stirring once halfway through, until tender and lightly browned, 40 to 50 minutes more.

Meanwhile, in a small bowl, whisk together the olives, the remaining 3 tablespoons olive oil, the lemon juice, shallot, and garlic. When ready to serve, transfer the vegetables to a platter and spoon the dressing on top. Sprinkle with the mint and cilantro. Serve warm or at room temperature.

---

196 CAL, 9 G FAT (1 G SATURATED), 2 G PROTEIN, 28 G CARB, 8 G SUGAR, 6 G FIBER, 271 MG SODIUM PER SERVING

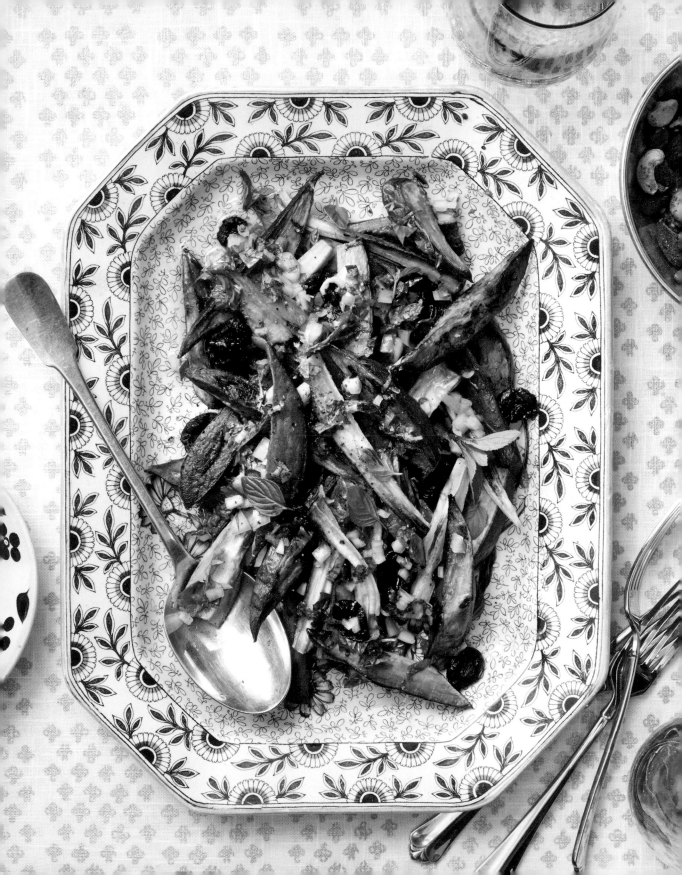

Lightened-Up Comfort Foods

These riffs on rich classics are healthified and rebooted with superfood ingredients.

Not-Fried Chicken with Buttermilk Slaw

SERVES 4

⅓ cup low-fat buttermilk

3 tablespoons finely chopped fresh chives or scallion greens

1 tablespoon mayonnaise

1 teaspoon honey

½ teaspoon Dijon mustard

½ teaspoon coarse salt

½ teaspoon freshly ground black pepper

1 (8-ounce) package shredded slaw

1½ cups cooked quinoa

¼ cup plus 1½ teaspoons olive oil

1 tablespoon finely grated Parmesan cheese

2 tablespoons chopped fresh flat-leaf parsley

1 pound chicken tenders (about 8 pieces)

1 large egg, lightly beaten

Preheat the oven to 350°F. Line a rimmed baking sheet with parchment paper.

In a small bowl, whisk together the buttermilk, chives, mayonnaise, honey, mustard, and ¼ teaspoon each salt and pepper. Toss with the slaw mix and refrigerate.

Toss the quinoa with the 1½ teaspoons olive oil. Spread the quinoa on the baking sheet and bake, stirring occasionally, until slightly dry and golden, about 20 minutes. (Keep the oven on.) Let the quinoa cool. Mix the quinoa with the cheese, parsley, and the remaining ¼ teaspoon each salt and pepper.

Dip the chicken, one piece at a time, into the beaten egg, then in the quinoa mixture, turning and pressing to coat both sides. Heat the ¼ cup olive oil in a large nonstick skillet over medium-high heat. Cook the chicken, in batches if necessary, until golden, 2 to 3 minutes per side. Transfer to a baking sheet and bake until cooked through, 3 to 5 minutes. Serve with the slaw.

See the photo on page 307.

---

330 CAL, 15 G FAT (3 G SATURATED), 29 G PROTEIN, 19 G CARB, 5 G SUGAR, 3 G FIBER, 413 MG SODIUM PER SERVING

Macaroni and Cheese with Butternut Squash

Preheat the oven to 375°F. Grease a 2- to 2½-quart shallow baking dish.

Bring a large saucepan of water to a boil. Add 1 teaspoon of the salt and the pasta. Cook according to the package directions until al dente, adding the squash for the last 4 minutes of the cooking time. Reserve ½ cup of the cooking water, then drain. Wipe the pan dry and set aside. Whisk together the milk, reserved cooking water, flour, mustard, Worcestershire sauce, and pepper in a measuring cup.

Meanwhile, heat the 2 teaspoons olive oil over medium heat in the dry saucepan. Add the onion and the remaining ½ teaspoon salt and cook, stirring, until softened, about 5 minutes. Add the milk mixture, raise the heat to medium-high, and cook until thickened slightly, 2 to 3 minutes. Remove from the heat. Add 2½ cups of the cheese and stir until smooth. Add the pasta and squash to the cheese mixture and toss gently. Spoon into the baking dish. Sprinkle the pasta with the remaining ½ cup cheese. Bake until golden and bubbling, 15 to 20 minutes.

---

396 CAL, 18 G FAT (10 G SATURATED), 18 G PROTEIN, 44 G CARB, 6 G SUGAR, 5 G FIBER, 518 MG SODIUM PER SERVING

SERVES 6

1 ½ teaspoons coarse salt

8 ounces whole wheat or quinoa pasta elbows, shells, or fusilli

3 cups diced (¼ inch) butternut squash

1 ½ cups 2% milk

2 tablespoons whole wheat flour (preferably white whole wheat)

1 teaspoon ground mustard

1 teaspoon Worcestershire sauce

½ teaspoon freshly ground black pepper

2 teaspoons olive oil, plus more for the baking dish

1 medium yellow onion, finely chopped

3 cups grated sharp cheddar (9 ounces)

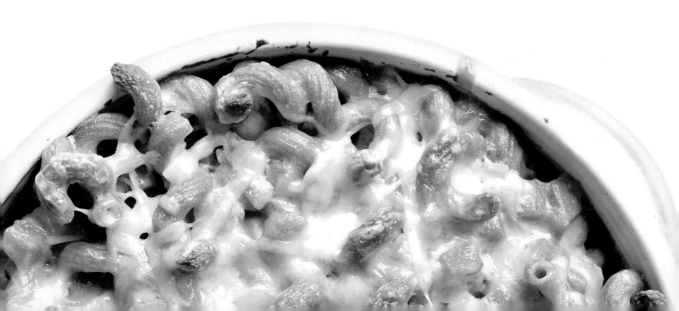

Ginger-Scallion Wings

SERVES 4

2 tablespoons safflower oil, plus more for the baking sheet

2 pounds chicken wingettes (tips removed) and drumettes

1 ¼ teaspoons coarse salt

6 scallions, finely chopped

1 tablespoon chopped fresh ginger

¼ teaspoon red pepper flakes

Preheat the oven to 450°F.

Lightly oil a rimmed baking sheet, then arrange the chicken on the sheet in a single layer. Season with ¼ teaspoon of the salt. Roast until golden brown and crisp, about 35 minutes. While the chicken roasts, in a food processor, combine the scallions, ginger, the remaining 1 teaspoon salt, the red pepper flakes, and the 2 tablespoons safflower oil until smooth. Remove the chicken from the oven and toss with the sauce in a large bowl. Return them to the baking sheet and roast until the sauce sets, about 15 minutes more.

291 CAL, 22 G FAT (5 G SATURATED), 21 G PROTEIN, 2 G CARB, 1 G SUGAR, 1 G FIBER, 689 MG SODIUM PER SERVING

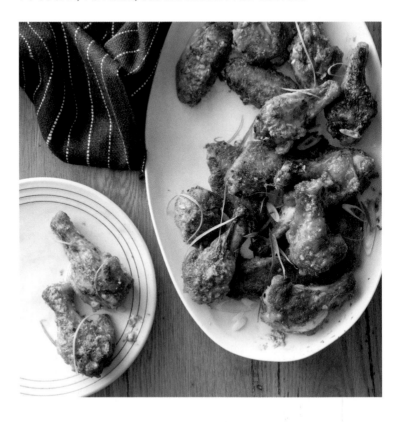

Baked Fries

Preheat the oven to 425°F.

Cut the potatoes into ½-inch-thick wedges. Spread on a nonstick baking sheet; toss with the olive oil, rosemary, and salt. Bake until golden brown on the bottoms, 30 to 35 minutes. Turn the fries and bake until golden brown all over, 10 to 15 minutes more.

389 CAL, 14 G FAT (2 G SATURATED), 7 G PROTEIN, 62 G CARB, 2 G SUGAR, 5 G FIBER, 258 MG SODIUM PER SERVING

SERVES 2

2 large Yukon Gold or baking potatoes (about 12 ounces each)

2 tablespoons olive oil

1 tablespoon chopped fresh rosemary

¼ teaspoon coarse salt

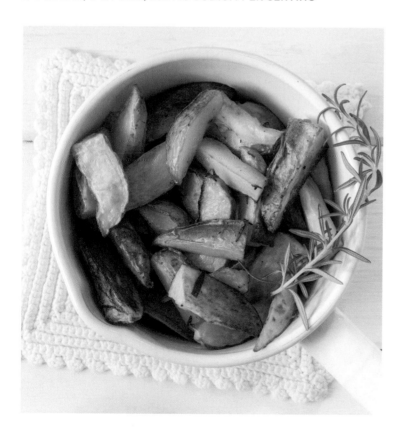

Superfood Treats

Much as I love a nice, juicy apple or pear for dessert, some-times a piece of fruit alone won't do the trick. Hence these crowd-pleasing goodies that you can feel good about. They include superfoods for nutritional oomph, and they'll satisfy your craving for a little something sweet.

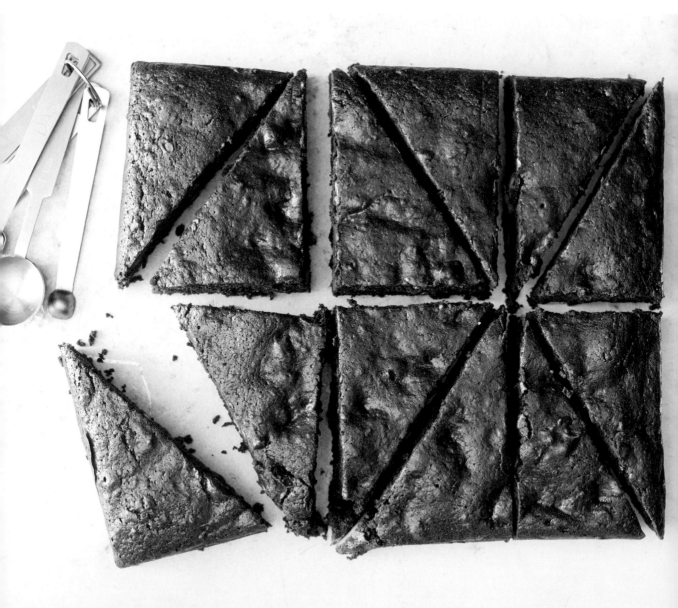

Dark Chocolate and Beet Brownies

Preheat the oven to 350°F. Grease an 8-inch square glass baking dish.

Puree the beets in a blender with orange juice until smooth, about 30 seconds. In a medium bowl, whisk together the flour, cocoa powder, baking powder, and salt.

Set a stainless-steel (or other heatproof) bowl over a saucepan of simmering water (be sure the bottom of the bowl does not touch the water). Put the butter and chocolate in the bowl and heat, stirring occasionally, until melted and smooth, 4 to 5 minutes. Remove from the heat and whisk in the sugar. Whisk in the eggs, one at a time, until each is incorporated. Stir in the beet mixture and vanilla. With a spatula, fold in the flour mixture and the nuts (if using) to just combine.

Pour the batter into the baking dish. Bake until slightly puffed and firm to the touch, 25 to 30 minutes. Let cool on a wire rack. Cut into 12 pieces.

---

191 CAL, 10 G FAT (7 G SATURATED), 3 G PROTEIN, 24 G CARB, 18 G SUGAR, 1 G FIBER, 111 MG SODIUM PER SERVING

SERVES 12

4 ounces precooked peeled whole beets (from an 8-ounce package), chopped

⅓ cup orange juice

½ cup whole wheat or all-purpose flour

¼ cup unsweetened cocoa powder

1 teaspoon baking powder

¼ teaspoon fine salt

4 tablespoons (½ stick) unsalted butter, plus more for the baking dish

6 ounces bittersweet chocolate (such as 70% cacao), finely chopped

½ cup firmly packed dark brown sugar

3 large eggs

2 teaspoons pure vanilla extract

1 cup chopped unsalted walnuts or pistachios, toasted (optional)

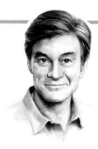

It's a Superfood

Beets are a good source of vitamin C, fiber, and potassium. Many of us are scarred by the tasteless sliver of beet on our elementary school lunch plate, but it's become my favorite veggie of all, roasted with a drizzle of olive oil, salt, and pepper.

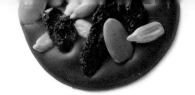

Chocolate Thins

MAKES 16; SERVING
SIZE 4 PIECES

4 ounces bittersweet
chocolate, finely chopped

½ teaspoon canola oil

1 tablespoon unsalted nuts

1 tablespoon pomegranate
seeds

1 tablespoon dried fruit
(chopped, if large)

1 tablespoon candied
ginger

Put the chocolate and canola oil in a microwave-safe bowl
and microwave on high for 1 minute. Stir until smooth
and cool to the touch. Line a baking sheet with parchment
paper. One teaspoon at a time, dollop the chocolate onto
the baking sheet, spreading each dollop out with the back
of a spoon.

In a small bowl, mix together the nuts, pomegranate seeds,
dried fruit, and candied ginger and spoon the mixture over
the rounds. Chill until firm, about 1 hour. Keep the choco-
lates refrigerated until ready to serve.

188 CAL, 15 G FAT, 4 G PROTEIN, 19 G CARB, 12 G SUGAR,
4 G FIBER, 2 MG SODIUM PER SERVING

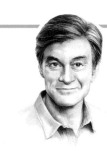

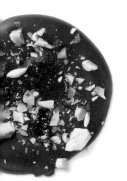

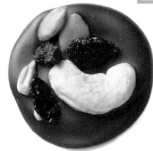

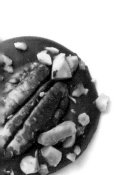

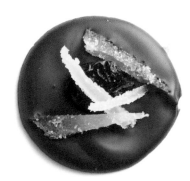

It's a Superfood

Recent research shows that
chocolate contains compounds that
could help lower your blood pressure
and "bad" cholesterol levels. (Experts
recommend the extra-dark kind.)

Banana "Ice Cream"

Puree the frozen bananas in a blender or food processor until creamy. Place in an airtight container and freeze for at least 1 hour. Scoop and serve.

Healthy Flavor-Upper: This one-ingredient dessert is great on its own, but if you're craving something fancier, you can mix in frozen berries as you blend. Or try topping with cocoa powder, cinnamon, or a drizzle of honey and some chopped nuts.

---

105 CAL, <1 G FAT, 1 G PROTEIN, 27 G CARB, 14 G SUGAR, 3 G FIBER, 1 MG SODIUM PER SERVING

SERVES 4

4 bananas, frozen

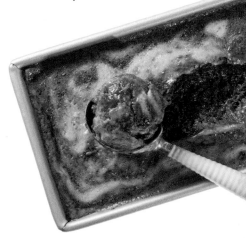

Chocolate-Dipped Clementines

Heat the chocolate and the canola oil in a microwave on high for 45 seconds. Stir until smooth. Line a baking sheet with parchment paper. Peel the clementines and separate into sections. Dip each section halfway into the chocolate, then into the pistachios, and arrange on the baking sheet. Chill until set, about 25 minutes. Keep refrigerated until ready to serve.

---

133 CAL, 8 G FAT (4 G SATURATED), 3 G PROTEIN, 17 G CARB, 11 G SUGAR, 3 G FIBER, 1 MG SODIUM PER SERVING

SERVES 4

2 ounces bittersweet chocolate, finely chopped

½ teaspoon canola oil

4 clementines

2 tablespoons shelled unsalted pistachios, finely chopped

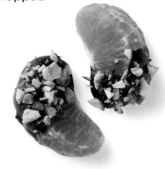

It's a Superfood

Clementines bring a nice helping of calcium, folate, and vitamin C to the table.

PUMP UP YOUR POPCORN

Make this whole-grain snack tastier with add-ins. Mist 5 cups of air-popped popcorn with cooking spray (so toppings stick) and dust on the fun flavorings here.

CURRY POWDER AND COCONUT SHAVINGS

(½ teaspoon + 2 tablespoons)

GRATED PARMESAN AND DRIED OREGANO

(2 tablespoons + ½ teaspoon)

MELTED DARK CHOCOLATE AND SEA SALT

(1 ounce + ½ teaspoon)

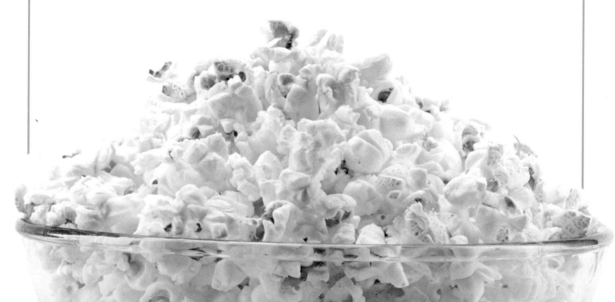

ACKNOWLEDGMENTS

Behind the simple title of this book lies an ambitious mission: to convince readers that food can nourish, heal, energize, and delight, all at the same time. I couldn't have pulled it off without the support of a squad of talented collaborators, and I am deeply grateful to every one of them. I must first thank Ted Spiker, who brings clarity, accuracy, and, crucially, humor to everything we write together. Also, enormous thanks go to Jill Herzig, who helped to create the concept behind *Food Can Fix It* and edited these pages along with the editors of my magazine, *Dr. Oz The Good Life*. Her staff leapt in to help, so additional thanks go to Lisa Bain and Rebecca Santiago, along with Margarita Bertsos, Abby Greene, Marty Munson, Allison Chin, and Miranda Van Gelder. Visual appeal plays a huge role in this book—would you eat a fix-it food if it didn't look delicious?—and for that I thank the magazine's photo director Bruce Perez and design director Jaclyn Steinberg, as well as the book's photo editor, Martha Corcoran. Every fact and study went through a triple-checking process led by Karen Jacob, along with Katherine Wessling and Joy Wingfield. Similarly, all recipes were developed by culinary pros including Christine Albano, Lori Powell, and Susan Spungen, and then tested by Maryann Pomeranz and Antonina Smith.

Numerous outside experts enriched this book with their deep knowledge. A few of those include Kristin Kirkpatrick, R.D.; Jacqueline Crockford, M.S., C.S.C.S.; Keri Gans, R.D.; and Dr. Michael Roizen.

My staff at *The Dr. Oz Show* also pitched in with this effort, so many thanks go to Amy Chiaro, Michael Crupain, Gretchen Goetz, Donna O'Sullivan, and Stacy Rader.

I am honored to work, once again, with Simon & Schuster, one of the great publishing houses, led by the visionary Carolyn Reidy. Thanks go to her and her talented and dedicated team at Scribner, including Susan

Moldow, Nan Graham, Roz Lippel, and Shannon Welch.

The management team at Hearst encouraged this project early on and boosted our efforts right through publication. I want to give special thanks to David Carey, Ellen Levine, Joanna Coles, and Fotoulla Damaskos. Also vital, from the Hearst marketing team: Jim Miller, Will Michalopoulos, and Michelle Spinale. And many thanks to the publishing group at *Dr. Oz The Good Life*, led by Jill Seelig.

For their help in spreading the word about *Food Can Fix It*, I want to thank several editors in chief at Hearst: Glenda Bailey, Rachel Barrett, Jane Francisco, Anne Fulenwider, Lucy Kaylin, Robbie Myers, Michele Promaulayko, Meredith Rollins, Susan Spencer, and Stellene Volandes.

Last but not least, I am indebted to Jacqueline Deval for expertly managing this project and organizing the efforts of all those mentioned above.

And finally, thanks to the master food fixer in my home and my life, Lisa Oz.

INDEX

Page numbers in *italics* refer to recipe photographs.

PHOTO CREDITS

David Lawrence/Studio D: 100
Stephen Lewis/Art + Commerce: 136
Ryan Liebe: 182, 202
Jeff Lipsky: 5, 51, 72, 75 (right)
Pernille Loof: 88, 184, 305
Cindy Luu: 18
Charles Masters: 60 (bottom), 193, 212, 217, 239
    (bottom), 240–241
Claire McCracken: 17, 19, 95
Kagan McLeod: 274–275 (logos)
Marko Metzinger: 24, 29
Johnny Miller: 135, 307, 323, 326
Mark Allen Miller: 91
Marcus Nilsson: 194, 222, 229
Courtesy of Dr. Mehmet Oz: 25, 74, 75 (left)
Bruce Peterson: 22 (avocado), 31 (bottom)
Con Poulos: 38, 44, 68, 76, 201, 215, 245, 311
Travis Rathbone: ix, 26, 99, 244, 246, 250–255, 257, 309
Peter Rees/StockFood: 128 (swordfish)
Emily Kate Roemer: 163, 269, 273

Matthew Rolston: 242
Tom Schierlitz: 154 (bottom), 310
Martin Schoeller: 276
Shutterstock: 128 (bluefish), 129 (mahimahi)
Paul Sirisalee/Offset: 290
Art Streiber: 6, 82
Christopher Testani: 63, 151 (top), 225, 227, 304, 319,
    321
Courtesy of *The Dr. Oz Show*: 14
Kenji Toma: 155
Marshall Troy: 35, 122, 256
Sarah Anne Ward: 12, 96, 187, 188, 190, 197, 199,
    206, 208, 210, 218, 221, 226, 230, 239 (top), 263,
    280–283, 285, 286, 288, 289, 291, 292
Luke Wilson (Dr. Oz illustration): 188, 195, 198, 207,
    209, 213, 224, 226, 231, 232, 248, 253, 254, 288,
    319, 327, 328
James Worrell/Studio D: 98, 148
Romulo Yanes: 32, 62, 178, 287, 324
Yasu + Junko: endpapers, 141

ABOUT DR. MEHMET OZ

Mehmet Oz, M.D., a cardiothoracic surgeon, has won nine Daytime Emmy Awards for *The Dr. Oz Show*. A professor of surgery at Columbia University, he directs the Complementary Medicine Program at NewYork–Presbyterian Hospital and performs more than fifty heart operations a year. Dr. Oz has written eight *New York Times* bestselling books, including *Food Can Fix It*, *YOU: The Owner's Manual*, *YOU: The Smart Patient*, *YOU: On a Diet*, *YOU: Staying Young*, and the award-winning *Healing from the Heart*. He hosts the internationally syndicated *Daily Dose* in numerous radio markets, syndicated through iHeartRadio, and his newspaper column is syndicated by Hearst in 175 markets around the world. He is the cofounder of Sharecare.com and its app AskMD, which won the Best Medical App award in 2014. Dr. Oz also has a regular column in *O, The Oprah Magazine*.

Dr. Oz belongs to every major professional society for heart surgeons and has been named one of *Time* magazine's 100 Most Influential People, *Forbes'* most influential celebrity, *Esquire* magazine's 75 Most Influential People of the 21st Century, a Global Leader for Tomorrow by the World Economic Forum, Harvard's 100 Most Influential Alumni, as well as receiving the Ellis Island Medal of Honor. He won the prestigious Gross Surgical Research Scholarship, and he has received an honorary doctorate from Istanbul University. Dr. Oz has been elected annually as a highest-quality physician by the Castle Connolly guide as well as other major ranking groups. He is also an honorary police surgeon for New York City. He lives in northern New Jersey with his wife of thirty-three years, Lisa; they have four children and three grandchildren.